# The Hip Handbook

# The Hip Handbook

Edited by

## Timothy L. Fagerson, M.S., P.T.

*Physical Therapy Private Practitioner and Consultant, Boston; Lecturer, Graduate Program in Physical Therapy, MGH Institute of Health Professions at Massachusetts General Hospital, Boston; Faculty and Consultant, Cross Country University, Boca Raton, Florida*

With a Foreword by

## David E. Krebs, Ph.D., P.T.

*Professor of Physical Therapy and Clinical Investigation, MGH Institute of Health Professions at Massachusetts General Hospital, Boston; Director, Biomotion Laboratory, Massachusetts General Hospital, Boston*

**Butterworth–Heinemann**
Boston Oxford Johannesburg Melbourne New Delhi Singapore

**Library of Congress Cataloging-in-Publication Data**
Fagerson, Timothy L.
　　The hip handbook / Timothy L. Fagerson; with a foreword by David
E. Krebs.
　　　　p. cm.
　　Includes bibliographical references and index.
　　ISBN 0-7506-9689-3
　　　1. Hip joint--Diseases--Physical therapy--Handbooks, manuals, etc.
I. Title.
　　[DNLM: 1. Hip joint. 2. Joint diseases--rehabilitation.
3. Wounds and Injuries--rehabilitation. 4. Lumbosacral Region.
5. Pelvis. WE 860 F153h 1997]
RD772.F34　1997
617.5'81--dc21
DNLM/DLC
for Library of Congress　　　　　　　　　　　　　97-34807
　　　　　　　　　　　　　　　　　　　　　　　　CIP


**British Library Cataloguing-in-Publication Data**
A catalogue record for this book is available from the British Library.

The publisher offers special discounts on bulk orders of this book.
For information, please contact:

Manager of Special Sales
Butterworth–Heinemann
225 Wildwood Avenue
Woburn, MA 01801-2041
Tel: 781-904-2500
Fax: 781-904-2620

For information on all Butterworth–Heinemann publications available,
contact our World Wide Web home page at: http://www.bh.com

10 9 8 7 6 5 4 3 2 1

Printed in the United States of America

*To Trudy*

Between the auricular appendages and at the distal extremities of forearm lies the most advanced technology in the world—wit and hand.

—Gregory P. Grieve.
(1983) The hip. *Physiotherapy* 69, 204.

# Contents

# Contributing Authors

**Timothy L. Fagerson, M.S., P.T.**
Physical Therapy Private Practitioner and Consultant, Boston; Lecturer, Graduate Program in Physical Therapy, MGH Institute of Health Professions at Massachusetts General Hospital, Boston; Faculty and Consultant, Cross Country University, Boca Raton, Florida

**Scott L. Jones, M.S., P.T., O.C.S.**
Physical Therapy Private Practitioner, Kansas City, Missouri

**Claire E. Robbins, M.S., P.T.**
Physical Therapist, New England Baptist Hospital, Boston

**Andrew A. Shinar, M.D.**
Orthopedic Surgeon, Associated Orthopedists of Detroit, St. Claire Shores, Michigan

# Foreword

Who needs this book? Like the ball joints of an automobile, most of us do not know exactly where the hip joint is, much less its function. When asked where, many people will point closer to their iliac crests than the greater trochanter. Indeed, most hip *specialists* will pause when asked how much pressure the acetabular cartilage may experience during daily activities such as chair rise or stair descent (about 5 megapascals [MPa] during normal walking, to 18 MPa—2,610 psi!—during chair and stair activities; by comparison, car tires use 29 psi).*

Tim Fagerson is supremely qualified to write this book. Tim began writing shortly after he finished his master's thesis in my lab. Despite the accumulated wisdom gained from thousands of hip patients treated by our staff, not to mention the technological marvels (the instrumented Austin-Moore prostheses we have implanted and subsequently studied) and a small library of books we have accumulated, we have not located what clinicians and researchers alike still need: an authoritative single-source reference book for hip rehabilitation. Data and theory need melding: We would probably need hundreds or even thousands of "million-dollar-man" implants before empirical evidence alone could be the determining factor in therapeutic decisions about hip rehabilitation. Tim has combined data and theory in this book.

Transferring research findings to the bedside is the gauntlet that Tim Fagerson has chosen to run. Many generations of researchers have toiled and found their data accepted in scientific journals but ultimately discarded by clinical practitioners. Tim took the time to write the "technology transfer"

---

*See Table 1-5 for details.

document that allows research to find its way directly into the clinic. This book is dedicated to clinicians who want to practice on the basis of data—to be scholarly clinicians.

David E. Krebs, Ph.D., P.T.

# Preface

The primary purpose of *The Hip Handbook* is to provide a clinical resource for physical therapists involved in hip rehabilitation. This book represents an essential body of knowledge for skilled rehabilitation of the hip. In addition to its use as a clinical resource, it should be helpful for research and teaching.

The alternative title considered for this work, *The Hip Complex*, encompasses two notions: (1) The hip is part of a *complex* of joints (i.e., the lumbopelvic region and the lower extremity kinetic chain). Because this book concerns the hip and not its joint partners, this title was not used; the *hip complex* concept holds true, however. I encourage readers to bear in mind this "big picture principle," whether the primary source of signs, symptoms, or both, is the lumbar spine, the hip, the foot, or anywhere in between. (2) The hip is a *complex* joint. Indeed, the hip is more complex than most rehabilitation professionals realize. I wrote *The Hip Handbook* because I sensed a void in the knowledge base of physical therapists.

The contents of *The Hip Handbook* are practical, evidence-based, and of use to both experienced and inexperienced clinicians. The evidence presented is primarily from peer-reviewed literature; where that is lacking, expert or the authors' opinions are given. Chapter 1 reviews important basic facts for clinical application. I urge readers to understand and learn the classic "balance of Pauwels" (Figure 1-13), which is one of the keys to hip joint function. Chapter 2 uses an easy-to-follow format that, in addition to the "hip tips," should make it immediately useful for clinical application. Chapter 3 is a detailed review of the examination process related to the hip, including some very useful tables and figures. The words *evaluation* and *assessment* are used in the chapter's title and subtitles, respectively, to indicate that during, and certainly after, the data-collection process, a clinical value judgment needs to be made. Chapter 4 first emphasizes the importance of thought process and formulation of a diagnosis, and then presents an eclectic review of treatment options used in hip rehabilitation. Chapter 5 provides a detailed look at total hip replacement especially—what Dr. Shinar calls "the approaches and the basics." The chapter eloquently presents the complexity of hip surgery from an orthopedic surgeon's perspective and what he thinks a physical therapist should know. Chapter 6 contains very important information for all physical therapists (e.g., weightbearing status, dislocation precautions, thrombosis prophylaxis). Without this knowledge, a physical therapist risks defying the first rule of medicine: *primum non nocere*—above all, do no harm. Chapter 6 also provides information about how a good surgical result can be transformed into an excellent result with appropriate postoperative management. The last two chapters, *Diagnostic Imaging* (Chapter 7) and *Outcomes Assessment* (Chapter 8), are crucial complements to the care of patients with hip dysfunction. These two fields span the spectrum of the disability model (see Figure 4-1). Diagnostic imaging detects and delineates a problem at the tissue level (e.g., fracture, pathology) and outcomes assessment detects and delineates a problem at the person level. Outcomes assessment gives us information about function as well as helps us gauge our success at making a difference for those who seek our help.

   Although this book is written for health professionals, I hope that it results in better conservative care for people with hip pain and dysfunction.

T.L.F.

# Acknowledgments

Putting this book together has not been a solo effort. I would like to acknowledge the contributions of the following people and in so doing express my heartfelt appreciation.

- My wife Trudy, for patience and understanding.
- Scott L. Jones, M.S., P.T., O.C.S.; Claire E. Robbins, M.S., P.T.; and Andrew A. Shinar, M.D., for the excellent chapters they contributed
- Barbara Murphy and Jana Friedman at Butterworth–Heinemann for assistance and support throughout the project, and Jane Bangley McQueen and Silverchair Science + Communications, Inc., for a very professional production process.
- David E. Krebs, Ph.D., P.T.; Bette Ann Harris, M.S., P.T.; Daniel Dyrek, M.S., P.T.; and Andrew Guccione, Ph.D., P.T., R.P., for teaching me much about writing, research, practice, and presentation.
- Many persons have reviewed chapters and the whole manuscript. Kim Amlong, M.S., P.T.; Mark Berenson, M.D.; Denis Byrne, M.D.; Dan Dyrek, M.S., P.T.; Jennifer Ellison, Ph.D., P.T.; Gwendolyn Fagerson, M.D.; Jonathan Fagerson, M.D.; Rev. Ladd Fagerson; Rebecca Fishbein, P.T., O.C.S.; Erin Gammell, M.S., P.T.; Norman Goguen, M.D.; Chris Goodyear, M.S., P.T.; Andrew Guccione, Ph.D., P.T.; April Guillet, M.S., P.T.; Bette Ann Harris, M.S., P.T.; Janet Hartley, P.T.A.; Scott L. Jones, M.S., P.T., O.C.S.; David E. Krebs, Ph.D., P.T.; Kate Maffa-Krailo, M.S., P.T., G.C.S.; Chris McGibbon, Ph.D.; Natasha Palatov, P.T.; Claire E. Robbins, M.S., P.T.; Andrew A. Shinar, M.D.; Peter von Lossnitzer, P.T.; Sumaya White, S.P.T.; Charles Wright, M.D.; and the anonymous reviewers obtained by the publisher. Your comments have greatly improved this work.
- Christine Creamer (a patient of mine) for drawing Figure 4-9 illustrations. Trudy Fagerson for typing in references and reformatting tables. Stefanie Oestreicher for the front cover idea. Jaime Paz for technical support. Karen Yuska for reformatting figures.

# 1

# Anatomy and Biomechanics

## Claire E. Robbins

The hip joint is a very strong articulation that connects the lower limb to the pelvis. The joint is widely classified as an ovoid (ball-and-socket) joint between the spherical head of the femur and the concave acetabulum. The spheroidal configuration allows for a wide range of mobility necessary for the body's daily locomotor activities. Incidentally, Rydell (1973) noted that the head of the femur is in fact not a perfect sphere, but is more ellipsoid.

## Anatomy

### Osteology

#### Os Coxae

In childhood, the os coxae (hip bone) consists of the following three individual bones:

- Ischium
- Ilium
- Pubis

Fusion of these bones takes place primarily within the acetabulum, between the ages of 15 and 25 years. The acetabulum serves as the concave receptor for the head of the femur. The ilium forms the superior portion of the acetabulum; the pubis forms the anteroinferior portion; and the ischium forms the posteroinferior portion.

#### Acetabulum

The cavity of the acetabulum faces anterior, lateral, and inferior. The amount of inferior tilt of the acetabulum is known as the *center edge angle*. The center edge angle is a line connecting the lateral rim of the acetabulum and the center of the femoral head and forms an angle with the

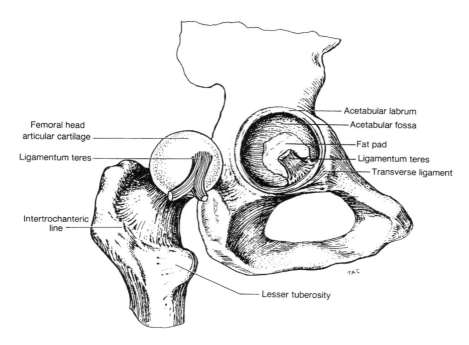

**Figure 1-1** The acetabulum and related hip-joint structures. (Reprinted with permission from CT Wadsworth. [1988] *Manual Examination and Treatment of the Spine and Extremities* [p. 161]. Baltimore: Williams & Wilkins.)

vertical (Norkin and Levangie 1992). A more vertical orientation of the acetabulum decreases the center edge angle and can also decrease the coverage of the head of the femur, thus increasing the risk of superior dislocation of the femoral head (Norkin and Levangie 1992).

The fibrocartilaginous acetabular labrum, whose circumference is smaller inferiorly, deepens the acetabulum from less than one-half of a sphere to greater than one-half of a sphere and gives added stability to the joint (Figure 1-1). The articular, or lunate, surface is horseshoe shaped and surrounds a nonarticular central depression known as the *acetabular fossa*. An articular fat pad occupies the fossa, which can become impinged in some patients. The acetabular notch is a gap in the articular surface inferiorly. The notch is traversed by the acetabular or transverse ligament (one of two intracapsular ligaments) converting it to a foramen. Vessels and nerves pass through this foramen with the ligamentum teres (the other intracapsular ligament at the hip).

The following are four types of cartilage in the acetabular area (LeVeau 1994):

- Physeal cartilage
- Undifferentiated hyaline cartilage
- Fibrocartilage of the labrum
- Articular cartilage

The articular cartilage of the acetabulum is thickest on the upper area of the horseshoe shape, the major weightbearing site, and at the outer periphery. The cartilage is thinnest toward the center and lower acetabulum (Figure 1-2).

Longmore and Gardner (1978) classified the curvatures, undulations, and irregularities of articular cartilage with respect to *dimension*. They are as follows:

- Primary anatomic contours (ovoid or sellar surfaces)
- Secondary undulations (100–500 μm crest to crest)
- Tertiary hollows (20–50 μm diameter; 0.5–2.0 μm deep)
- Quaternary ridges (1–4 μm diameter; 130–275 μm deep)

The undulations of articular surfaces deepen and develop minute, ragged projections with advancing age.

Macirowski et al. (1994) also reported on cartilage *thickness* measured from intact natural acetabular cartilage of a 78-kg man. The topographies in their study were measured using a noncontact ultrasonic technique. Cartilage thicknesses by acetabular location were as follows:

- Superior (1,750–2,500 μm)
- Anteromedial (1,250–2,250 μm)
- Posteromedial (750–1,250 μm)

### Femur

The femur, one of the strongest bones in the body, is divided into thirds (particularly for purposes of fracture classification):

- Proximal third: femoral head and neck, greater trochanter, lesser trochanter, intertrochanteric line, and crest (Hip fractures are defined as occurring in the proximal third of the femur.)
- Middle third: shaft of femur and linea aspera
- Distal third: medial and lateral condyles, medial and lateral supracondylar lines, adductor tubercle, and intercondylar notch

The head of the femur forms two-thirds of a sphere and is the convex component of the hip joint. Articular cartilage completely covers the femoral head with the exception of a slight depression called the *fovea centralis*, to which the ligament of the head of the femur (ligamentum teres) is attached. The cartilage is thickest on the medial central surface, where it makes con-

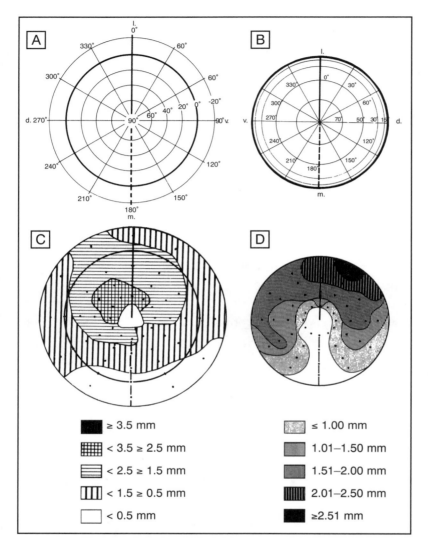

**Figure 1-2** Thickness variation of articular cartilage of the femoral head (A and C) and the acetabular lunate surface (B and D). A and B are designated reference grids. The distance and angular direction of sampling points are measured from the center of the femoral head (A) and the acetabulum center (B). C and D show average contours of the thickness ranges indicated by the shaded codes below the diagrams. Black dots (in C and D) represent sampling points, and they indicate the intersections of latitude and longitude lines. (d = dorsal; v = ventral; l = superolateral points on the articular surface of the femoral head; m = inferomedial points on the articular surface of the femoral head.) (Reprinted with permission from PL Williams, R Warwick, M Dyson, LH Bannister. [1989] *Gray's Anatomy* [37th ed] [p. 522]. Edinburgh, UK: Churchill Livingstone.)

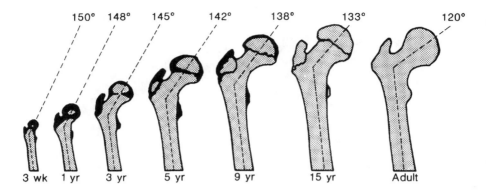

**Figure 1-3** Angle of inclination varies in the life cycle from 150 degrees at 3 weeks of age to approximately 120 degrees in the adult. (Reprinted with permission from DC Reid. [1992] *Sports Injury Assessment and Rehabilitation* [p. 613]. New York: Churchill Livingstone.)

tact with the acetabulum and is thinnest on the periphery (see Figure 1-2). The head of the femur faces the acetabulum in a medial, cranial, and slightly ventral position.

The diameter of most femoral heads are in the range of 45–56 mm, and, before acetabular contact pressure studies, replacement femoral heads were manufactured in 0.25-in. increments. However, following the work of Harris and colleagues (1975) and Rushfeldt and colleagues (1981), femoral hemiarthroplasties were manufactured in 1-mm increments, because it was discovered that a more intimate fit of the femoral head to the acetabulum results in lower peak articular contact pressures.

The femoral head is connected to the shaft of the femur by the neck of the femur, which is approximately 5 cm long. The neck of the femur forms an angle with the shaft, known as *the angle of inclination*, in the frontal plane (Figure 1-3). The angle varies in the life cycle but is approximately 125 ± 5 degrees in the adult. Coxa valga is present when the angle exceeds 130 degrees. A decrease in the angle below 120 degrees is called *coxa vara*. An angle less than 100 degrees may need surgical correction. The angle of torsion in the frontal plane is formed by the neck of the femur and the transverse axis of the femoral condyles (Figure 1-4). The angle is approximately 14 degrees anterior in the average adult, but it can vary. Anteversion is a pathologic increase in the angle of torsion; retroversion is a pathologic decrease in the angle of torsion (Norkin and Levangie 1992).

The neck of the femur widens at its attachment with the femoral shaft. The greater trochanter projects laterally and superiorly just above the junc-

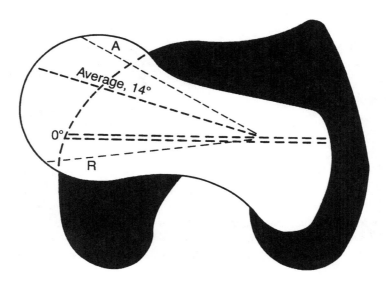

**Figure 1-4** The angle of torsion. The angle is 14 degrees on average. It can be anteverted (A) or retroverted (R). (Reprinted with permission from M Harty. [1991] Anatomy. In ME Steinberg [ed], *The Hip and Its Disorders* [p. 29]. Philadelphia: Saunders.)

tion of the neck and the shaft of the femur. The lesser trochanter, a smaller prominence, is located posteromedially at the junction of the neck and shaft. Anterior and posterior intertrochanteric ridges connect the greater and lesser trochanters in the front and the back. The intertrochanteric crest is found on the posterior surface, and the intertrochanteric line is located on the anterior surface. The quadrate tubercle, which serves as the attachment for the quadratus femoris muscle, is posterior on the crest. The femoral tubercle, which serves as an attachment for the ischiofemoral ligament, is located anterior on the intertrochanteric line.

The shaft of the femur is cylindrical in shape at the top. It narrows in the middle and becomes triangular in shape just above the medial and lateral femoral condyles. The posterior surface of the shaft has several crests and prominences that serve as attachment sites for musculature of the hip. The most notable prominence is the linea aspera.

### Trabeculae

The trabecular patterns of the upper femur are designed to resist the forces of tension and compression that occur at the hip joint. Sources differ when reporting the number of trabecular systems. A frequently used classification organizes trabecular structure into three systems (Kessler 1983; Lhowe 1990; Saudek 1985):

- Arcuate system (primary tensile): projects medially and resists a bending moment or tension forces brought about by the neck of the femur. It runs from the lateral cortex of the shaft of the femur and then extends superior and medial to the inferior border of the head and neck of the femur.
- Medial system (primary compressive): also known as the *vertical bundle*. Resists compressive forces through the head of the femur. The medial system runs along the medial cortex of the shaft and neck and continues upward to the superior surface of the head of the femur.
- Lateral system (secondary compressive): runs from the base of the neck at the lesser trochanter to the greater trochanter. The lateral system is believed to resist tension and compressive forces produced by the hip musculature.

The trabecular patterns reflect the normal stresses sustained by the hip. The areas of the femoral neck that provide the greatest strength are those in which trabecular systems intersect at right angles to one another. Distal to the intersection is an area of weakness in the neck where the trabeculae do not cross and are thin. This area is known as *Ward's triangle* and is prone to fracture when forces are excessive or the femoral neck undergoes osteoporotic changes associated with aging (Figure 1-5). Ward's triangle is prominent in coxa vara, when the neck-shaft angle is less than normal and tensile forces are more pronounced.

The calcar femorale is a dense vertical bone plate in the interior of the femur that originates in the posteromedial shaft (under the lesser trochanter) of the femur and radiates laterally toward the greater trochanter (Harty 1991). The calcar femorale blends with the posterior neck cortex proximally and fuses distally with the posteromedial shaft deep to the lesser trochanter (Harty 1991). It is known for its strength to resist compression and prevent collapse of the femoral neck (Weissman and Sledge 1986). The calcar is said to be the most highly stressed region of the human body (Kyle 1994).

## Capsule and Ligaments

The articulating surfaces of the hip joint and the majority of the femoral neck are enclosed by a strong fibrous capsule. Proximally, the capsule attaches to the rim of the acetabulum, the acetabular labrum, and the transverse ligament. The capsule runs distally and attaches anteriorly to the intertrochanteric line and the root of the greater trochanter. The capsule

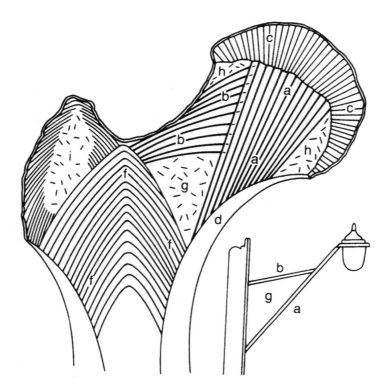

**Figure 1-5** Ward's original picture of compression and tension trabecular patterns. (g = Ward's triangle.) (Reprinted with permission from M Harty. [1991] Anatomy. In ME Steinberg [ed], *The Hip and Its Disorders* [p. 31]. Philadelphia: Saunders.)

attaches on the femoral neck, just proximal to the intertrochanteric crest posteriorly. Most of the fibers of the capsule run longitudinally. They are parallel to the neck of the femur. A smaller portion of the fibers, the zona orbicularis, run circularly around the neck of the femur. These fibers help to hold the head of the femur in the acetabulum.

Three strong extracapsular longitudinal ligaments reinforce the capsule (Figure 1-6). The ligaments originate on the pelvis and terminate on the femur and are named for their bony attachments (Table 1-1). In the neutral position, the ligaments are coiled and twisted as they pass from the origin on the pelvis to the femur. They tighten in extension or hyperextension. The combined position of flexion, abduction, and lateral rotation make the ligaments slack (Norkin and Levangie 1992). The three extracapsular longitudinal ligaments are:

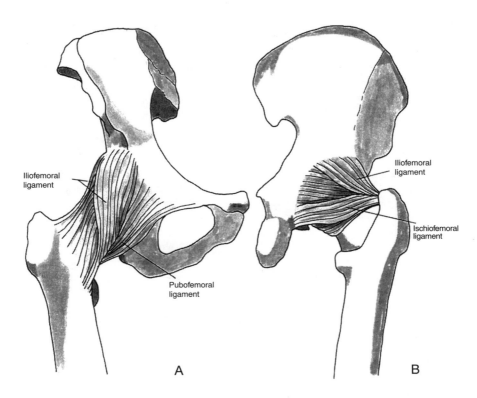

**Figure 1-6** Anterior (A) and posterior (B) views of the three extracapsular ligaments of the hip joint. (Reprinted with permission from RM Kessler. [1983] The Hip. In RM Kessler, D Hertling [eds], *Management of Common Musculoskeletal Disorders: Physical Therapy Principles and Methods* [p. 374]. Philadelphia: Harper & Row.)

- Iliofemoral ligament: also referred to as the *Y ligament* or the *ligament of Bigelow*. It is the strongest ligament. The ligament splits into two bands, forming an inverted Y shape. It helps to maintain erect posture and strengthen the anterior capsule of the hip joint.
- Pubofemoral ligament: strengthens the anterior and inferior aspects of the capsule of the hip joint.
- Ischiofemoral ligament: a thin and weaker ligament that helps to reinforce the posterior capsule of the hip joint.

A fourth ligament, the ligament of the head of the femur, also known as the *ligamentum teres*, is intracapsular and surrounded by synovial membrane (see Figure 1-1). Mechanically, this ligament is of little importance in

**Table 1-1** Ligaments of the Hip

| Ligament | Proximal attachment | Insertion | Function |
|---|---|---|---|
| Iliofemoral | Anterior inferior iliac spine and the acetabular rim | Intertrochanteric line of the femur | Chief stabilizer of the hip in the erect position<br>Prevents hyperextension<br>Posterior portion resists internal rotation |
| Ischiofemoral | The ischium Posteroinferior to the acetabular rim | Posterior aspect of the neck of the femur at the greater trochanter, just posterior to the iliofemoral ligament | Resists hip extension and internal rotation |
| Pubofemoral | Pubic aspect of acetabular rim and iliopubic eminence | Anterior to the lesser trochanter of the femur<br>Blends with medial portion of iliofemoral ligament | Resists external rotation and abduction of the hip |
| Ligament of the head of the femur | Nonarticular area of the inferior acetabulum near the acetabular notch<br>Both sides of the notch<br>Deep to the transverse ligament | Fovea of the femoral head | Provides vascularization to the head of the femur |

stability of the hip joint. It provides vascularization to the head of the femur. If the ligament of the head of the femur is ruptured, aseptic necrosis of the femoral head can occur.

## Synovium

The internal surface of the fibrous capsule is lined by the synovium. The synovium also lines the acetabular fossa, the surfaces of the acetabular labrum, and the portion of the head and neck of the femur that is contained within the hip-joint capsule. The synovium forms a sleeve for the ligament of the head of the femur and covers the acetabular fat pad. The synovial capsule is attached to the transverse acetabular ligament and the edges of the acetabu-

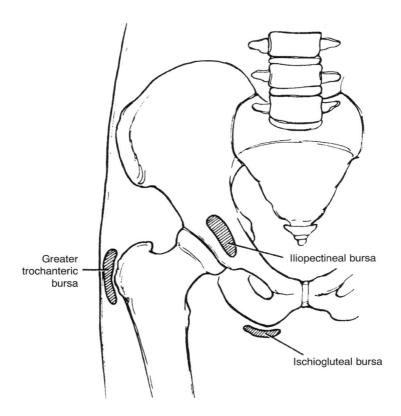

Greater
trochanteric
bursa

Iliopectineal bursa

Ischiogluteal bursa

**Figure 1-7** Anterior view of the hip, showing the three most commonly inflamed bursae. (Reprinted with permission from P Beattie. [1997] The Hip. In TR Malone, T McPoil, AJ Nitz [eds], *Orthopaedic and Sports Physical Therapy* [3rd ed] [p. 498]. St. Louis: Mosby–Year Book.)

lar fossa. Also, the synovial membrane protrudes inferior to the fibrous capsule and forms a bursa to protect the tendon of the obturator externus muscle.

### Bursae

Bursae reduce friction as muscle passes over bone or tendon. There are many bursae at the hip joint. Wadsworth (1988, p. 162) described as many as 18 bursae that exist in the hip region, "but only three appear to have clinical significance." The following are the most commonly inflamed and described bursae of the hip (Figure 1-7):

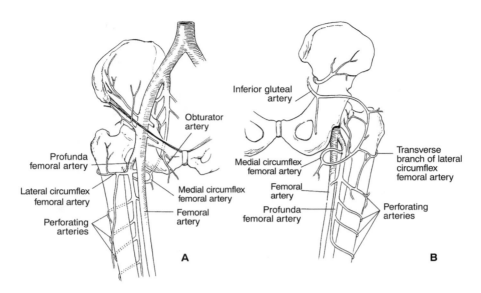

**Figure 1-8** A. Arterial supply of the anterior view of the lower limb. B. Arterial supply of the posterior view of the lower limb. (Reprinted with permission from P Beattie. [1997] The Hip. In TR Malone, T McPoil, AJ Nitz [eds], *Orthopaedic and Sports Physical Therapy* [3rd ed] [p. 469]. St. Louis: Mosby–Year Book.)

- The trochanteric bursae lie between the tendon of the gluteus maximus muscle and the posterolateral surface of the greater trochanter. Additional trochanteric bursae lie between the gluteus maximus and gluteus medius tendon and between the gluteus medius muscle and the greater trochanter.
- The ischiogluteal bursa lies over the ischial tuberosity and deep to the gluteus maximus muscle. Prolonged periods of sitting can irritate this bursa.
- The iliopectineal bursa is deep to the iliopsoas muscle as it crosses in front of the hip joint. This bursa communicates with the joint space in 15% of persons (Chandler 1934).

Reference can be made to Chapter 2 for additional information on bursae of the hip.

## Blood Supply

The hip joint receives its blood supply from several sources (Figure 1-8). It is important to understand these arterial sources and their relationship in pathologic conditions such as fractures and avascular necrosis.

The internal iliac artery branches into the superior and inferior gluteal arteries. These arteries supply the upper portion of the acetabulum, the inferior portion of the acetabular rim, and the posterior portion of the acetabular rim. The obturator artery is a branch of the superior gluteal artery. A branch of the obturator artery, known as the acetabular branch, supplies blood to the medial aspect of the acetabular rim, the surface of the acetabulum, and the transverse acetabular ligament. A small terminal branch traverses from the acetabulum to the femoral head with the ligament of the head of the femur and supplies a small area of the head just adjacent to the fovea.

The medial and lateral circumflex arteries, which are branches of either the femoral artery or profunda femoris artery, supply most of the head and neck of the femur. They surround the neck and ascend along it, forming rings around the upper region of the neck and the subcapital sulcus. Alternative blood supply is provided to the femoral neck through several anastomoses. However, anastomotic flow between the neck and head is limited.

Branches of the medial circumflex artery include the lateral, superior, and inferior epiphyseal arteries. The lateral epiphyseal artery is of particular importance, as it supplies more than half of the femoral head. Branches of the lateral circumflex artery, known as the *ascending arteries*, pierce the joint capsule close to its distal femoral attachment. They run proximally along the neck of the femur intracapsularly and deep to the synovial lining of the neck. These arteries are likely to experience an interruption of flow in the case of femoral neck fracture or increased intracapsular pressure.

## Nerve Supply

The skin over the hip region (see Chapter 3; Figure 3-6), the hip joint itself, and the muscles responsible for movement at the hip are richly innervated. It is important for the physical therapist to understand the innervation of the hip, as it can explain the source of evaluative findings such as pain and weakness. Hilton's law, as reported by Harty (1991, p. 42), states, "the same trunks of nerves, whose branches supply the groups of muscles moving a joint, furnish also a distribution of nerves to the skin over the insertion of the same muscles; and what at this moment more especially merits our attention—the interior of the joint receives its nerves from the same source."

Cutaneous nerve supply to the anterior region of the hip is often divided by the position of the nerve relative to the inguinal ligament (i.e., superior or inferior to the ligament). The iliohypogastric nerve innervates the area superior to the inguinal ligament. The subcostal nerve, the femoral branch of the genitofemoral nerve, and the ilioinguinal nerve innervate the inferior region.

Posteriorly, skin over the gluteal region is innervated by the dorsal primary rami of L1, L2, and L3; the dorsal primary rami of S1, S2, and S3; and cutaneous branches of the posterior femoral cutaneous nerve. Collectively, these nerves are often referred to as the *clunial nerves*. Also supplying posterior cutaneous innervation are the subcostal and iliohypogastric nerves. The lateral femoral nerve provides cutaneous nerve supply to both the anterolateral and posterolateral aspect of the thigh. Entrapment of the lateral femoral cutaneous nerve, known as *meralgia paresthetica*, can result in tingling and numbness at the nerve's sensory distribution on the anterolateral thigh.

The superior aspect of the joint capsule is innervated by the superior gluteal nerve (L4, L5, and S1). The anterior joint capsule receives innervation from the femoral nerve (L2, L3, and L4). The medial articular nerve, which arises from the anterior division of the obturator, supplies the anteromedial and inferior aspects of the joint capsule. The most extensive nerve supply to the joint is the posterior articular nerve to the quadratus femoris muscle. Branches of this nerve supply the posterior joint capsule, inferior regions of the joint capsule, and the ischiofemoral ligament. The obturator nerve also supplies the posterior aspect of the capsule.

Nerve supply to muscles of the hip can be found in Table 1-2. Several nerves of the hip are susceptible to injury or irritation, which frequently results in hip pain, radiating pain to the thigh, or both. The sciatic nerve is a primary source of involvement. The sciatic nerve, a continuation of the sacral plexus, passes between the obturator internus muscle and the piriformis muscle before it descends along the back of the thigh, deep to the hamstring muscles. Irritation of this nerve can be a result of inflammation of the hamstring muscles, contracture or overstretch of the piriformis muscle, or ischial bursitis. Traumatic crushing of the nerve can occur secondary to a posterior dislocation of the femoral head. There have been reports of nerve palsy of the sciatic nerve or peroneal division of the sciatic nerve after a total hip replacement (Schmalzried et al. 1991).

Irritation of the obturator nerve can also cause hip pain and refer pain to the medial thigh. The obturator nerve leaves the pelvis via the obturator foramen and is susceptible to entrapment. Obturator neuropathy can occur as a result of intrapelvic extension of cement during total hip replacement surgery (Siliski et al. 1985). Injury to the femoral nerve can affect both cutaneous nerve supply of the hip and quadriceps femoris muscle function.

The greater sciatic foramen is an important anatomic landmark in the gluteal region. The greater sciatic notch forms the roof of the foramen. The following structures exit through it (Burgess and Tile 1991):

**Table 1-2** Nerve Supply to Muscles of the Hip

| *Nerve* | *Muscle* |
|---|---|
| Femoral | Iliopsoas |
| | Rectus femoris |
| | Sartorius |
| Inferior gluteal | Gluteus maximus |
| Obturator | Adductor brevis |
| | Adductor longus |
| | Adductor magnus |
| | Obturator externus |
| Sciatic | Adductor magnus |
| | Biceps femoris |
| | Semimembranosus |
| | Semitendinosus |
| Superior gluteal | Gluteus medius |
| | Gluteus minimus |
| | Tensor fascia latae |
| Nerve to obturator internus | Gemellus superior |
| | Obturator internus |
| Nerve to quadratus femoris | Gemellus inferior |
| | Quadratus femoris |
| Ventral rami of S1 and S2 | Piriformis |

Source: Modified from JM Cuckler. (1991) Surgical Approaches. In ME Steinberg (ed), *The Hip and Its Disorders*. Philadelphia: Saunders.

One muscle
    Piriformis
Three vessel sets
    Superior gluteal artery and vein
    Inferior gluteal artery and vein
    Internal pudendal artery and vein
Seven nerves
    Sciatic
    Superior gluteal
    Inferior gluteal
    Internal pudendal
    Posterior femoral cutaneous
    Nerve to quadratus femoris
    Nerve to obturator externus

## Muscles

Almost two dozen muscles act on the hip joint. These muscles produce movements of the joint as well as provide stability. Movement around the transverse axis in the sagittal plane is provided by the hip flexors and extensors. Hip abductors and adductors provide movement in the frontal plane about a dorsal-ventral axis. The medial and lateral rotators are responsible for motion about a longitudinal axis in the transverse plane. For standardization, hip movements are commonly described as occurring in cardinal planes, but functionally the joint does not behave in cardinal planes. A summary of the origins, insertions, and innervations of the muscles providing movement at the hip joint are summarized in Table 1-3.

### Flexors

The psoas minor and major muscles combine with the iliacus muscle to provide the strongest hip flexor, known as the *iliopsoas*. The common tendon of the iliopsoas muscle inserts at the lesser trochanter of the femur. It is especially active with movements such as kicking. The rectus femoris is also a hip flexor. Being a two-joint hip flexor, the rectus femoris makes its best contribution to hip flexion when the knee is also in flexion. Considerable shortening of the rectus femoris muscle occurs with simultaneous hip flexion and knee extension. Minor contributions include lateral rotation and abduction of the hip. The sartorius, a hip flexor, is a straplike muscle that runs obliquely down the anterior aspect of the thigh and is the most superficial of the thigh muscles. Similar to the rectus femoris, it assists with lateral rotation and abduction of the hip. It also acts on the knee as a flexor and medial rotator. The tensor fascia latae works as a hip flexor and stabilizer of the pelvis. Clinically, a patient may present with adaptive shortening of the tensor fascia latae from habitual W sitting (reverse tailor position) or sartorius shortening from a tailor or yoga position (Kendall et al. 1993).

### Extensors

The gluteus maximus, a large and powerful muscle, is the chief extensor of the hip. It also assists with lateral rotation of the hip. The gluteus maximus muscle, when assisted by superior fibers of the adductor magnus muscle, extends the hip while a person climbs stairs or gets up from a seated position. The three hamstring muscles, biceps femoris, semimembranosus, and semitendinosus, are also hip extensors. These are two joint muscles and their strength as a hip extensor increases when the knee is extended; hence, when testing gluteus maximus strength, the knee should be flexed. Collectively, the hamstring muscles also flex the knee.

**Table 1-3** Muscles of the Hip: Origin, Insertion, and Nerve Supply

| Action | Muscle | Origin | Insertion | Nerve supply |
|---|---|---|---|---|
| Hip flexion | Iliopsoas | Transverse processes T12–L5 Iliac crest Sacrum | Lesser trochanter | Branches of femoral nerve |
| | Rectus femoris | Anterior and inferior iliac spine Groove superior to acetabulum | Base of patella via quadriceps tendon | Femoral nerve (L2, L3, and L4) |
| | Tensor fasciae latae | ASIS External lip iliac crest | Iliotibial tract | Superior gluteal nerve (L4 and L5) |
| | Sartorius | ASIS | Superior aspect of medial surface of tibia | Femoral nerve (L2 and L3) |
| Hip extension | Gluteus maximus | External surface ilium Dorsal surfaces of sacrum and coccyx Sacrotuberous ligament | Posterior iliotibial tract Gluteal tuberosity | Inferior gluteal nerve (L5, S1, and S2) |
| | Biceps femoris (long head) | Ischial tuberosity | Head of fibula Lateral condyle of tibia | Tibial branch of sciatic nerve (L5, S1, and S2) |
| | Semimembranosus | Ischial tuberosity | Posteromedial condyle tibia | Tibial branch of sciatic nerve (L5, S1, and S2) |
| | Semitendinosus | Ischial tuberosity | Medial flare of tibia | Tibial branch of sciatic nerve (L5, S1, and S2) |
| Hip adduction | Adductor magnus | Inferior ramus of pubis ramus of ischium | Gluteal tuberosity Medial femur | Obturator nerve (L2 and L3) |

**Table 1-3** *Continued*

| Action | Muscle | Origin | Insertion | Nerve supply |
|---|---|---|---|---|
| | | Ischial tuberosity | Adductor tubercle | Sciatic nerve (L2, L3, and L4) |
| | Adductor longus | Body of pubis, inferior to pubic crest | Middle third of linea aspera | Obturator nerve (L2, L3, and L4) |
| | Adductor brevis | Inferior ramus and body of pubis | Proximal linea aspera and pectineal line | Obturator nerve (L2, L3, and L4) |
| Hip abduction | Gluteus medius | Anterior gluteal line | Lateral surface of greater trochanter | Superior gluteal nerve (L5 and S1) |
| | Gluteus minimus | External surface of ilium | Anterior surface of greater trochanter | Superior gluteal nerve (L5 and S1) |
| | Tensor fasciae latae | ASIS External lip iliac crest | Iliotibial tract | Superior gluteal nerve (L4 and L5) |
| Hip medial rotation (secondary action) | Gluteus minimus | External surface of ilium | Anterior surface of greater trochanter | Superior gluteal nerve (L5 and S1) |
| | Gluteus medius | Anterior gluteal line | Lateral surface of greater trochanter | Superior gluteal nerve (L5 and S1) |
| | Tensor fasciae latae | ASIS External iliac crest | Iliotibial tract | Superior gluteal nerve (L4 and L5) |
| Hip lateral rotation | Obturator internus | Pelvic surface of obturator membrane | Medial surface of greater trochanter | Nerve to obturator internus (L5 and S1) |
| | Obturator externus | External surface obturator membrane Rami of pubis and ischium | Trochanteric fossa | Obturator nerve (L3 and L4) |

| Action | Muscle | Origin | Insertion | Nerve supply |
|--------|--------|--------|-----------|--------------|
| | Gemellus superior | Spine of ischium | Greater trochanter | Nerve to obturator internus |
| | Gemellus inferior | Tuberosity of ischium | Greater trochanter | Nerve to quadratus femoris |
| | Quadratus femoris | Lateral border of ischial tuberosity | Quadrate tubercle | Nerve to quadratus femoris |
| | Piriformis | Anterior surface of sacrum Sacrotuberous ligament | Superior border of greater trochanter | Ventral rami of S1 and S2 |

ASIS = anterior superior iliac spine.
Sources: Modified from CR Saudek. (1985) The Hip. In JA Gould III, GG Davies (eds), *Orthopaedic and Sports Physical Therapy.* St. Louis: Mosby; and KL Moore. (1985) *Clinically Oriented Anatomy.* Baltimore: Williams & Wilkins.

### Adductors

The adductor muscles of the hip form most of the muscle mass along the medial aspect of the thigh. The primary adductors (see Table 1-3) are the adductor longus, adductor brevis, and adductor magnus (Reid 1992). As a group, these adductor muscles originate from both the inferior ramus and body of the pubis and insert along the linea aspera of the femur. The gracilis and pectineus muscles are also adductors of the hip. Each hip adductor muscle also performs one or more secondary actions at the hip. Sources agree the adductor longus, adductor brevis, gracilis, and pectineus can assist with flexion and medial rotation of the thigh, depending on the position of the hip (Grabiner 1989; Kapandji 1970; LeVeau 1994). Anterior fibers of the adductor magnus muscle assist with hip flexion, and posterior fibers of the same muscle assist with hip extension. The gracilis is a two-joint muscle and also assists with flexion of the leg.

### Abductors

The gluteus medius and gluteus minimus are prime movers for the motion of abduction. The gluteus minimus, a fan-shaped muscle, lies deep to the gluteus medius. The tensor fascia latae also provides assistance with abduction of the hip. However, the contribution of this muscle as an abductor is dependent on position of the hip. Most sources agree that maximum power of the tensor fascia latae is generated when the hip is in the neutral position (Kapandji 1970; Magee 1992), but some argue that the muscle is effective as an abductor only when the hip is in flexion (Norkin and Levangie 1992).

The gluteus medius is a three-part muscle that inserts at the outer aspect of the greater trochanter. It has anterior, middle, and posterior fibers. The anterior portion flexes and medially rotates the hip, and the posterior portion acts during extension and lateral rotation. All muscle fibers abduct the hip. The gluteus medius plays an important role in stabilizing the pelvis and prevents dropping of the pelvis, known as the *Trendelenburg sign*, contralateral to the support leg during gait.

The more superior fibers of the gluteus maximus muscle and sartorius muscle can also assist in active abduction against strong resistance.

Kapandji (1970, p. 54) described the deltoid of the hip as "a wide muscular fan covering the external aspect of the hip joint." The two muscular parts of the triangular deltoid are the tensor fascia latae and the superior fibers of the gluteus maximus. The tensor fascia latae is anterior. It arises from the anterosuperior iliac spine and runs obliquely inferior and posterior. Posteriorly, the superior fibers of the gluteus maximus arise from the dorsum of the coccyx and sacrum and from the posterior third of the iliac crest. They also run obliquely, but in an inferior and anterior direction. Both muscles, the tensor fascia latae and the superior fibers of the gluteus maximus, insert into the anterior and posterior borders of the iliotibial tract, respectively. Pure abduction is produced when both muscles of the deltoid contract in a balanced fashion (Kapandji 1970).

### Medial Rotators

There are no muscles of the hip that act as primary movers for medial rotation. Several muscles produce medial rotation as a secondary action, and these include the following:

- Tensor fascia latae
- Gluteus medius
- Gluteus minimus

### Lateral Rotators

The six primary lateral rotators are noted in Table 1-3. Due to their anatomic position, these deep, one-joint muscles are difficult to study using electromyography surface or wire electrodes.

The superior and inferior gemelli accompany the obturator internus muscle. The gemellus superior runs along the superior border of the obturator internus, and the gemellus inferior runs along the inferior border.

The three muscles share a common insertion at the greater trochanter of the femur via the tendon of the obturator internus. The obturator externus lies behind the adductor muscles and winds its way around the femoral neck. It acts as a lateral rotator when the hip is flexed. The quadratus femoris is a short, flat, and quadrilateral muscle that is located inferior to the obturator internus and gemelli muscles. The piriformis muscle occupies a key position in the gluteal region. The superior gluteal vessels and nerve emerge superior to the piriformis, and the inferior gluteal vessels and nerve emerge inferior to it. The sciatic nerve passes anterior to the piriformis in 85% of cases as it travels through the greater sciatic notch. However, there are variations in this anatomic relationship (Figure 1-9). In approximately 10% of the population, the sciatic nerve divides before entering the gluteal region, where the common peroneal division passes through the piriformis muscle, and the tibial division passes anterior to piriformis (Beaton and Anson 1937; Travell and Simons 1992).

The sciatic nerve is vulnerable to compression or irritation from the piriformis muscle, whether it passes anterior, posterior, or through the muscle and whether divided or undivided.

The piriformis performs lateral rotation when the hip is extended, abducts at approximately 60 degrees flexion, and performs medial rotation at 90 degrees flexion (Kapandji 1970)—this is an example of inversion of muscle action (see "Inversion of Muscular Action"). As a group, the lateral rotator muscles lie almost perpendicular to the shaft of the femur and parallel to the head and neck. This orientation allows them to function effectively as lateral rotators of the hip and, theoretically, as compressors of the joint to provide stabilization, much as the rotator cuff does in the shoulder. The piriformis and obturator externus, in combination with the gluteus minimus and medius are called *muscles of apposition of the hip* (Kapandji 1970).

### Inversion of Muscular Action

The "inversion of muscular action" concept, discussed by Kapandji (1970), explains that the muscles of the hip joint can have different actions depending on the position of the joint. This results from a change in the relationship of the line of action of a muscle to the axis of rotation of the hip joint. It is most common with the secondary actions of muscles. An example of inversion of muscular action at the hip occurs with the flexor component of the adductor muscle group. All hip adductors are flexors when the hip is in neutral (zero-degrees flexion), except the posterior fibers of the abductor magnus (Kapandji 1970). As the hip changes position, the following inversion of muscular action occurs with the adductors:

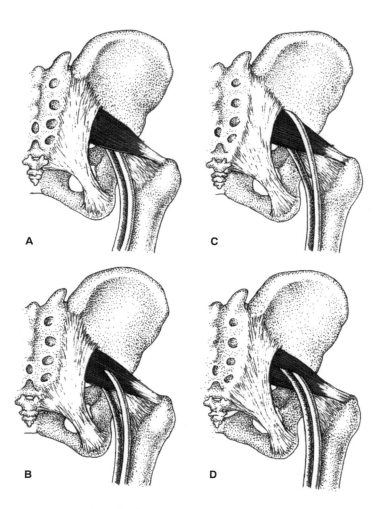

**Figure 1-9** Four routes by which portions of the sciatic nerve may exit the pelvis. A. The usual route, in which all fibers of the nerve pass anterior to the piriformis between the muscle and the rim of the greater sciatic foramen, seen in about 85% of cadavers. B. The peroneal portion of the nerve passes through the piriformis muscle and the tibial portion travels anterior to the muscle, as seen in more than 10% of cadavers. C. The peroneal portion of the sciatic nerve loops above and then posterior to the muscle, and the tibial portion passes anterior to it; both portions lie between the muscle and the upper or lower rim of the greater sciatic foramen, as seen in 2–3% of cadavers. D. An undivided sciatic nerve penetrates the piriformis muscle in less than 1% of cadavers. (Reprinted with permission from JG Travell, DG Simons. [1992] *Myofascial Pain and Dysfunction. The Trigger Point Manual. Volume 2, The Lower Extremities* [p. 201]. Baltimore: Williams & Wilkins.)

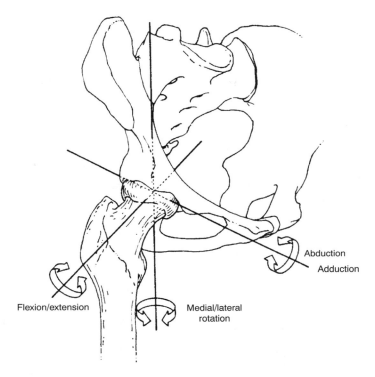

**Figure 1-10** Three degrees of freedom. Flexion and extension occur in the sagittal plane. Abduction and adduction occur in the frontal plane. Medial and lateral rotation occur in the transverse plane. (Reprinted with permission from D Lee. [1989] *The Pelvic Girdle* [p. 54]. New York: Churchill Livingstone.)

- The adductor longus is a flexor at 50 degrees but an extensor at 70 degrees.
- The adductor brevis is a flexor up to 50 degrees and then becomes an extensor.
- The gracilis is a flexor up to 40 degrees.

## Biomechanics

The hip joint possesses three degrees of freedom. Motion occurs in the sagittal, frontal, and transverse planes (Figure 1-10). Three degrees of freedom allow for the movement of circumduction to occur at the hip joint. Kapandji (1970, p. 22) defines circumduction as, "the combination of elementary movements occurring simultaneously around the three axes."

The clinician should be familiar with the following positions of the hip (note that *open-packed* and *closed-packed* are jargon terms used by physical therapists):

- Open-packed position (loose-packed position, resting position): for comfort and to accommodate swelling, a position of 10 degrees flexion, 10 degrees abduction, and 10 degrees external rotation of the hip is commonly observed (Wadsworth 1988); for joint mobilization purposes, a position of 30 degrees flexion, 30 degrees abduction, and slight lateral rotation is described (Kaltenborn 1989); the true physiological position of the hip is approximately 55 degrees flexion, 55 degrees abduction, and 5 degrees external rotation (Kapandji 1970). Norkin and Levangie (1992) noted that the hip is one of the few joints in which the position of optimal articular contact is the open-packed position rather than the close-packed position. The open-packed position allows for ligamentous laxity and the greatest amount of joint play in all directions.
- Close-packed position: full extension with medial rotation and abduction.
- Capsular pattern: a capsular pattern exists when the loss of joint motion demonstrates a characteristic pattern. There is variation in the literature as to how the capsular pattern for the hip is described. However, from clinical experience and from forming a general consensus of the literature, the most limited motions in a hip capsular pattern are medial rotation, extension, and abduction.

The articular surfaces of the hip do not maintain optimal congruence in the standing or erect position. This is a particular concern with pediatric conditions of the hip such as developmental dysplasia, congenital coxa vara, and Legg-Calvé-Perthes disease. To improve the congruence of the joint surfaces, the containment of the femoral head within the acetabulum, and the coverage of the joint surfaces with articular cartilage, the pediatric hip is often positioned in the "frog-leg" position of flexion (55 degrees), abduction (55 degrees), and slight external rotation (5 degrees).

### Kinematics

The hip joint allows for a large degree of mobility despite the strong articular capsule and ligamentous stability. Range of motion (ROM) at the hip joint should be interpreted as movement of the femur relative to the pelvis.

The largest ROM at the hip joint occurs in the sagittal plane. Flexion and extension occur around a left-right axis, and movement takes place in the sagittal plane. Generally, active movements of flexion and extension at the hip joint are of a lesser value than passive movements. Active hip flexion reaches 120 degrees when the knee is flexed either due to capsular restriction or contact with the trunk and 90 degrees when the knee is extended secondary to hamstring tension. Passive flexion can reach 140 degrees with the knee flexed. Hip extension reaches 10–20 degrees actively and 30 degrees passively with the knee extended. Passive tension of the rectus femoris muscle can lessen active hip extension when the knee is flexed. The iliofemoral ligament can also limit hip extension. The clinician should recall that anterior pelvic tilting on a fixed femur produces hip flexion, and posterior tilting results in hip extension. See Table 3-6 for anatomic structures limiting hip motion.

Movements of abduction and adduction at the hip occur around an anteroposterior axis, and movement takes place in the frontal plane. Abduction of the lower extremity is the lateral movement directly away from the midline of the body. Average hip abduction is 50 degrees (Oatis 1990). The movement is limited by adductor muscle tightness, the pubofemoral ligament, and the iliofemoral ligament. Pure adduction, from a neutral position, is limited by the presence of the opposite lower extremity. The hip can adduct up to 30 degrees and is limited by tightness of the tensor fascia latae muscle. See Table 4-3 for normative hip ROM values by age.

Hip rotation occurs about a vertical axis when the hip joint is in neutral. However, hip ROM is usually assessed with the hip in 90 degrees flexion, in either supine or sitting. It is also assessed in prone with the knees bent. Medial rotation is restricted by the external rotator muscles and the ischiofemoral ligament. A restriction in lateral rotation can be secondary to the following:

- The lateral band of the iliofemoral ligament
- The pubofemoral ligament
- Tension in the medial rotator muscles
- Femoral anteversion

Design and implementation of hip rehabilitation programs requires the therapist to be aware of mobility required to complete functional activities. Average hip ROM required for common functional activities is as follows (Johnston and Smidt 1970):

- Ascending stairs: 67 degrees flexion
- Descending stairs: 36 degrees flexion

## NORMAL GAIT

| SWING 40% | | | STANCE 60% | | | | |
|---|---|---|---|---|---|---|---|
| INITIAL SWING | MIDSWING | TERMINAL SWING | INITIAL CONTACT | LOADING RESPONSE | MIDSWING | TERMINAL STANCE | PRESWING |
| | | | | | | | |

| HIP | FLEXION 20° NEUTRAL ROTATION ABDUCTION ADDUCTION | FLEXION 20°-30° NEUTRAL ROTATION ABDUCTION ADDUCTION | FLEXION 30° NEUTRAL ROTATION ABDUCTION ADDUCTION | FLEXION 30° NEUTRAL ROTATION ABDUCTION ADDUCTION | FLEXION 30° NEUTRAL ROTATION ABDUCTION ADDUCTION | EXTENDING TO NEUTRAL NEUTRAL ROTATION ABDUCTION ADDUCTION | APPARENT HYPEREXT 10° NEUTRAL ROTATION ABDUCTION ADDUCTION | NEUTRAL EXTENSION NEUTRAL ROTATION ABDUCTION ADDUCTION |
|---|---|---|---|---|---|---|---|---|

**Figure 1-11** Gait cycle. Swing phase (40%) and stance phase (60%) of one complete gait cycle with motion at the hip joint noted for each phase. (Hyperext = hyperextension.) (Reprinted with permission from J Perry. [1981] *Pathokinesiological Service and Physical Therapy Department, Normal and Pathological Gait Syllabus* [p. 11]. Downey, CA: Ranchos Los Amigos Medical Center.)

- Putting on trousers: 90 degrees flexion
- Squatting: 122 degrees flexion, 26 degrees medial rotation, and 28 degrees abduction
- Sitting: 104 degrees flexion (for average-height chair)
- Tying shoes with foot on floor: 124 degrees flexion, 19 degrees abduction, and 15 degrees lateral rotation

### Gait

The hip joint plays a primary role in lower-extremity advancement during gait activities. To have a better understanding of this role, the therapist needs to recall the gait cycle. One gait cycle, or stride, is described as the point of initial contact to the next point of initial contact of the same lower extremity. One complete cycle is recognized as 100%. The gait cycle is divided into stance and swing periods (Figure 1-11).

The Ranchos Los Amigos gait syllabus and Perry's text on gait analysis further subcategorize gait into eight phases (Adkins et al. 1981; Perry 1992). The eight phases and percent of the gait cycle they represent are found in Table 1-4.

Kinematics of the hip during gait are easily understood with reference to Table 1-4 for percent of the gait cycle. During a normal stride, the hip rotates approximately 40 degrees in the sagittal plane. Maximum hip extension of

**Table 1-4** Eight Phases of the Gait Cycle

| Phase | Percent of cycle |
|---|---|
| Initial contact | 0–2% |
| Loading response | 0–10% |
| Midstance | 10–30% |
| Terminal stance | 30–50% |
| Preswing | 50–60% |
| Initial swing | 60–73% |
| Midswing | 73–87% |
| Terminal swing | 87–100% |

Sources: Modified from HV Adkins, L Baker, J Campbell, et al. (1981) *Normal and Pathological Gait Syllabus*. Downey, CA: Professional Staff of Ranchos Los Amigos Hospital; and W Perry. (1992) *GAIT ANALYSIS: Normal and Pathological Function*. Thorofare, NJ: Slack.

10 degrees occurs at about 50% of the gait cycle, and maximum flexion of 30–35 degrees is reached at approximately 85% of the cycle. Hip adduction occurs through early stance's loading response and reaches a maximum of 5 degrees at 80% of the stance phase. Hip abduction reaches a peak of 5–7 degrees in early swing. Maximal medial rotation occurs at the end of the loading response. The hip laterally rotates during swing phase (Chao and Cahalan 1990; Giannini et al. 1994; Oatis 1990; Perry 1992).

Muscles of the hip provide control in advancement of the lower extremity during gait. Initial contact is marked by activity of the hamstrings and gluteus maximus musculature, which aid in hip extension. In midstance, the abductors stabilize the pelvis. The gluteus minimus and medius continue to provide lateral stabilization in terminal stance. Muscles active in late stance and preswing hip flexion are the iliacus and anterior fibers of the tensor fascia lata. The gluteus maximus and hamstrings are strongly active in terminal swing to decelerate hip flexion.

The average ROM and muscle activity occurring at the hip during the eight phases of gait are summarized as follows (Perry 1992):

Initial contact
    ROM: 30 degrees flexion
    Muscle activity: hamstrings, gluteus maximus
Loading response
    ROM: 30 degrees flexion, 5–10 degrees adduction, maximal medial
        rotation

Muscle activity: hamstrings, gluteus maximus

Midstance

ROM: hip extends toward 0 degrees flexion and to neutral abduction

Muscle activity: gluteus medius, gluteus minimus, tensor fascia lata

Terminal stance

ROM: 10 degrees extension

Muscle activity: iliacus

Preswing

ROM: hip returns to 0 degrees flexion, maximal lateral rotation

Muscle activity: iliacus, adductor longus

Initial swing

ROM: 20 degrees flexion, 5 degrees abduction

Muscle activity: iliopsoas, rectus femoris, gracilis, sartorius, tensor fascia lata

Midswing

ROM: 20–30 degrees flexion

Muscle activity: iliopsoas, gracilis, sartorius

Terminal swing

ROM: 30 degrees flexion

Muscle activity: hamstrings, gluteus maximus

A decrease in ROM, muscle weakness, or other hip-joint pathology can alter the gait pattern at any of the eight phases of gait. The physical therapist commonly terms this alteration in biomechanics as a *gait deviation*. Common gait deviations are as follows:

Antalgic gait (analgesic gait)

Primarily due to pain

Decreased or avoidance of weightbearing on the involved side

Shortened stance

Unloading of involved limb

Trendelenburg gait (uncompensated)

Contralateral pelvic drop during stance phase of affected limb

Weakness of the gluteus medius muscle

Possible congenital hip dislocation

Apparent lateral protrusion of stance hip

Compensated Trendelenburg gait (gluteus medius lurch or Duchenne sign)

Trunk shift or lean toward involved limb during stance phase to decrease force required of ipsilateral hip abductor muscles and to maintain center of gravity over base of support

Extreme weakness of gluteus medius muscle

Can increase stance time on involved limb

Duck waddle (bilateral compensated Trendelenburg gait)

  Rolling of hips or shifting of trunk from side to side during stance phase with each step, essentially a bilateral compensated Trendelenburg gait

  Significant waddling element

  Exaggerated lumbar lordosis in walking

  Difficulty with running or climbing stairs

  Typical with muscular dystrophy diagnosis, bilateral hip abductor weakness, and children with bilateral congenital coxa vara

Gluteus maximus (hip extensor gait)

  Weakness of gluteus maximus muscle

  Possible hip flexion contracture

  Increased lumbar lordosis

  Backward lean of trunk with loading response and during stance phase

  Slightly elevated hip of involved limb in midstance secondary to knee extension

Scissors gait

  Excessive hip adduction during swing phase

  Swing limb crosses stance limb

  Narrow base of support

  Often unable to advance limbs secondary to "crossing" of knees and feet

Short leg gait

  Ipsilateral pelvic drop in stance to accommodate a decrease in leg length

  Wide-based gait

  Possible circumduction of longer limb during swing phase

Psoas gait

  Weakness of psoas muscle

  Hip held in external rotation, flexion, and adduction during swing phase

  Adductors compensate for weakness of hip flexors

  Exaggerated trunk and pelvis motion

Stiff hip gait

  Patient lifts the lower extremity higher than normal to clear ground

  Characterized by excessive lumbar and trunk motion

  Compensated for by increased pelvic and lumbar motion and increased contralateral hip and ipsilateral knee motion (Gore et al. 1975)

### Bilateral Stance

The line of gravity falls just posterior or through the axis of the hip joint in the sagittal plane during erect bilateral stance. This position creates a slight posterior tilt of the pelvis on the femoral head, which is opposed by passive tension of the hip-joint ligament and joint capsule. As long as the line of gravity remains in the posterior or neutral position, an anterior-posterior equilibrium is maintained with little or no muscle activity.

Additionally, little or no muscle activity is required to maintain equilibrium in the frontal plane when bilateral stance remains symmetrical. The joint axis of each hip is equidistant from the line of gravity, and the body weight on each femoral head is the same. The gravitational torques around each hip are also the same but occur in opposite directions. Therefore, the pelvis is maintained in equilibrium secondary to the opposing gravitational torques of equal magnitude. Active muscle contraction of the contralateral hip abductors and adductors is required to return to a neutral position from a nonsymmetric bilateral stance (Figure 1-12).

### Unilateral Stance

In unilateral stance, significant hip-joint muscle forces are required to maintain equilibrium in the frontal plane. As reported by Paul (1966), Fischer (1895–1904) was one of the first investigators to recognize that muscle forces were largely responsible for the high forces generated during unilateral stance. The hip abductor muscles must respond to the natural tendency of the pelvis and trunk to drop toward the side of the unweighted limb. Since the lever arm from the hip-joint center to the line of gravity of body weight is about 2.5 times greater than the lever arm for hip abduction force, a force 2.5 times body weight must be generated by the abductor muscles to balance the pelvis in the frontal plane (Figure 1-13). This is a classic example of a first-order lever system. This example represents a static model, but to understand the loads on the hip with dynamic activity requires measurement in vivo (i.e., directly from within the body).

Rydell (1966) was the first to study hip forces in vivo, and he reported total hip-joint force during unilateral stance to be as high as 3.3 times body weight. More recent in vivo force studies have obtained similar results (Bergmann et al. 1993).

In patients with diseases and disorders of the hip (e.g., osteoarthritis), an appropriate intervention may be to teach the patient methods of reducing hip abductor muscle force. The following are treatment options:

- Ipsilateral trunk and pelvis lean: a compensatory lateral lean of the trunk toward the osteoarthritic or painful hip decreases the length of the moment arm (OC) of the body-weight force. In turn, this decreases the force of the hip abductor muscles on the involved side during

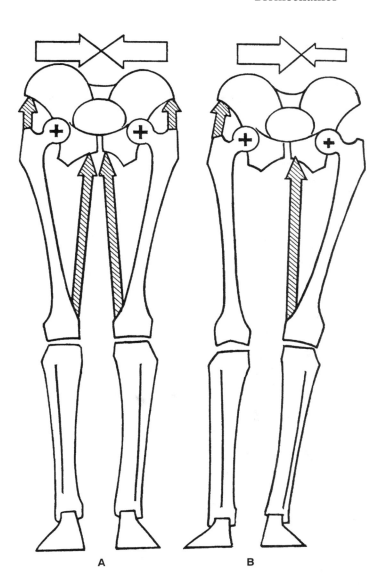

A                                B

**Figure 1-12** Pelvic stability. A. Neutral bilateral stance or symmetry. B. Non-symmetric bilateral stance in which the pelvis tilts laterally toward the side of the adductor prominence (left). (Reprinted with permission from IA Kapandji. [1970] *The Physiology of the Joints: Volume 2: The Lower Extremity* [p. 57]. Edinburgh, UK: Churchill Livingstone.)

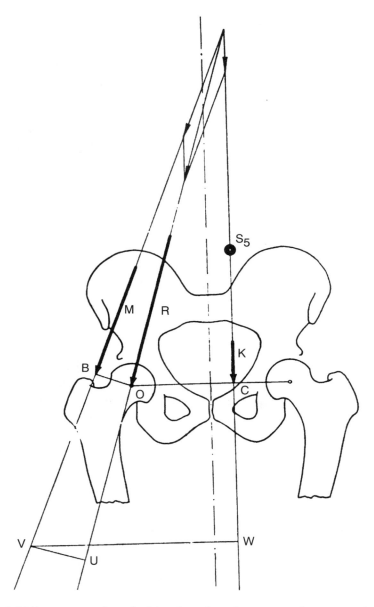

**Figure 1-13** Forces exerted on the hip when the subject is standing on one leg. ($S_5$ = center of gravity of the mass of the body acting on the hip [i.e., head, trunk, upper limbs, and opposite leg] K = force exerted by the partial body mass; OC = lever arm of force K; M = force exerted by the abductor muscles to counterbalance K; OB = lever arm of force M; R = resultant of forces K and M.) (Reprinted with permission from F Pauwels. [1976] *Biomechanics of the Normal and Diseased Hip: Theoretical Foundation, Technique and Results of Treatment.* Berlin: Springer-Verlag.)

es the force of the hip abductor muscles on the involved side during single-limb support and decreases the joint reaction force.

- Weight loss: using the equation $K \times OC = M \times OB$ used in Figure 1-13, a decrease in 1 lb of body weight theoretically decreases the force of the hip abductor muscles on the involved limb by 2.5 lb for each pound of weight loss (given that the OB to OC ratio equals 1 to 25).
- Contralateral cane use: provides a "sharing" of the counterclockwise hip moment that is required to maintain frontal-plane equilibrium in unilateral stance. The hip abductor muscles also share in producing the counterclockwise hip moment (Neumann 1989). The required hip-abductor force is reduced when a cane is held contralateral to the painful or osteoarthritic hip.
- Ipsilateral load carry: if the patient situation necessitates carrying a load, it should be carried ipsilateral to the side of the affected hip (Neumann and Hase 1994). Similar to contralateral cane use, an ipsilateral load also creates a counterclockwise hip moment that is shared with the hip-abductor muscles on the involved side. Thus, the hip-abductor force is reduced.

### Lumbar-Pelvic-Hip Relationship

When observing the gait pattern of a patient with a known or suspected hip pathology, the therapist must be careful to observe the motion occurring at the pelvis and the lumbar spine, in addition to the hip joint. Compensatory patterns of the hip, pelvis, and lumbar spine can influence the evaluative findings. It is important to understand the compensatory relationship of the three. The motions that can occur at the pelvis, hip joint, and lumbar spine in each of three planes during *right unilateral stance* are as follows (Norkin and Levangie 1992):

- Sagittal plane: (1) anterior pelvic tilt, hip flexion, and lumbar extension or (2) posterior pelvic tilt, hip extension, and lumbar flexion
- Frontal plane: (1) lateral pelvic tilt (right pelvic drop), right hip adduction, and right lateral lumbar flexion or (2) lateral pelvic tilt (right pelvic hike), right hip abduction, and left lateral lumbar flexion
- Transverse plane: (1) forward pelvic rotation, right hip medial rotation, and left lumbar rotation or (2) backward pelvic rotation, right hip lateral rotation, and right lumbar rotation

## Forces and Pressures

In vivo hip joint forces during exercise, gait, and other functional activities have been studied by several researchers (Table 1-5). Rydell

**Table 1-5** Range of In Vivo Forces and Pressures at the Hip for Various Activities

|  | Activity | Force range (×BW) | | Pressure range (MPa) | |
|---|---|---|---|---|---|
|  |  | Min max | Max max | Min max | Max max |
| **Exercise** | Passive hip ROM | 0.30[a] | 0.50[a] | — | 1.7[b] |
|  | Stationary bicycling | 0.5[c] | 1.40[c] | 1.6[b] | 5.8[d] |
|  | Active exercises | 0.46[e] | 3.0[f] | — | — |
|  | Supine hip abduction | 0.46[e] | 0.77[e] | 1.69[g] | 3.5[d] |
|  | Straight leg raise | 0.97[e] | 2.0[h] | 1.85[g] | 5.9[i] |
|  | Lifting opposite leg | 0.4[e] | 2.6[j] | — | — |
|  | Isometric quadriceps | — | — | 2.13[i] | 3.44[k] |
|  | Bridging | 2.10[a] | 3.0[f] | 2.1[d] | 3.8[d] |
|  | Prone hip extension | 1.25[e] | 2.11[e] | 3.4[d] | 4.9[d] |
|  | Isometric hip extension | — | — | 3.1[d] | 6.2[d] |
|  | Resisted hip extension (supine) | — | 2.70[f] | — | — |
|  | Sidelying hip abduction | — | — | 3.78[k] | 6.3[d] |
|  | Isometric hip abduction | — | — | 4.14[g] | 12.9[d] |
|  | Standing on operated leg, abducting non-operated hip | — | — | 5.9[d] | 12.6[d] |
|  | Standing on non-operated leg, abducting operated hip | — | — | 7.8[d] | 9.8[d] |
| **Gait** | Free speed gait | 1.51[e] | 4.64[l] | 3.69[g] | 6.7[d] |
|  | Slow gait | 1.8[j] | 2.93[l] | 5.2[d] | 7.8[d] |

| | Activity | Force range (×BW) | | Pressure range (MPa) | |
|---|---|---|---|---|---|
| | | Min max | Max max | Min max | Max max |
| | Fast gait | 2.7[j] | 4.71[l] | 4.4[m] | 7.7[d] |
| | Walking at various speeds, (no aid) | 1.51[e] | 4.71[l] | 3.69[g] | 7.8[d] |
| | NWB (crutches or walker) | — | — | 1.08[i] | 2.4[b] |
| | TWB (crutches or walker) | — | — | 2.0[n] | 6.5[n] |
| | PWB (crutches or walker) | 1.82[o] | — | 1.39[p] | 3.5[b] |
| | Bilateral crutch walking | 0.6[j] | 3.1[j] | 1.39[p] | 6.5[n] |
| | Ipsilateral crutch walking | 1.5[j] | 2.4[j] | — | — |
| | Contralateral crutch walking | 1.4[j] | 2.8[j] | — | — |
| | Contralateral cane walking | 1.9[j] | 2.9[j] | 3.8[m] | 5.4[b] |
| **Other** | Chair-rise | 0.8[j] | 1.6[j] | 1.21[p] | 18.0[b] |
| | Stairs-up (with and without aid) | 0.5[j] | 6.11[q] | 2.39[p] | 13.75[p] |
| | Stairs-down | 1.29[e] | 5.95[q] | — | 18.2[r] |
| | Accidental stumble | 7.2[l] | 8.7[l] | — | — |
| | Jogging | 4.33[e] | 5.84[l] | — | 7.7[b] |
| | Jumping | — | — | 7.8[b] | 16.2[r] |
| | Double-leg stance | 0.5[s] | 2.42[o] | 0.8[d] | 1.4[d] |
| | Single-leg stance | 2.0[j] | 5.4[j] | 7.2[d] | 9.7[d] |
| | Single-leg stance on opposite leg | 0.4[e] | 0.94[e] | 4.2[d] | 9.8[d] |

**Table 1-5** *Continued*

| | Force range (×BW) | | Pressure range (MPa) | |
|---|---|---|---|---|
| *Activity* | *Min max* | *Max max* | *Min max* | *Max max* |
| Ischial weightbearing brace (walking) | 2.36[t] | 2.48[t] | — | 3.6[b] |

[a]Bergmann et al. (1989)  
[b]Hodge et al. (1989)  
[c]Wolff et al. (1989)  
[d]Tackson (1996)  
[e]Rydell (1966)  
[f]Bergmann et al. (1990a)  
[g]Krebs et al. (1991)  
[h]Davy (1994)  
[i]Behr (1994)  
[j]Kotzar et al. (1991)  
[k]Strickland et al. (1992)  
[l]Bergmann et al. (1993)  
[m]Robbins (1995)  
[n]Givens-Heiss et al. (1992)  
[o]English and Kilvington (1979)  
[p]Fagerson et al. (1995)  
[q]Bergmann et al. (1995)  
[r]Carlson (1993)  
[s]Davy et al. (1988)  
[t]Bergmann et al. (1990b)  

ROM = range of motion; NWB = nonweightbearing; TWB = touch weightbearing; PWB = partial weightbearing; Min max = lowest reported maximum; Max max = highest reported maximum; ×BW = a multiple of body weight; MPa = megapascals.
Source: TL Fagerson. (May 1997) Presented at American Physical Therapy Association Annual Conference, San Diego.

(1966) was the first to study in vivo joint forces using a noncemented endoprosthesis instrumented with strain gauges in the femoral neck. Additional researchers have used force-instrumented total hip replacements (Bergmann et al. 1993; Davy et al. 1988; English and Kilvington 1979), and others have used implanted hip nails that broadcast the bending moment at the nail-plate junction (Brown et al. 1988; Frankel et al. 1971). Recent in vivo hip studies have examined acetabular contact pressures collected from two separate pressure-instrumented femoral head endoprostheses (Fagerson et al. 1995; Krebs et al. 1991). Recall, that force equals mass times acceleration, and pressure equals force over unit area.

Most in vivo hip-force studies report the measured force as a multiple of body weight (×BW). Studies measuring in vivo acetabular contact pressures report results in megapascal (MPa). One MPa is equal to 145 psi. Because acetabular contact pressures cannot be expressed in terms of a body weight multiple (×BW), the analogy of car tire pressure is helpful. An average car tire pressure is 29 psi. During walking, acetabular contact pressures in the hip are about 5 MPa, which is 25 times the amount of pressure in a car tire. During sit-to-stand transfers, acetabular contact pressures can be as high as 18 MPa, which is 90 times the amount of pressure in a car tire. It is believed that, in normal hip joints, hydrostatic pressure in the fluid between the articulating surfaces withstands more than 90% of the load so that the cartilage matrix does not have to withstand such tremendously high pressure loads (Macirowski et al. 1994).

Table 1-5 documents the range of maximum forces (×BW) and pressures (MPa) reported in the literature for various activities. "Min max" is the lowest reported maximum, and "Max max" is the highest reported maximum for a given activity. The table demonstrates that a wide range of loads occur at the hip between different activities and within the same activity. This suggests that there must be variables other than different activities that contribute to loads at the hip. The following variables have been identified in the studies reported in Table 1-5:

1. Instructions to the patient
2. Weightbearing status
3. Use of assistive device
4. Length of time postsurgery
5. Exercise speed
6. Exercise effort
7. Gait speed
8. Height of stairs
9. Height of chairs
10. Use of chair armrests
11. Cortical preprogramming
12. Accidental loss of balance or stumbling

Stair climbing and rising from a chair can cause very high acetabular contact pressures (see Table 1-5). They also induce a high "out-of-plane" load component that has been identified as a potential precipitating factor for loosening of hip replacements (Burke et al. 1991; Harrigan et al. 1992; Phillips et al. 1990).

## Summary

The stability and mobility properties of the hip are diverse. The clinician who lacks in anatomic and biomechanical knowledge of hip-joint function is also likely to be deficient in evaluation and treatment.

> *Nowhere is the knowledge of anatomy more essential and the ignorance of it more apparent than in the examination of the musculoskeletal system.*
>
> —Sir Sydney Sunderland (1978)

# 2

# Diseases and Disorders of the Hip

## Timothy L. Fagerson

In addition to a good foundation in anatomy and biomechanics, a good understanding of the many diseases and disorders that affect the hip is required for accurate diagnosis and effective management. Even though the hip is not as commonly injured as the knee or low back (Cunningham and Kelsey 1984), a poor understanding of hip details places many clinicians at risk for misdiagnosing some serious conditions.

A large number of conditions affect the hip (Table 2-1). It is important to grasp the big picture, as well as details of each condition, so that all factors can be considered in formulating a diagnosis and making clinical decisions. Note from Table 2-1 the strong developmental disposition for hip disorders as evidenced by their relationship to age.

Diseases and disorders of the hip are presented in this chapter based on type of condition: (1) arthritis, (2) bone disorders, (3) fractures and dislocation, (4) soft tissue disorders, (5) nerve entrapment syndromes, and (6) pediatric hip disorders. A bulleted, quick reference style is used, making it easy for the clinician to find a topic when a condition is suspected. Most conditions are presented using the following outline:

Definition
Epidemiology
Clinical features
Radiologic features
Diagnosis (classification)
Management (treatment)
Hip tip(s)

Additional factors are included for some conditions when warranted, such as risk factors and prevention of risk factors for osteoporosis, red flags for avascular necrosis (AVN), and hip involvement for diseases that affect multiple joints and for which the hip problem is secondary (e.g., rheumatoid arthritis, ankylos-

**Table 2-1** Hip Disorders and Their Relationship to Age

| Disorder | Age |
| --- | --- |
| Developmental dysplasia of the hip | Newborn through infancy |
| Congenital coxa vara | 1–3 yrs |
| Acute transient synovitis | 2–10 yrs |
| Legg-Calvé-Perthes disease | 2–10 yrs |
| Slipped femoral capital epiphyses | 10–16 yrs |
| Avulsed ASIS, AIIS, lesser trochanter | 12–16 yrs |
| Osteoid osteoma (femoral neck) | 5–30 yrs |
| Malignancy | Any age |
| Stress fractures | 14–25 yrs |
| Avascular necrosis | 20–40 yrs |
| Rheumatoid arthritis | 35 yrs and older |
| Paget's disease | 40 yrs and older |
| Osteoarthritis | 45 yrs and older |
| Hip fracture | 65 yrs and older |

ASIS = anterior superior iliac spine; AIIS = anterior inferior iliac spine.

ing spondylitis). General points are provided for factors of importance that do not easily fit a specific grouping. Similarly, some conditions are less common or less serious and do not warrant the same depth of description or do not fit easily in to the outline. These conditions are presented as prose (e.g., nerve entrapment syndromes, hip dislocation, acetabular fracture, stress fracture).

The "Hip Tips" at the end of each section are important points related to physical therapy evaluation or management.

Illustrations are limited in this chapter because of the large number of conditions described. The pediatric section is the exception, in which the fine drawings of the late Frank Netter are used. The rationale for this is that the rest of the book deals primarily with the adult hip; these illustrations help to do justice to pediatric problems.

## Arthritis

### Osteoarthritis or Degenerative Joint Disease

#### Definition

Osteoarthritis (OA), or degenerative joint disease, is a noninflammatory disorder of movable joints characterized by deterioration of articular cartilage and new bone formation.

### Epidemiology

- OA is the most common joint disease, with more than 50 million Americans affected.
- By 40 years of age, 90% of all persons have some degenerative change in weightbearing joints, although symptoms usually are not present.
- More than 120,000 hip replacements are performed in the United States every year (National Institutes of Health 1994).
- Both men and women are equally prone to hip disease, whereas, for example, knee and hand OA are more common in older women.
- Chronic obesity correlates with development of osteoarthritis.
- Heredity is a determinant in secondary OA but not in idiopathic OA (Mankin 1993).
- In more than 80% of cases, hip OA is the end result of other hip diseases, such as developmental dysplasia of the hip (DDH), slipped capital femoral epiphyses (SCFE), and Legg-Calvé-Perthes disease (LCP) (Harris 1986).

### Clinical Features

*General*
The following are signs and symptoms of OA:

- Typically pain on movement
- Rest pain and night pain later in course
- Sometimes referred pain
- Muscle spasm
- Progressive loss of range of motion (ROM)
- Joint stiffness after rest
- Moderate effusion
- Thickened joints
- Crepitus, sometimes audible
- Limp with walking when weightbearing joint affected

*Hip Related*
The following are specific clinical features of *hip* OA:

- Hip pain on movement and walking
- Loss of hip motion
- Hip joint contracture most frequently in adduction, flexion, and outward rotation

- Occasional deformity as a result of incongruity of the femoral head and acetabulum
- Antalgic gait; Trendelenburg gait
- Leg length discrepancy from subchondral collapse

### Radiologic Features
Radiographic findings correlated with likely pathologic abnormalities are as follows:

| Radiographic findings | Pathologic abnormalities |
| --- | --- |
| Loss of joint space | Cartilage erosion |
| Bone eburnation | Increased cellularity and deposition of subchondral bone |
| Subchondral cysts | Synovial fluid intrusion into bone |
| Osteophytes | Revascularization of remaining cartilage causing traction on the capsule |
| Osteophytes | Stimulation of the synovial membrane |
| Bone collapse | Compression of weakened bone |
| Loose bodies | Osteochondral bone fragmentation |
| Deformity | Deterioration of capsular ligaments coupled with bone collapse |

Note that fewer than one-half of all patients with radiographically identifiable OA have symptoms. OA of the hip most often causes joint space narrowing along the superior (horizontal) aspect of the hip joint, which is best seen on an anterior-posterior radiograph. Osteophytes, loose bodies, and sclerosis are also common features.

### Diagnostic Classification
OA can be classified as either primary (idiopathic) or secondary. It is likely that primary OA of the hip is rare. Most authorities agree that the most common clinical pattern of OA represents a "final common pathway" for a number of different primary conditions (e.g., DDH, SCFE, LCP, AVN). Primary OA is divided into localized and generalized OA. Secondary OA is further divided into the following groupings

**Table 2-2** American College of Rheumatology Combined Clinical (History, Physical Examination, Laboratory) and Radiographic Criteria for the Classification and Reporting of Osteoarthritis of the Hip (Traditional Format)*

Hip pain

> and

At least two of the following three features:

> $ESR < 20$ mm/hr
>
> Radiographic femoral or acetabular osteophytes
>
> Radiographic joint space narrowing (superior, axial, medial, or any combination of these)

ESR = erythrocyte sedimentation rate (Westergren).
*This classification method yields a sensitivity of 89% and a specificity of 91%.
Source: Reprinted with permission from R Altman, G Alarcon, D Appelrouth, et al. (1991) The American College of Rheumatology Criteria for the Classification and Reporting of Osteoarthritis of the Hip. *Arthritis and Rheumatism* 34, 511.

depending on primary cause: trauma, congenital, metabolic, endocrine, other bone and joint disease, and diseases of obscure etiology (Mankin 1993).

Table 2-2 is a recognized diagnostic classification scheme for reporting OA of the hip. Table 2-3 is a functional classification for arthritis, which can be usefully applied to clinical outcomes research and, ultimately, to help predict and direct treatment.

### Management

- Exercises
- Weight reduction
- Bracing or walking aids
- Drugs
- Surgery

### Hip Tips

- Encourage the patient to maintain function.
- Prevent deformity.
- Relieve symptoms.
- The patient should use a cane in the opposite hand.

**Table 2-3** American College of Rheumatology Revised Criteria for Classification of Functional Status in Rheumatoid Arthritis*

| Class | Description |
|-------|-------------|
| I | Completely able to perform usual activities of daily living (self-care, vocational, and avocational) |
| II | Able to perform usual self-care and vocational activities, but limited in avocational activities |
| III | Able to perform usual self-care activities, but limited in vocational and avocational activities |
| IV | Limited in ability to perform usual self-care, vocational, and avocational activities |

*Usual self-care activities include dressing, feeding, bathing, grooming, toileting. Avocational (recreational or leisure, or both) and vocational (work, school, homemaking) activities are patient-desired and age- and gender-specific.
Source: Reprinted with permission from MC Hochberg, RW Chang, I Dwosh, et al. (1992) The American College of Rheumatology 1991 Revised Criteria for the Classification of Global Functional Status in Rheumatoid Arthritis. *Arthritis and Rheumatism* 35, 499.

## Rheumatoid Arthritis

### Definition
Rheumatoid arthritis (RA) is a systemic autoimmune disorder of unknown etiology. Its distinctive feature is chronic, symmetric, and erosive synovitis of peripheral joints.

### Epidemiology
- Female to male prevalence is 2.5 to 1.0.
- The incidence of RA increases with age for both men and women.

### Clinical Features

*General*

- The majority of patients have elevated titers of serum rheumatoid factor.
- The severity of RA ranges from a few mildly affected joints to complete ankylosis of many joints.
- The severity of the disease can vary over time, but the most common course is progressive joint destruction, deformity, and disability.
- Associated nonarticular manifestations can include subcutaneous nodules, vasculitis, pericarditis, lung nodules, and mononeuritis.

- Sjögren's syndrome (dry eyes and mouth) and Felty's syndrome (splenomegaly, leukopenia, leg ulcers) can occur in conjunction with RA.

### Hip Related

- The hip joint is commonly involved in RA.
- Early involvement is often asymptomatic; however, subtle reductions of ROM may be observed.
- Difficulty putting on shoes and socks is usually an early sign of hip involvement.
- Hip symptoms characteristically occur in the groin or thigh but may be felt in the lumbar spine or knee.
- Hip replacement is required in severe cases, even in young patients.

### Radiologic Features

- Periarticular soft tissue swelling
- Juxta-articular osteoporosis progressing to generalized osteoporosis
- Uniform loss of joint space
- Marginal erosions progressing to severe erosions of subchondral bone
- Synovial cyst formation
- Subluxations
- Bilateral symmetrical distribution

### Diagnosis

- For diagnosis of RA, there must be evidence of an inflammatory synovitis by any of the following means: (1) synovial fluid leukocytosis (white blood cell count >2,000/mm$^3$), (2) histologic demonstration of a chronic synovitis, and (3) radiologic evidence of characteristic erosions (Anderson 1993).
- A signs and symptom pattern consistent with RA is also diagnostic (Table 2-4).
- Ruling out other causes of synovitis (e.g., systemic lupus erythematosus [SLE], psoriatic arthritis) is important before diagnosis of RA is made.

### Management

- Patient education
- Balance of rest with activity and exercise
- Physical and occupational therapy
- Use of aspirin and other nonsteroidal anti-inflammatory drugs (NSAIDS)
- Use of disease-altering drugs (e.g., gold salts, penicillamine, hydroxychloroquine, methotrexate)

**Table 2-4** American Rheumatism Association 1987 Revised Criteria for the Classification of Rheumatoid Arthritis (Traditional Format)*

| Criterion | Definition |
|---|---|
| 1. Morning stiffness | Morning stiffness is observed in and around the joints, lasting at least 1 hour before maximal improvement. |
| 2. Arthritis of three or more joint areas | At least three joint areas simultaneously have had soft tissue swelling or fluid (not bony overgrowth alone) observed by a physician. The 14 possible areas are the PIP, MCP, wrist, elbow, knee, ankle, and MTP joints on the right or left side. |
| 3. Arthritis of hand joints | At least one area is swollen (as defined in 2, above) in wrist, MCP, or PIP joint. |
| 4. Symmetric arthritis | Simultaneous involvement of the same joint areas (as defined in 2, above) occurs on both sides of the body. (Bilateral involvement of PIPs, MCPs, or MTPs is acceptable without absolute symmetry.) |
| 5. Rheumatoid nodules | Subcutaneous nodules, over bony prominences or extensor surfaces or in juxta-articular regions, observed by a physician. |
| 6. Serum rheumatoid factor | Abnormal amounts of serum rheumatoid factor are demonstrated by any method for which the result has been positive in <0.5% of normal control subjects. |
| 7. Radiographic changes | Radiographic changes typical of rheumatoid arthritis on posteroanterior wrist and hand radiographs, which can include erosions or unequivocal bony decalcification localized in or most marked adjacent to the involved joints (osteoarthritis changes alone do not qualify). |

PIP = proximal interphalangeal; MCP = metacarpophalangeal; MTP = metatarsophalangeal.
*For classification purposes, a patient is said to have rheumatoid arthritis if he or she has satisfied at least four of these seven criteria. Criteria 1–4 must have been present for at least 6 weeks. Patients with two clinical diagnoses are not excluded. Designation as classic, definite, or probable rheumatoid arthritis is *not* to be made.
Source: Reprinted with permission from FC Arnett, SM Edworthy, DA Bloch, et al. (1988) The American Rheumatism Association 1987 Revised Criteria for the Classification of Rheumatoid Arthritis. *Arthritis and Rheumatism* 31, 319.

Hip Tips

The patient should be educated regarding the following hip-joint protection principles (Liang and Logigian 1992; Neumann and Hase 1994):

- Decrease body weight
- Carry lightest loads possible
- Carry loads between sides (If one hip is affected, load should be carried on that side.)
- Carry loads close to the body (Posterior carrying [e.g., knapsack] creates less hip load than anterior carrying.)
- Avoid standing over one side
- Use cane on the opposite side

## Ankylosing Spondylitis

### Definition

Ankylosing spondylitis (AS) is a chronic, systemic, inflammatory disorder primarily affecting the spine with sacroiliitis as a distinguishing feature.

### Epidemiology

- The male to female ratio is 3 to 1.
- Approximately 0.5–1.0% of the white population develop AS, which is a similar prevalence to RA.
- The incidence is less in blacks and Japanese, who have a lower prevalence of human leukocyte antigen (HLA)-B27.
- Approximately one-third of patients with ankylosing spondylitis have hip involvement, which is bilateral in 75% of cases (Forrester and Brown 1987).
- Other than hip and shoulder involvement, limb joints are rarely affected.
- AS has a strong association with the antibody HLA-B27.
- Clinical manifestations of AS usually begin in late adolescence or early adulthood.

### Clinical Features

*General*

- Low back pain
- Pain and stiffness after rest
- Sacroiliac joints tender to forced movement

- Stiff back
- Loss of lumbar lordosis
- Progressive kyphosis
- Forward head posture
- Reduced chest expansion
- Sunken chest and pot belly
- Hip and shoulder involvement
- Plantar fasciitis
- Achilles' tendinitis

### Hip Related
- The hip is involved in 17–36% of cases; involvement is usually bilateral, of insidious onset, and potentially crippling.
- The hip can be the site of initial symptoms.
- Hip-flexion contractures can develop later in the disease course and result in a rigid gait with compensatory knee flexion.

### Radiologic Features

- Sacroiliac erosion and later fusion
- Arthritic changes in facet joints
- Ligamentous ossification (bamboo spine)
- Squaring of vertebral bodies
- New bone growth between vertebrae (syndesmophytes)
- Peripheral joint erosions

### Diagnosis

Table 2-5 is an internationally accepted criteria for AS. In addition to this criteria, an elevated erythrocyte sedimentation rate, an elevated serum immunoglobulin A (IgA) concentration, and the presence of the genetic marker HLA-B27 are laboratory findings that help confirm the diagnosis.

### Complications

- Reduced chest expansion and vital capacity
- Atlantoaxial subluxation
- Possible spinal cord damage
- Fractures of rigid spine with frequent resulting spinal cord damage
- Iritis

**Table 2-5** Modified New York Criteria for Ankylosing Spondylitis

A. Diagnosis

    1.   Clinical criteria

        a.   Low back pain and stiffness for more than 3 months that improves with exercise, but is not relieved by rest.

        b.   Limitation of motion of the lumbar spine in both the sagittal and frontal planes.

        c.   Limitation of chest expansion relative to normal values corrected for age and gender.

    2.   Radiologic criterion: Sacroiliitis grade $\geq$ 2 bilaterally or sacroiliitis grade 3–4 unilaterally.

B. Grading

    1.   Definite ankylosing spondylitis if the radiologic criterion is associated with at least one clinical criterion.

    2.   Probable ankylosing spondylitis if

        a.   Three clinical criteria are present.

        b.   The radiologic criterion is present without any signs or symptoms satisfying the clinical criteria. (Other causes of sacroiliitis should be considered.)

Source: Reprinted with permission from S Van Der Linden, HA Valkenburg, A Cats. (1984) Evaluation of diagnostic criteria for ankylosing spondylitis: A proposal for modification of the New York criteria. *Arthritis and Rheumatism* 27, 366.

- Can occur in association with reactive arthritis, psoriasis, or chronic inflammatory bowel disease (secondary AS)

**Objective Measures**

- Finger-floor, standing with knees straight (flexion and side flexion)
- Chest expansion at nipple line
- Occiput-wall distance, standing with heels to wall
- Schroeder's test (Mark fourth and fifth lumbar vertebra joint space and 10 cm proximal in standing upright, measure distance between the two marks at extreme of forward flexion.)
- Vital capacity
- Range of extremity joint motion (hip and shoulder especially)
- Spondylometer

### Management

The following are principles of management of AS (adapted from Khan 1993):

- There is no cure, but most patients can be well managed.
- Educating patients about the disease helps increase compliance.
- Early diagnosis is very important, as is the early recognition and treatment of extraskeletal manifestations (e.g., acute iritis) and of the associated diseases or complications.
- NSAIDs can be used to control pain and suppress inflammation.
- Daily exercises preserve good posture, minimize deformity, and maintain chest expansion. Swimming is probably the best overall exercise.
- Surgical measures, such as hip arthroplasty or correction of spinal deformity, can be helpful.
- Psychosocial and vocational supportive measures and counseling, family and genetic counseling, and patient support groups are sources of help and information for patients.
- Thorough family history and, if possible, physical examination of the patient's relatives can sometimes disclose remarkable disease aggregation and many undiagnosed or misdiagnosed affected relatives.

### HIP TIPS

According to Khan (1993), "regular therapeutic exercise to minimize and prevent deformity and disability is the single most important measure in AS management." The following recommendations should be incorporated into a physical therapy program:

- Encourage regular exercise (swimming is ideal) and stretching (especially spine and hip extension).
- Maintain and increase spinal and hip mobility.
- Prevent deformity and correct if possible.
- Maintain and increase chest expansion and vital capacity.
- Emphasize maintenance of good posture.

## Bone Disorders

### Osteoporosis

#### Definition

Osteoporosis is a metabolic disorder characterized by decreased bone mass that results in a weak bony skeleton susceptible to fractures. It is characterized by decreased bone-mineral density at the endosteal surface of bone. The disease is associated with age, inactivity, and especially gender. Osteoporosis is the most common metabolic bone disease.

### Classification
Osteoporosis can be classified as

- Primary
  Type I (postmenopausal)
  Type II (age related)
  Idiopathic
- Secondary to a disease process or drugs (see next section)

### Epidemiology (Risk Factors)

- Gender. The prevalence of Type I (postmenopausal [hormone-related]) osteoporosis is 6 to 1 for women to men. The prevalence of Type II (age-related) osteoporosis for women to men is 2 to 1.
- Age. The risk of sustaining an osteoporotic fracture doubles every decade for women after the age of 40 years. Women experience a rapid loss of bone for about 6 years after menopause. This is not usually evident in men until after the age of 50 years.
- Heredity. Heredity accounts for 80% of an individual's peak bone mass. Black people have a higher bone density and therefore a lower incidence.
- Hormonal factors. Decreased estrogen (particularly after menopause) and decreased testosterone are major factors in the development of osteoporosis.
- Surgery. Women who have undergone oophorectomy (removal of the ovaries) are at greater risk.
- Associated diseases. Renal and hepatic disorders, myeloma, and hypercalciuria are associated with osteoporosis.
- Drugs. Steroids, thyroid drugs, and heparin are thought to contribute to osteoporosis.
- Nutritional factors include decreased lifelong calcium intake and decreased vitamin D.
- Weight. Increased body fat is probably protective against osteoporosis.
- Inactivity. Maintaining weightbearing activity, exercising, and doing back-extension exercises are preventative measures.
- Cigarette smoking and heavy alcohol intake contribute to bone loss.

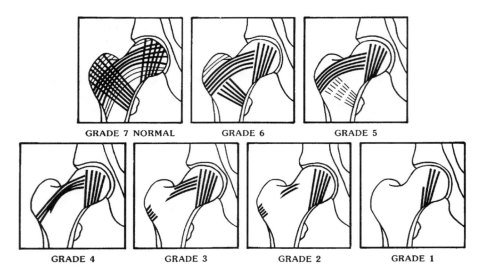

GRADE 7 NORMAL     GRADE 6     GRADE 5

GRADE 4     GRADE 3     GRADE 2     GRADE 1

**Figure 2-1** The Singh index of osteopenia. The Singh index describes the trabecular groups that are present. As osteopenia develops, trabeculae disappear in sequence, with the least-stressed areas disappearing earliest. Patients with grade 4 or less are considered to have abnormally reduced amounts of bone. (Reprinted with permission from BNW Weissman, CB Sledge. [1986] *Orthopedic Radiology* [p. 405]. Philadelphia: Saunders.)

### Hip Involvement
Because of decreased bone strength, the likelihood for hip fracture after minor falls or trauma is increased in the person with osteoporosis.

### Radiologic Features

- The radiographic hallmark of osteoporosis is osteopenia, which is characterized by increased radiolucency of bone. Osteopenia is not usually visible on radiographs until there has been a 30–50% loss of bone mineral (Chew 1989).
- The Singh index uses trabecular patterns seen on radiographs to classify the degree of osteopenia of the proximal femur (Figure 2-1). It is mostly used by orthopedic surgeons for hip surgery planning. If the Singh index is grade IV or less, the surgeon may opt for femoral head replacement instead of internal fixation—one of many decision-making factors.
- Fractures are a common feature in the osteoporotic population, particularly vertebral compression fractures, Colles' fracture, and hip

fractures. This same population falls at a much greater rate and is more susceptible to fractures with each fall.

- Bone densitometry is a method of radiographically measuring bone-mineral content and is often performed on patients who exhibit risk factors for osteoporosis. The techniques used to measure integral bone density at the hip are computed tomography with automated image analysis and dual photon absorptiometry with either a radionuclide or a dual-energy x-ray source. Bone densitometry can be used to aid diagnosis and severity of osteoporosis, identify areas of bone at risk for fracture, and monitor efficacy of estrogen replacement treatment and the course of the disease (Chew 1989).

### Management
Conservative management includes the following:

- Minimization of risk factors
- Exercise, especially weightbearing activity
- Empowerment of patients with information that can be used to counteract the pain, postural changes, weakness, and loss of flexibility associated with osteoporosis

Preventative measures for high-risk patients include the following:

- Calcium supplementation
- Adequate vitamin D
- Maintenance of weightbearing activity
- Hormone replacement therapy—usually estrogen supplementation
- Calcitonin
- Biphosphonates (i.e., etidronate [Didronel] and alendronate [Fosamax])
- Minimization of associated risk factors

Considerable research is being performed on osteoporosis, including the effect of daily injections of parathyroid hormone in stimulating osteoblasts, which can possibly reverse osteoporosis.

### Hip Tips

- Minimize the bone-weakening effects of osteoporosis with regular, active weightbearing exercise, in addition to dietary measures and supplementation.
- Prevent falls with education, home modifications, and balance training and exercise, as well as with the appropriate use of assistive devices (e.g., walker), hip pads, and physician-ordered restraints.

## Avascular Necrosis

### Definition

AVN is a condition in which progressive ischemia of the femoral head leads to bone collapse and eventual degenerative arthritis. This condition should be viewed as a multifactorial, heterogeneous group of disorders that lead to a final common pathway of mechanical failure of the femoral head and arthritis (Mont and Hungerford 1995). It is also termed *osteonecrosis, ischemic necrosis,* and *aseptic necrosis.*

### Epidemiology

- AVN occurs most frequently in the femoral head.
- The prevalence ratio of men to women is 4 to 1.
- AVN usually occurs in the 30- to 70-year age range.
- Sudden onset of hip pain without trauma is a common presentation.
- AVN is bilateral in 50% of patients; involvement of both hips is usually asymmetric.
- Bo Jackson (American football and baseball star) was a publicized case of AVN that occurred as a complication of a hip fracture-dislocation sustained in a football tackle.

### Clinical Features

The following combination of clinical features are red flags for AVN of the hip:

- Groin or thigh pain
- Hip joint tender to palpation
- Antalgic gait
- Hip ROM painful and often decreased in flexion, internal rotation, and abduction
- History of alcohol or corticosteroid use

### Diagnosis

- Early diagnosis has been cited as the single most important factor in treatment.
- The early stages of the disease are not identifiable from plain radiographs. Once radiographic changes are evident, the disease is often far advanced. The earliest radiographic sign of mechanical failure is the crescent sign, which represents separation of the subchondral plate from the underlying necrotic cancellous bone.

**Table 2-6** Association Research Circulation Osseous International Staging System: Osteonecrosis of the Femoral Head

| Stage | Diagnostic imaging findings |
|---|---|
| Stage 0 | All diagnostic studies normal |
| | Diagnosis by history only |
| Stage 1 | Plain radiographs and computed tomography normal |
| | Magnetic resonance imaging +/or scintigraphy + |
| | Biopsy + |
| | Extent of involvement A, B, or C (<15%, 15–30%, or >30%, respectively) |
| Stage 2 | Radiographs +, but no collapse |
| | Extent of involvement A, B, or C |
| Stage 3 | Early flattening of dome, crescent sign |
| | Computed tomography or tomograms possibly needed |
| | Extent of involvement A, B, or C |
| | Further characterization by amount of depression (in mm) |
| Stage 4 | Flattening of femoral head with joint space narrowing |
| | Other signs of early osteoarthritis possible |

+ = positive.
Source: Reprinted with permission from BN Stulberg. (1997) Editorial comment. *Clinical Orthopaedics and Related Research* 334, 4.

- It is important that patients with hip pain who fit an etiologic pattern (e.g., past or present alcoholism or corticosteroid use) be evaluated by an orthopedist for the possibility of AVN.
- Patients with symptomatic herniation pit (Daenen et al. 1997) and transient osteoporosis (Daniel et al. 1992) are sometimes misdiagnosed with AVN and vice versa.
- Early AVN is best demonstrated by intramedullary pressure measurement or magnetic resonance imaging (MRI); there are no early x-ray findings of osteonecrosis.
- Table 2-6 is the international staging system for AVN proposed by the Association Research Circulation Osseous (ARCO).

### Etiology

The following are the currently held views on causative agents of AVN:

- Interruption of blood supply to the femoral head is the precipitating factor.
- There are a number of reasons why osteonecrosis can occur and occasionally it occurs idiopathically.
- The most common cause of *unilateral* AVN is complication of surgery or trauma.
- The most common cause of *bilateral* AVN is alcoholism or corticosteroid use (*not* anabolic steroids).

### Pathogenesis

There is still uncertainty about the pathologic mechanisms that cause AVN. However, multiple theories have been presented for the pathogenesis of nontraumatic AVN of the femoral head, including thromboemboli in the blood supply, bone resulting from circulating fat, nitrogen bubbles, sickle cell red blood cells, and increased bone-marrow pressure (Mont and Hungerford 1995). Most of the theories are mutually supportive and not exclusive.

A possible theory as to the mechanism for blood-flow restriction is an increase in femoral head intraosseous pressure to levels exceeding perfusion pressure. The ensuing ischemic necrosis of marrow and bone is often accompanied by pain, intramedullary pressure measurements are raised, and x-rays can demonstrate a wedge-shaped area of infarction in the weightbearing region of the femoral head. Articular cartilage remains healthy because its nutrition is obtained from the synovial fluid. Following infarction, the bone becomes revascularized from the periphery.

### Management

- Methods of treatment for AVN span most options available for treatment of the hip. Which method is used is dependent on the stage of progression, age, activity level, presence of other conditions, and use of corticosteroids.
- For *mild* cases, core decompression or electromagnetic stimulation is indicated. For *intermediate* disease, bone grafting and osteotomy may be indicated. For *advanced* disease, total hip replacement (THR) is required.

## HIP TIPS

- Always include questions about past or present use of alcohol and corticosteroids in the subjective exam. Steroids are often given for the medical conditions asthma, brain or spinal cord trauma, inflammatory arthritis (e.g., RA, SLE), and autoimmune conditions.
- Also inquire about trauma or fracture of the hip.

## *Heterotopic Ossification*

### Definition

Bone formed in soft tissues without a well-defined cause is referred to as *heterotopic ossification* (HO), whereas bone formed in muscle as a result of inflammation is referred to as *myositis ossificans*. HO has been described after injuries and surgeries to the spinal cord, elbow, and hip.

### Epidemiology

- The incidence of HO after hip replacement is about 53% but usually does not present a clinical problem (Naraghi et al. 1996).
- Risk factors include patients with previous ectopic ossification, ankylosing spondylitis, transtrochanteric and anterior surgical approaches, and concurrent head trauma.

### Classification

HO is most commonly classified by the Brooker classification:

- Class I:  Islands of ectopic bone
- Class II: Ectopic bone with a space of greater than 1 cm between opposing surfaces
- Class III:  Bone spurs that reduce the opposing space to less than 1 cm
- Class IV:  Bony bridging or apparent radiographic fusion

### Management

- Prevention of HO includes nonsteroidal anti-inflammatory medication and radiotherapy. Such prophylaxis is recommended in at-risk groups.
- Surgical resection is the only option when heterotopic bone interferes with mobility and function. This is usually delayed for a minimum of 6 months postoperation to ensure bone maturation.
- Physical therapy with recent postoperative hip patients should avoid passive stretching methods, especially in the at-risk group, because passive ROM has been associated with formation of HO in elbow and hip patients (Naraghi et al. 1996).

### HIP TIP

Avoid forceful passive stretching after hip surgery, especially if HO risk is suspected.

## Fractures and Dislocation

### Hip Fracture

#### Definition

A hip fracture is generally defined as any fracture of the proximal third of the femur. Hip fractures should be described like other fractures in terms of displaced or nondisplaced and open or closed. Hip fractures should also be defined as intracapsular and extracapsular, as follows:

Intracapsular
  Femoral head
  Femoral neck
Extracapsular
  Intertrochanteric
  Trochanteric
  Subtrochanteric

Each subcategory has its own classification; for example, the Garden classification of femoral neck fractures (Garden 1964), the Kyle classification of intertrochanteric fractures (Kyle et al. 1979), and the Seinsheimer classification of subtrochanteric fractures (Seinsheimer 1978).

#### Epidemiology and Societal Impact

Hip fracture is a problem of high incidence, high cost, and high risk, as outlined in the following section (Guccione et al. 1996).

##### Incidence

- After 50 years of age, the incidence of hip fracture rises considerably (Zuckerman 1996).
- In patients older than 65 years of age, 79% of hip fractures occur in women, and 93% occur in whites (Craik 1994).
- A U.S. Congress document reported that there were more than 300,000 hip fractures in the United States in 1991, with 94% of these occurring in people older than 50 years of age. Note that 55% occurred in people age 80 years and older (U.S. Congress, Office of Technology Assessment 1994).

##### Cost

The 1992 United States cost per year in medical bills and lost income from hip fracture was $9.8 billion, this is equivalent to $35,000 per hip fracture (Adams 1993).

*Risk*

- The 1-year mortality rate after hip fracture is approximately 20% (Craik 1994).
- The rate of failure to return to prefracture level of functional mobility (i.e., functional morbidity) 1 year after the event is about 50% (Craik 1994; Koval et al. 1995; Magaziner et al. 1990), and it may be considerably worse than this (U.S. Congress, Office of Technology Assessment 1994).

### Etiology

- In the elderly, hip fracture usually results after a fall. Less frequently, it occurs spontaneously (pathologic fracture).
- In the elderly, hip fracture is often part of a downward spiral of health.
- In young persons, hip fracture is most often the result of high-impact trauma (e.g., car accident, fall from a height).

### Classification
The Garden scale (Garden 1961) is the most widely used classification system for femoral neck fractures. The following is a modification of the Garden classification:

- Garden I: Incomplete or impacted fractures
- Garden II: Complete fracture *without* displacement
- Garden III: Complete fracture with partial displacement
- Garden IV: Complete fracture with full displacement

There are multiple classification systems for intertrochanteric fractures and subtrochanteric fractures. Factors comprising classification systems include anatomic location, fracture configuration, fracture fragments (i.e., two-part, three-part, or comminuted with four or more parts), ability to reduce the fracture, and prognosis.

### Management
All but stable, nondisplaced fractures should be internally fixed.

### Surgical Fixation
See Chapter 5 for an additional discussion of surgical fixation of hip fractures.

The following are methods of surgical fixation of hip fractures:

- Pins and screws
- Sliding screw and plate

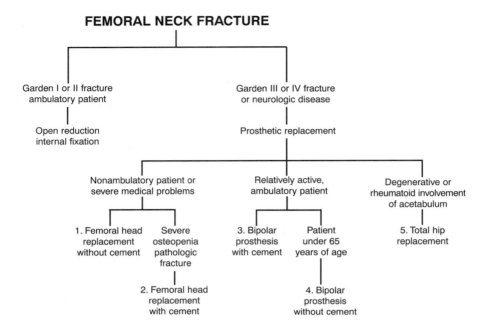

**Figure 2-2** Algorithm of options for treatment of femoral neck fractures. (Reprinted with permission from RN Stauffer. [1990] Prosthetic Hip Replacement for Femoral Neck Fractures. In CM Evarts [ed], *Surgery of the Musculoskeletal System* [2nd ed] [p. 2600]. New York: Churchill Livingstone.)

- Hemiarthroplasty
- THR

Reduction and fixation of displaced intracapsular hip fractures within 12 hours has been correlated with lower rates of osteonecrosis and nonunion. The most likely explanation being the restoration of blood supply through stretched or compressed blood vessels. As displaced femoral neck fractures often result in disruption of blood supply to the femoral head, they usually require hemiarthroplasty, whereas intertrochanteric fractures can be managed with plate and screw fixation. Most intertrochanteric fractures are internally fixed because pull of the hip musculature can lead to further displacement (Lhowe 1990). Figure 2-2 is an algorithm of orthopedic treatment options for femoral neck fracture.

### Postoperative Physical Therapy

See Chapter 6 for an additional discussion of postoperative physical therapy for hip fractures.

In a review, Craik (1994) raised the issue that physical therapy intervention following hip fracture really has not changed since the 1970s. Improved means of reducing residual disability after hip fracture is a clinical challenge. Rapid remobilization is encouraged. A team approach is essential.

### Prevention

In large part, preventing hip fractures means preventing falls. The following are hip fracture prevention methods:

- Modification of the home environment
- Improving balance and gait speed with physical therapy and exercise
- Educating those at risk
- Decreasing osteoporosis
- Use of walkers, wearing hip pads, or both for those with irreversibly poor balance
- Reducing the amount of sedative drugs taken by the elderly

### HIP TIPS

- Prevent falls.
- Ensure rapid remobilization after surgery.
- Develop a good understanding of the hip-fracture problem (see Chapters 5 and 6).
- Above all, give every patient the individual attention and time needed to listen to his or her problem and to tailor treatment to his or her specific needs. Not least, take time to educate the patient and family.

Innovative methods to provide quality care and at the same time contain costs should be developed, proven, and promoted.

## Hip Dislocation

Dislocation of the hip occurs when the femoral head dislodges from the acetabulum. In nonhip replacement cases, dislocation usually occurs as a result of trauma (e.g., car accident). Posterior dislocation occurs in 85–90% of cases (Brown and Neumann 1995), and it can be associated with an acetabular fracture. Dislocation is a potential complication after hip replacement and usually occurs in the direction of surgical approach. Table 2-7 presents the likely position of the lower extremity after different types of dislocation or fracture. Refer to Chapter 6 for details on physical therapy education.

### HIP TIP

Apply dislocation precautions to the individual patient's situation and give the patient examples of functional activities to modify or avoid.

**Table 2-7** Lower-Extremity Position After Hip Dislocation or Fracture

| Hip position (patient supine) | Possible explanation |
|---|---|
| Flexed, adducted, internally rotated and limb shortened, pain | Posterior dislocation |
| Abducted, externally rotated, limb short Often cyanosis and swelling of extremity from compression of femoral vein, pain | Anterior dislocation |
| Shortened extremity, 45 degrees external rotation, pain (capsule prevents further rotation) | Intracapsular fracture |
| Shortened extremity, 90 degrees external rotation, pain | Extracapsular fracture |

## Acetabular Fracture

### Definition

Any fracture involving the acetabulum can be defined as an acetabular fracture. Such a fracture should not be defined as a hip fracture or pelvic fracture, although it can occur with either of these.

### Etiology

Fractures of the acetabulum are usually caused by high-energy trauma (e.g., car and motorcycle accidents, fall from heights). They are often associated with multiple injuries, some of which can be life threatening.

### Radiology

Radiographic evaluation for acetabular fractures should include an anteroposterior (AP) view of the pelvis and hip and 45-degree oblique views of the pelvis. Computerized tomography scans prove useful for evaluation of displaced or comminuted fractures.

### Diagnostic Classification

There is no perfect classification for acetabular fractures because of the wide variations in fracture type. A detailed system of classification has been proposed that captures the wide variety of acetabular fracture presentations (Table 2-8).

### Management

Nondisplaced and some minimally displaced fractures are treated nonoperatively with traction or nonweightbearing for 4–8 weeks,

**Table 2-8** Comprehensive Anatomic Classification of Acetabular Fractures

Type A: *Partial articular* fractures, one column involved

| | |
|---|---|
| A1 | Posterior wall fracture |
| A2 | Posterior column fracture |
| A3 | Anterior wall or anterior column fracture |

Type B: *Partial articular* fractures (transverse or T-type fracture, *both columns involved*)

| | |
|---|---|
| B1 | Transverse fracture |
| B2 | T-shaped fracture |
| B3 | Anterior column plus posterior hemitransverse fracture |

Type C: *Complete articular* fracture (both column fracture; floating acetabulum)

| | |
|---|---|
| C1 | Both-column fracture, high variety |
| C2 | Both-column fracture, low variety |
| C3 | Both column fracture involving the sacroiliac joint |

Qualifiers: Additional information can be documented concerning the condition of the articular surfaces to further define the prognosis of the injury. The information should, as additional qualifiers, be identified by Greek letters.

| | |
|---|---|
| α1 | Femoral head subluxation, anterior |
| α2 | Femoral head subluxation, medial |
| α3 | Femoral head subluxation, posterior |
| β1 | Femoral head dislocation, anterior |
| β2 | Femoral head dislocation, medial |
| β3 | Femoral head dislocation, posterior |
| γ1 | Acetabular surface, chondral lesion |
| γ2 | Acetabular surface, impacted |
| δ1 | Femoral head, chondral lesion |
| δ2 | Femoral head, impacted |
| δ3 | Femoral head, osteochondral fracture |
| ε1 | Intra-articular fragment requiring surgical removal |
| φ1 | Nondisplaced fracture of the acetabulum |

Source: Reprinted with permission from M Tile. (1995) *Fractures of the Pelvis and Acetabulum* (2nd ed) (p. 260). Baltimore: Williams & Wilkins.

especially when the weightbearing dome of the acetabulum has not been affected. Open reduction and internal fixation is usually required for displaced fractures.

Postoperative physical therapy involves teaching touchdown weight-bearing gait (or nonweightbearing if patient cannot maintain touch weightbearing), gentle passive or active-assisted ROM of the hip, and submaximal isometrics. There may be dislocation precautions (usually posterior) and limitation of ROM (usually flexion) to prevent stress on the fractured wall (usually posterior) of the acetabulum.

**HIP TIP**

Incorporate findings of in vivo acetabular contact pressure studies in rehabilitation program (Fagerson et al. 1995; Givens-Heiss et al. 1992; Krebs et al. 1991; Hodge et al. 1989; Strickland et al. 1992).

### Stress Fracture

Nonspecific hip pain with insidious onset in athletic (especially distance runners) and osteoporotic populations should be evaluated by radiographs for suspected stress fracture. Other terms for stress fracture are *fatigue fracture, insufficiency fracture,* and *occult fracture.* A bone scan or MRI may be necessary in the early stages, because the problem is not always evident on plain films. Most common sites at the hip for stress fracture are the femoral neck and inferior pubic ramus. Differential diagnosis includes AVN and SCFE in adolescents. This problem should be managed by an orthopedic surgeon. If not detected early, not managed properly, or both, a patient with a stress fracture could end up with a THR because of AVN or progression of the fracture. Conservative treatment involves rest for 6–8 weeks and using crutches for restricted weightbearing (Satterfield et al. 1990).

**HIP TIPS**

- MRI is emerging as the diagnostic tool of choice for this problem as it is more specific than a bone scan (Shin et al. 1996).
- Allowing sufficient rest is important if stress fracture is diagnosed or suspected.

### Avulsion Fracture

**Definition**

An avulsion fracture is a fracture that occurs at the attachment of tendon or ligament to bone. It is usually caused by strong and rapid muscular contraction.

**Table 2-9** Avulsion Fracture Classification

| Bony prominence | Muscle |
|---|---|
| ASIS | Sartorius |
| Lesser trochanter | Iliopsoas |
| AIIS | Rectus femoris |
| Ischial tuberosity | Hamstrings |
| Iliac crest | ITB and external oblique |
| Pubis | Adductors |
| Greater trochanter | Gluteus maximus |

ASIS = anterior superior iliac spine; AIIS = anterior inferior iliac spine; ITB = iliotibial band.

### Epidemiology

Avulsions of bony prominences around the hip most commonly occur in the *adolescent* during sporting activity from excessive muscular force.

### Diagnosis

Differentiating from contusion is usually clear with localized tenderness and pain at a muscle's bony attachment. A weak and painful response to muscle contraction is produced. Tenderness at one of the locations listed in Table 2-9 associated with a forcible muscle contraction should signal to the clinician the need for x-rays.

Often mimicking an avulsion fracture is apophysitis, which is inflammation at the tenoperiosteal junction but with no avulsion of bone. Apophysitis is usually the result of aggressive training and presents with pain at the same sight as a suspected avulsion. Apophysitis is differentiated from an avulsion based on history and radiology. An avulsion is associated with a violent pull of the myotendinous unit, whereas apophysitis is usually from overuse. An avulsion fracture should be apparent on appropriate plain films, whereas x-rays would be negative for apophysitis.

Common locations for avulsions are listed in Table 2-9 in order of decreasing frequency.

### Management

Most avulsions are managed conservatively with at least 3 weeks of rest, using crutches for partial weightbearing, and avoiding or minimizing contraction of the involved muscle. Once radiographs show the fracture has healed and the patient is pain free, ROM and strengthening exercises are instituted.

Avulsion of a large bone fragment can require prompt reduction and surgical fixation.

### HIP TIP
Always suspect avulsion fracture possibility in nontraumatic athletic injuries to the hip or pelvis.

## Soft Tissue Disorders

The relatively low incidence of hip and pelvis soft tissue injuries compared with the incidence in other regions of the body (e.g., knee, shoulder) is probably reason for the limited literature on the topic. A survey of overuse running injuries determined that only 5% were to the hip and pelvis (Clement et al. 1981). However, soft tissue disorders of strains, tears, ruptures, and tendinitis have been described as common to the hamstring, quadriceps, and gluteus medius muscles (Geraci 1994). Lloyd-Smith and colleagues (1985) documented that the three most common soft tissue injuries of the hip and pelvis in athletes are gluteus medius strain or tendinitis, trochanteric bursitis, and hamstring strain.

### Bursitis

Bursae are fluid-filled sacs with a synovium-like inner membrane found between tendon or muscle and bone. Their function is to reduce friction between adjacent structures. As many as 21 bursae have been described in the hip region (Shbeeb and Matteson 1996). Some of these communicate with the joint itself. Bursae can become inflamed as a result of trauma, repetitive activity, or as a part of inflammatory arthritis. The most commonly involved bursae at the hip are the trochanteric, iliopectineal, and ischiogluteal. Bursitis about the hip should be considered a clinical, rather than an anatomic diagnosis, as in most cases there is no objective evidence of bursitis by diagnostic tests (Traycroff 1991).

#### Trochanteric Bursitis
Trochanteric bursitis is sometimes called *gluteal bursitis.*

*Definition*
There are three trochanteric bursa: one between gluteus maximus and gluteus medius tendon, one between gluteus maximus and the greater trochanter, and one between gluteus medius and the greater trochanter.

*Epidemiology*

- Middle-aged and elderly people are most commonly affected.
- It occurs slightly more often in women.
- In the athletic community, long-distance runners present more commonly with trochanteric bursitis.

*Clinical Features*

- Aching over trochanteric area and sometimes down lateral thigh
- Worse with walking or running and on contraction, stretch, or both of the lateral and posterior hip muscles
- Onset is usually gradual but can be sudden

*Diagnosis*

- Sharply localized tenderness over the greater trochanter and usually most intense in the posterior region of the trochanter.
- Relief of pain following injection with corticosteroid and local anesthetic confirms the diagnosis (Traycroff 1991).
- Resisted abduction and external rotation of the hip are usually painful.
- Passively flexing of the hip then adducting and internally rotating should elicit pain.
- Ober test may be positive.
- Differentiate from tensor fascia lata syndrome, piriformis syndrome, abductor muscle strain or tendinitis, and from lumbar or sacroiliac (SI) referral.
- Trochanteric bursitis can arise in many cases at the insertions of the gluteus maximus and medius.
- X-rays are usually negative but can be valuable as a means of ruling out skeletal problems, such as avulsion or stress fracture.

*Management*
The following are options for management:

- Corticosteroid or local anesthetic injection (which can often prove diagnostic)
- Nonsteroidal anti-inflammatory medication
- Ice massage and heat contrasts followed by stretching the hamstrings and tensor fasciae latae, strengthening exercises, phonophoresis, and iontophoresis

- Correcting posture, correcting muscle imbalances, correcting leg length discrepancy, and weight loss are important features of long-term relief

### Iliopectineal Bursitis

*Definition*

The iliopectineal bursa lies deep to the iliopsoas tendon over the front of the hip joint and is just lateral to the femoral vessels. It communicates with the joint in 15% of cases. It is thought to be one of the largest bursae in the body.

*Epidemiology*

Iliopectineal bursitis is common in patients with OA or RA.

*Clinical Features*

- Groin pain
- Lower abdominal pain
- Anterior thigh pain (sometimes)

With severe pain, the patient may exhibit a psoatic gait (see Chapter 1) in which the hip is externally rotated and adducted with the knee slightly flexed, which seems to give some relief by presumably relieving tension of the iliopsoas muscle on the bursa. Overuse or direct trauma are often the cause of iliopectineal bursitis.

*Diagnosis*

- Passive hip flexion and adduction are painful, especially if combined.
- Isometric hip flexion and passive hip extension can also be painful, as they compress the iliopectineal bursa.
- Palpation of the bursa is painful just lateral to the femoral artery where it goes under the inguinal ligament.
- Differentiating other causes of groin pain (particularly hip OA) can necessitate radiologic work-up.

*Management*

- Injection of a corticosteroid or local anesthetic mix is often relieving.
- Phonophoresis and cold and hot contrasts have also been advocated.

**Ischiogluteal Bursitis**
Ischiogluteal bursitis is also called *weaver's bottom*.

*Definition*
The ischiogluteal bursa, which is not always present, lies between the ischial tuberosity and gluteus maximus.

*Epidemiology*

- Usually occurs in persons with sedentary occupations.
- The term *weaver's bottom* refers to the fact that weavers tended to be sitting most of the time and developed this bursitis.

*Clinical Features*

- Pain over the ischial tuberosity, worse when sitting
- Occasionally, there can be referral into the posterior thigh
- Can be of gradual or sudden onset

*Diagnosis*

- Pain occurs on deep palpation over the ischial tuberosity.
- Stretch of the hamstring by forward flexion or straight-leg raise is typically painful.
- Stride is usually short on the involved side.
- Patrick's test should be negative.
- Rule out lumbar or SI referral.
- Rule out rectal or abdominal pathology.
- Rule out infection (more likely with this superficial bursa).

*Management*

- The patient should avoid sitting.
- When patient sits, he or she should use a well-cushioned chair.

**HIP TIPS**

- For successful treatment of bursitis, it is important that the intervention be directed at the lesion itself and not merely at the location of the pain complaint.
- For long-term success, determine all of the possible contributing factors and address these (e.g., leg length discrepancy, repeated movement pattern, sustained posture, muscle imbalance, pelvic contracture).

## Tendinitis

### Definition

Inflammation of tendons about the hip are often the source of pain. Due to deep location, the exact diagnosis can be difficult to determine and to differentiate from bursitis. Tendon injuries usually occur at stress risers (i.e., musculotendinous junction or tenoperiosteal junction).

### Clinical Features

- In the older individual, the tendinous inflammation can be of a chronic nature associated with fibrous reaction. Onset of pain is usually gradual.
- In active persons, overuse syndrome causing microrupture can also result in gradual onset of pain.
- Athletic individuals are more prone to acute tears from a sudden change in direction or speed or from direct trauma.
- In the adolescent, the possibility of avulsion fracture from forceful muscle contraction should be considered.

### Diagnosis

- Movements of the hip that stress the involved tendon (contraction or stretch) elicit pain and are used to implicate the injured tissue.
- Pain on palpation of the suspected tendon is also useful at arriving at the diagnosis.

### Management

- Acute tendon injuries should be treated for the first 5 days with rest, ice, and compression, then with progressive remobilization and strengthening.
- Included in treatment of chronic tendinitis should be deep friction massage, stretching, and eccentric exercise.

### HIP TIPS

- Consider biomechanical cause of the problem and address if such a cause is found.
- Apply the recommendations of Curwin and Stanish (1984) in retraining: stretching, progressive eccentric exercising, and ice after exercise.

## *Muscle Strain*

### Definition

Strains or tears of muscles about the hip are fairly common athletic injuries. The musculotendinous junction, midbelly, and site of previous strains are stress risers and more prone to breakdown under load.

### Clinical Features

- Muscle injuries can be caused by direct (external) trauma or by indirect (internal) stress.
- Of the classic signs of inflammation, pain and loss of function are almost always present with a hip muscle strain. Swelling, redress, and increased local temperature are not easily detected around the hip unless the muscle tear is severe.

### Diagnosis

As with diagnosing a tendon injury, the following are important diagnostic variables for muscle strain:

- History of the injury
- Location within a muscle belly
- Pain on palpation (sometimes palpable and visible defect in the case of a complete rupture [i.e., grade III tear])
- Weak and painful response to contraction
- Pain on stretch

### Diagnostic Classification

Muscle, tendon, and ligament injuries can be classified according to the extent of the tear:

- Grade I: Microscopic tearing of fibers. Pain occurs on stress tests without loss of stability.
- Grade II: Significant tearing of fibers but not complete rupture. Pain is considerable. Of ligamentous damage, there is joint laxity but still a firm end point.
- Grade III: Complete rupture of fibers. Muscles and tendon can show a palpable or visible defect, and there will be loss of function of that structure. Ligament rupture results in instability and empty end-feel.

The following are commonly strained hip muscles:

- Adductors

- Hamstrings
- Rectus femoris
- Iliopsoas
- Tensor fascia lata
- Gluteus maximus

### Management

- Use first aid measures in the acute phase (see Figure 4-4).
- After 5 days of rest, start progressive remobilization.
- Gradually, as tolerated, increase stretch, increase resistance, increase speed, and increase repetitions.
- Use eccentric and functional activities.
- Use soft tissue mobilization techniques in addition to passive stretching to prevent a permanent stress riser that is prone to reinjury.
- Ideally, before returning to sport, the tissue should exhibit normal strength, normal length, normal density, and normal flexibility.

### Hip Tip

The single most important factor with a recent soft tissue injury is application of first aid measures (i.e., rest and ice) started immediately and continued for at least 48 hours. At a cellular level, as much damage can be caused by failure to treat an injury as was caused by the injury itself (Evans 1980).

## Osteitis Pubis

### Definition

Osteitis pubis is a chronic inflammation at the pubic symphysis caused in athletes by repetitive stress of muscles that attach there (i.e., rectus abdominus, gracilis, adductor longus).

### Epidemiology

Osteitis pubis is common in distance running, soccer, and American football. It is also common after urologic surgery.

### Clinical Features

- The primary symptom is groin pain with possible referral to the lower abdomen, the inner thigh, or both.
- There is usually localized tenderness over the pubic tubercle, and the adductors may spasm.
- Severe pain can result in a waddling gait.

### Radiologic Features

In nonresolving cases, further work-up reveals a hot bone scan, and there can be some x-ray changes, including loss of bone definition and widening of the symphysis.

### Management

- Treatment is usually rest, ice, NSAIDs initially, and then slowly progressive strengthening and stretching of the lumbo-pelvic-hip region.
- Osteitis pubis is frequently chronic and recurrent; therefore, early diagnosis and adequate rest are essential, as is flexibility training and warm-up before return to sporting activity.

### HIP TIPS

- Allow sufficient rest.
- Address posture and correct muscle imbalances.

## Hip Pointer

A direct blow sustained to or near the anterosuperior iliac spine (ASIS) can result in a painful contusion termed *hip pointer*. It is common in American football, ice hockey, and rugby from a tackle or a direct kick. X-rays are required to rule out a fracture. Avulsion of the iliac crest is possible. Visceral injury must be ruled out. Numbness of the lateral buttock and hip can result from injury to lateral cutaneous nerves (T12–L3). Initial treatment includes ice and NSAIDs with remobilization as tolerated.

### HIP TIPS

- To prevent reinjury, a "donut" pad can be fashioned to protect the ASIS.
- For symptomatic relief, athletic taping is sometimes helpful for limiting motion.

## Snapping Hip Syndrome

A snapping or clicking sensation or sound during hip motion, physical activity, or both, often with associated pain, is termed *snapping hip syndrome*. It is most common in athletes, especially gymnasts. Potential causes include the following, organized by location (Reid 1992):

Hip joint
    Suction phenomenon (most common cause)
    Iliofemoral ligaments on femoral head
    Subluxation
    Torn acetabular labrum
    Loose body
    Osteochondromatosis
Iliopsoas tendon
    Lesser trochanter
    Iliopectineal eminence
Symphysis pubis
    Postpartum
    Post-traumatic
    Generalized ligament laxity
Iliotibial band
    Greater trochanter
Biceps femoris tendon
    Ischial tuberosity

Localizing the source of the snapping should be attempted by careful palpation during active and passive hip ROM. Possibility of hip instability should be considered, especially if the patient has a history of dislocation. Possible contributing factors are muscle imbalance, muscle tightness, narrow iliac width, training technique, lower extremity alignment, and systemic disease.

**HIP TIP**
Identify the cause and contributing factors of the patient's complaint of "snapping hip" and address these in treatment.

### Hernia

A hernia is the protrusion of internal tissues through a weak section of muscle and peritoneum. Inguinal hernia is the most common type in the hip region. It occurs mostly in men. The inguinal canal is the normal opening in the abdominal wall for the spermatic cord, blood vessels, and nerves. A small enlargement of the canal permitting a small herniation can produce subtle anterior hip region pain. A larger herniation is visibly obvious. Varying presentation features can make hernias difficult to diagnose. History may reveal a contusion or strain in the area. Coughing, sneezing, and exercise usually increase the pain. A femoral hernia can occur in the proximal anterior thigh, and these are most often seen in athletic women.

Hernias usually require surgical repair, because, if left untreated, the protruding contents can become strangled and cut off the blood supply.

HIP TIP
Avoid always thinking musculoskeletal. Internal organs can be a source of pain, of which hernia is a good example.

## Nerve Entrapment Syndromes

The most common nerve entrapment syndromes encountered in the hip region are described in this section. It should be realized, however, that any nerve coursing from the spine into the leg is capable of yielding symptoms, signs, or both in the hip region when abnormally compressed or stretched or due to ischemia or inflammation. When inflamed, a nerve's threshold of excitation is lowered, so that a facilitated response occurs to functionally normal loads (Korr 1977).

### Piriformis Syndrome

Prolonged spasm, inflammation, or both of the piriformis muscle, often caused by a twisting injury on a fixed leg, can present as posterior thigh and calf pain in the sciatic nerve distribution or as deep buttock pain known as *piriformis syndrome*. The sciatic nerve runs adjacent to the piriformis through part of its course and in some individuals actually pierces the muscle belly (Figure 2-3; see also Figure 1-9). Persons with this syndrome report pain when walking, climbing stairs, and when rotating the trunk.

Chapter 3 provides details about testing for piriformis syndrome. However, the suggestion by Kapandji (1972) that piriformis acts as an internal rotator of the hip at 90 degrees flexion should make the clinician question the validity of resisting external rotation of the hip at 90 degrees flexion as a test for piriformis. A positive piriformis stress test produces buttock pain with possible radiation into the leg. Travell and Simons (1992) described piriformis as the "double devil," because it can refer pain from (1) irritation of the sciatic nerve or (2) irritation of the piriformis trigger points. Localized buttock pain can be a primary piriformis muscle strain. L4 to S3 distribution referred pain is likely propagated by sciatic nerve irritation.

Treatments for piriformis syndrome can include the following:

- Gentle, static stretching
- Ice massage
- Vapo coolant spray and stretch technique
- Ultrasound

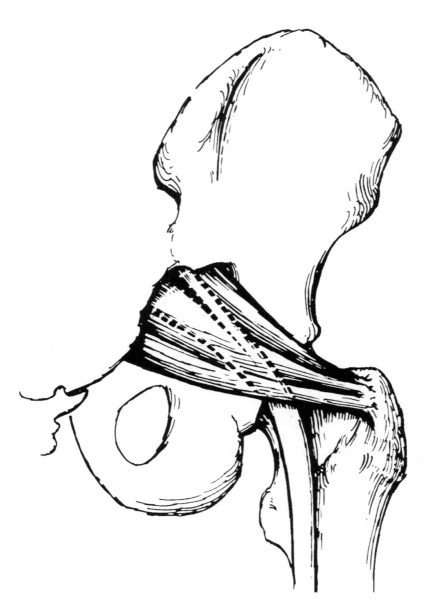

**Figure 2-3** The intimate relationship between the piriformis muscle and the sciatic nerve, which in most cases runs directly anterior to the muscle. (Reprinted with permission from A Conti. [1994] Hips and Pelvis. In RM Buschbacher [ed], *Musculoskeletal Disorders: A Practical Guide for Diagnosis and Rehabilitation* [p. 189]. Boston: Butterworth–Heinemann.)

- NSAIDs
- A heel insert of up to 0.25 in. on the nonaffected side, which can take tension off the piriformis
- Rest from sporting activity for 3 weeks (often necessary)

HIP TIP

Do not assume that buttock tenderness in the region of the piriformis muscle is piriformis syndrome. Assess all possibilities, including "referred tenderness" from the lumbar spine.

## Meralgia Paresthetica

Entrapment of the lateral femoral cutaneous nerve of the thigh as it emerges from the pelvis adjacent to the ASIS can result in tingling and numbness at the nerve's sensory distribution on the anterolateral thigh. This condition is termed *meralgia paresthetica*. It can present during pregnancy, in obese persons, in laborers who carry heavy tool bags around their waists, and from direct trauma near the ASIS during sports. Sensory testing can confirm the diagnosis, and there may be a positive Tinel sign to tapping adjacent to the ASIS and inguinal ligament. The diagnosis should not be made before ruling out other hip, lumbar, or intrapelvic pathology. The following treatments can be beneficial:

- Rest
- Ultrasound
- NSAIDs
- Injection with analgesic and corticosteroid (sometimes warranted)
- Surgical release of the nerve (rarely, when conservative measures have failed)

HIP TIP

Remember the characteristic superficial anterolateral thigh distribution of symptoms (i.e., tingling, numbness, or pain) that suggests meralgia paresthetica.

## Hamstring Syndrome

Hamstring syndrome occurs when the sciatic nerve becomes entrapped as a result of chronic strain to the proximal hamstrings. Pain can be worse with sitting, stretching, and during athletic activity. Hamstring syndrome appears to be most common in sprinters and hurdlers. Conservative interventions generally provide only temporary relief. Surgical release of adhesions in the proximal hamstrings, particularly biceps femoris (ventral to the sciatic nerve), usually provides lasting relief (Puranen and Orava 1988).

**HIP TIP**
Warm-up, stretching, eccentric exercise, and ice are advocated in the retraining phase of hamstring injuries (Stanish et al. 1986; Stanton and Purdam 1989).

## Superior Gluteal Nerve Entrapment Syndrome

A less common nerve entrapment syndrome is that of the superior gluteal nerve being compressed by the piriformis muscle in the greater sciatic notch (Reid 1992). Deep gluteal aching pain and tenderness to palpation just lateral to the greater sciatic notch are the usual symptoms. Pain is usually increased by hip internal rotation. Lack of hip internal rotation and anterior innominate rotation on the involved side have been correlated with impingement of the superior gluteal nerve (Turner 1996). Treatment is similar to that for piriformis syndrome.

**HIP TIPS**

- Assess pelvic alignment, stability, and mobility.
- Assess hip ROM.
- Have patient position hip in abduction at rest to prevent stretch weakness if gluteus medius and minimus weakness results from the superior gluteal nerve entrapment.

## Nerve Palsy After Hip Replacement

The rate of nerve palsy as a complication following THR has been reported in between 0.6% and 3.7% of cases. A study from the Joint Replacement Institute in Los Angeles on 3,126 consecutive THRs found the overall incidence of nerve palsy was 1.7% (Schmalzried et al. 1991). However, there was a considerably higher prevalence of nerve palsy after hip replacement in the following two population groups (making them risk factors for postoperative nerve palsy):

- Patients with congenital hip dysplasia had a nerve palsy incidence of 5.2%.
- Patients undergoing revision THR had a nerve palsy incidence of 3.2%.

The sciatic nerve (in particular the peroneal division) is involved in more than 80% of post-THR nerve palsy cases (Schmalzried et al. 1991).

## Less Common Entrapment Syndromes

The following nerve syndromes have also been described (see references for further description):

- Ilioinguinal nerve (Koppell et al. 1962)
- Femoral nerve (Miller and Benedict 1985)
- Obturator nerve (Siliski and Scott 1985)
- Genitofemoral nerve (Ingber 1989)
- Lateral cutaneous branches of the subcostal and iliohypogastric nerves (Maigne et al. 1986)

### HIP TIPS

- If possible, identify cause of entrapment.
- Correct any mechanical contributor or cause of the entrapment.
- Recognize the natural history (time span) for recovery from nerve injury.
- Prevent secondary problems such as stretch weakness or contracture.
- Compensate for irreversible damage (e.g., ankle-foot orthosis in cases of drop-foot from sciatic nerve palsy).

## Pediatric Hip Disorders

### Developmental Dysplasia of the Hip

#### Definition

*Dysplasia* is a term for abnormal development or growth. The term *developmental dysplasia of the hip* (DDH) is replacing the term *congenital dysplasia of the hip*, because it includes hips that were normal at birth but subsequently developed dysplasia.

#### Epidemiology

- The incidence of DDH in the United States is 1 in 100 live births with dysplasia (subluxatable), but only 1–2 cases in 1,000 live births that are dislocated or dislocatable (Mubarek et al. 1987).
- Dysplasia is six times more common in girls than in boys and more than 30 times more common in whites than in blacks.
- The left side is involved one and one-half times more often than the right.
- When the disease is bilateral, it is more severe on the left in approximately 30% of cases.

### Etiology

- The etiology of DDH is multifactorial.
- Dislocated fetal hips tend to appear only in the last trimester.
- The following can be predisposing factors:
    Mechanical. Small intrauterine space, tight abdominal wall of a primipara mother, breech presentation, and positioning of the fetal hip against the mother's sacrum in utero
    Physiologic. Ligamentous laxity in the female infant caused by the maternal hormones estrogen and relaxin
    Environmental (e.g., Eskimos and Lapps who carry children on cradle boards where the hips are strapped in extension have a greater incidence of DDH than cultures in which children are carried with the hips in flexion and abduction).

### Clinical Features

- Most infants have 75–90 degrees hip abduction. If there is significant limitation in this ROM or an asymmetry of even 5–10 degrees, further diagnostic studies should be performed for the possibility of hip dysplasia. Additional clinical indicators are asymmetric thigh folds, pistoning, positive Galeazzi sign (apparent femoral shortening with uneven knee heights), positive Barlow sign, or positive Ortolani sign (Figure 2-4).
- Ortolani and Barlow signs of instability usually disappear by 2–3 months after birth as the hip improves in stability or becomes fixed in a dislocated position. When performing the maneuvers, the infant must be completely relaxed, because slight muscle contraction can nullify the test.
- Limited hip abduction is often the only evident clinical sign of dysplasia in the infant older than 1 month.

### Radiologic Features

- Ultrasonography is a useful method of examining the hips of newborns and infants up to 6 months of age. The secondary ossification center is usually present by 6 months of age, and the deep cartilaginous structures are then obscured by the femoral head.
- Radiography becomes useful after 6 months of age and provides bilateral comparison. Many parameters of hip development can be measured on radiographs (Figure 2-5).

### Clinical Classification

The following is a clinical classification of newborn hips (Mubarek et al. 1987):

**Ortolani (reduction) test**
With baby relaxed and content on firm surface, hips and knees flexed to 90 degrees. Hips examined one at a time. Examiner grasps baby's thigh with middle finger over greater trochanter and lifts thigh to bring femoral head from its dislocated posterior position to opposite the acetabulum. Simultaneously, thigh gently abducted, reducing femoral head into acetabulum. In positive finding, examiner senses reduction by palpable, nearly audible "clunk."

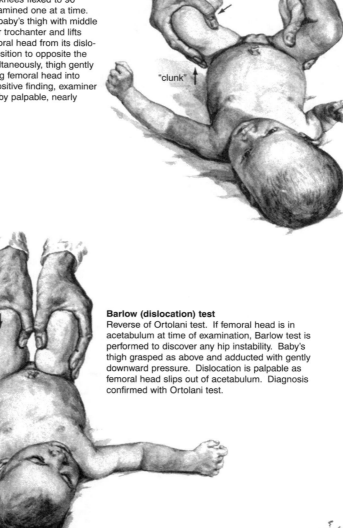

"clunk"

**Barlow (dislocation) test**
Reverse of Ortolani test. If femoral head is in acetabulum at time of examination, Barlow test is performed to discover any hip instability. Baby's thigh grasped as above and adducted with gently downward pressure. Dislocation is palpable as femoral head slips out of acetabulum. Diagnosis confirmed with Ortolani test.

**Figure 2-4** Recognition of developmental (congenital) dislocation of the hip. (Reprinted with permission from FH Netter. [1990] *The CIBA Collection of Medical Illustrations, Volume 8: Musculoskeletal System* [p. 52]. West Caldwell, NJ: CIBA-GEIGY Corporation.)

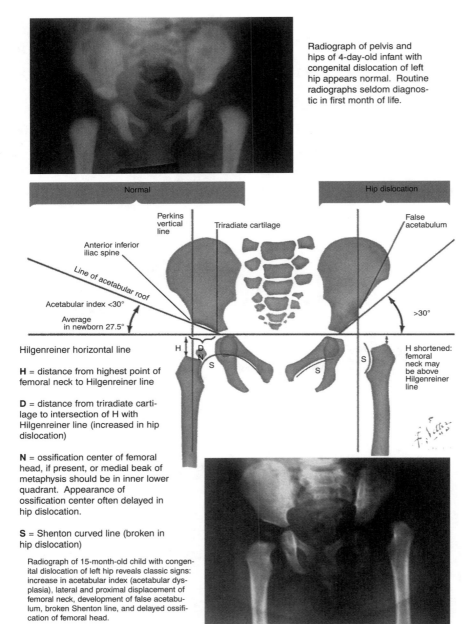

Radiograph of pelvis and hips of 4-day-old infant with congenital dislocation of left hip appears normal. Routine radiographs seldom diagnostic in first month of life.

Normal

Hip dislocation

Perkins vertical line

Triradiate cartilage

False acetabulum

Anterior inferior iliac spine

Line of acetabular roof

Acetabular index <30°

Average in newborn 27.5°

>30°

Hilgenreiner horizontal line

H = distance from highest point of femoral neck to Hilgenreiner line

D = distance from triradiate cartilage to intersection of H with Hilgenreiner line (increased in hip dislocation)

N = ossification center of femoral head, if present, or medial beak of metaphysis should be in inner lower quadrant. Appearance of ossification center often delayed in hip dislocation.

S = Shenton curved line (broken in hip dislocation)

H shortened: femoral neck may be above Hilgenreiner line

Radiograph of 15-month-old child with congenital dislocation of left hip reveals classic signs: increase in acetabular index (acetabular dysplasia), lateral and proximal displacement of femoral neck, development of false acetabulum, broken Shenton line, and delayed ossification of femoral head.

**Figure 2-5** Radiographic evaluation of developmental dysplasia of hip. (Reprinted with permission from FH Netter. [1990] *The CIBA Collection of Medical Illustrations, Volume 8: Musculoskeletal System* [p. 54]. West Caldwell, NJ: CIBA-GEIGY Corporation.)

- Normal: No instability is noted.
- Subluxatable (9.2 of 1,000): Femoral head is in acetabulum but can be partially displaced out to the acetabular rim.
- Dislocatable (1.3 of 1,000): Femoral head is in the hip socket but can be dislocated with the Barlow maneuver.
- Dislocated but reducible (1.2 of 1,000): Femoral head is out of the acetabulum at rest but can reduced by the Ortolani maneuver.
- Dislocated but not reducible: This usually occurs prenatally from a neurologic or muscular abnormality such as myelomeningocele or arthrogryposis.

### Radiographic Classification

- Acetabular dysplasia (without subluxation or dislocation)
- Subluxated (with associated acetabular dysplasia)
- Dislocated

### Management and Treatment

The goal of treatment for infants with DDH is to achieve a concentric reduction of the femoral head in the acetabulum to prevent abnormal wear. Treatment options are dependent on the etiology of the dysplasia, degree of dislocation, and the age of the child. There are also considerable variations in practice patterns between centers.

*Management of Developmental Dysplasia of the Hip:*
*Birth to 9 Months of Age*

A commonly used protocol suggests abduction diapers be used for 1 month. If the hip is stable after this time, the child should be re-evaluated at 3 and 12 months to ensure maintained stability and adequate acetabular development.

If the hip is still unstable after 1 month in abduction diapers, then a Pavlik harness is fitted. It is important that the Pavlik harness maintain the hip in the safe zone of Ramsey (Figure 2-6). It is worn at all times for 2–3 weeks until the hip is demonstrated to be reduced both clinically and by ultrasonography or radiography. Once reduced and stabilized, the harness is worn for an additional 3 months. It can be taken off only for a total of 1 hour per day to enable cleaning and changing of the child. It is then worn for 12 hours per day for another 3–6 months or until clinical and diagnostic examinations are normal. Parental education is key to successful use of the Pavlik harness.

If the Pavlik harness does not reduce the hip after 3 weeks of use, surgical treatment is indicated. The child is first placed in skin traction at home

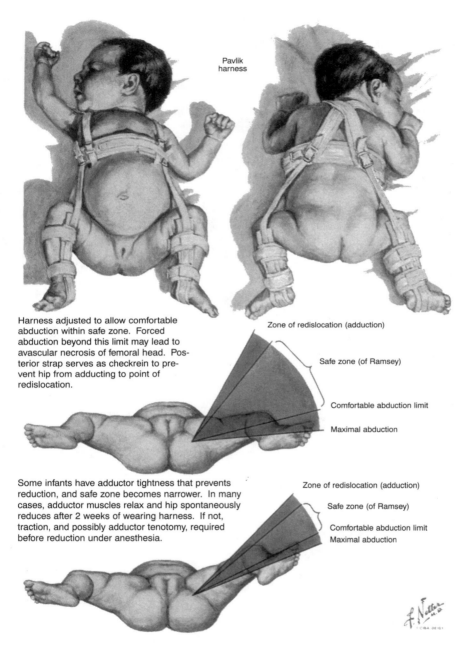

Pavlik harness

Harness adjusted to allow comfortable abduction within safe zone. Forced abduction beyond this limit may lead to avascular necrosis of femoral head. Posterior strap serves as checkrein to prevent hip from adducting to point of redislocation.

Zone of redislocation (adduction)

Safe zone (of Ramsey)

Comfortable abduction limit

Maximal abduction

Some infants have adductor tightness that prevents reduction, and safe zone becomes narrower. In many cases, adductor muscles relax and hip spontaneously reduces after 2 weeks of wearing harness. If not, traction, and possibly adductor tenotomy, required before reduction under anesthesia.

Zone of redislocation (adduction)

Safe zone (of Ramsey)

Comfortable abduction limit

Maximal abduction

**Figure 2-6** Device for treatment of clinically reducible dislocation of hip. (Reprinted with permission from FH Netter. [1990] *The CIBA Collection of Medical Illustrations, Volume 8: Musculoskeletal System* [p. 57]. West Caldwell, NJ: CIBA-GEIGY Corporation.)

for 2–3 weeks to reduce the incidence of femoral head AVN. Surgery then consists of an arthrogram to identify anatomic landmarks, percutaneous adductor tenotomy, closed or, if necessary, open reduction of the hip, and application of a spica cast.

*Management of Developmental Dysplasia of the Hip:*
*9 Months of Age and Older*
Figure 2-7 illustrates the likely findings in a child with developmental dysplasia that has not been treated successfully or that only became apparent when the child started walking. For the child 9 months of age and older, an abduction orthosis that enables walking is a first-line treatment for persistent acetabular dysplasia. If this fails, surgical treatment is usually required with either a closed or an open reduction.

In children not diagnosed until about 2 years of age, open reduction is often indicated, sometimes with femoral shortening to reduce compressive forces on the reduced femoral head. Children who continue to have acetabular dysplasia at age 4 years and older benefit from pelvic osteotomy (acetabuloplasties). Mild dysplasia often goes unnoticed for decades until the patient develops osteoarthritis of the hip.

**Hip Tips**

- Diagnosis in the newborn is most important for an excellent result. A positive Barlow sign and Ortolani "click" are important tests in the diagnostic process.
- It has been suggested that too frequent or too forcible examination of infants' hips can induce or worsen hip instability. Therefore, it is recommended that a gentle examination of an infant's hip be performed only once by a skilled examiner (Moore 1989).
- Parental education is the key to successful Pavlik harness management.
- Asymmetric hip abduction is an indicator that a more in-depth examination should be performed.

## Slipped Capital Femoral Epiphysis

### Definition
SCFE is a displacement of the femoral head in relationship to the femoral neck, which is caused by a slip at the proximal femoral epiphysis. SCFE is sometimes known as *epiphyseal* or *adolescent coxa vara* or *proximal femoral epiphysiolysis.*

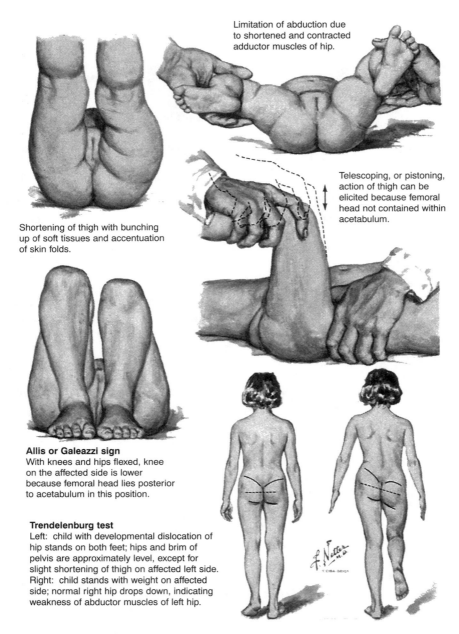

Limitation of abduction due to shortened and contracted adductor muscles of hip.

Telescoping, or pistoning, action of thigh can be elicited because femoral head not contained within acetabulum.

Shortening of thigh with bunching up of soft tissues and accentuation of skin folds.

**Allis or Galeazzi sign**
With knees and hips flexed, knee on the affected side is lower because femoral head lies posterior to acetabulum in this position.

**Trendelenburg test**
Left: child with developmental dislocation of hip stands on both feet; hips and brim of pelvis are approximately level, except for slight shortening of thigh on affected left side. Right: child stands with weight on affected side; normal right hip drops down, indicating weakness of abductor muscles of left hip.

**Figure 2-7** Clinical findings in developmental dislocation of the hip (if untreated, signs become more obvious with growth and weightbearing). (Reprinted with permission from FH Netter. [1990] *The CIBA Collection of Medical Illustrations, Volume 8: Musculoskeletal System* [p. 53]. West Caldwell, NJ: CIBA-GEIGY Corporation.)

### Epidemiology

- SCFE is more common in boys than girls by a 2 to 1 ratio.
- SCFE is most common in adolescents from 10 to 16 years of age (the proximal femoral epiphyseal line must be open for a slip to occur) and is often associated with periods of rapid growth.
- Approximately 50% of cases are bilateral, with one side slipping before the other.
- Two body types seem to be more commonly affected: (1) the short, obese child with poorly defined secondary sex characteristics and (2) the very tall, thin child.

### Etiology

Between the ages of 16 and 19 years, the proximal femoral (capital) epiphysis unites to the neck of the femur. However, in the 12–18 months before this event, the epiphyseal plate can become susceptible to shear, and the head can slip posteriorly and medially in relation to the femoral shaft, producing an adduction, external rotation, and extension deformity.

### Clinical Features

- The obese or tall adolescent reports gradually increasing hip pain and limp.
- Internal rotation in extension and abduction ROMs are decreased.
- When the hip is passively flexed, it often also abducts and externally rotates (Figure 2-8).
- An acute slip, which occurs in less than 10% of cases, can be associated with trauma. This is an orthopedic emergency, as AVN could result.
- A chronic slip can be present for 3–12 months or longer. It involves a gradual development of coxa vara with posterior medial position of the proximal femoral epiphysis. The patient usually has a short and externally rotated leg.

### Radiologic Features

- Radiographic studies include an AP view of each hip, AP view of the pelvis, and a frog-leg lateral view.
- Based on the radiographs, there are three grades of slip (see Figure 2-8).

### Management

- Reduction of the acute slip can be achieved by traction or gentle manipulation under anesthesia.

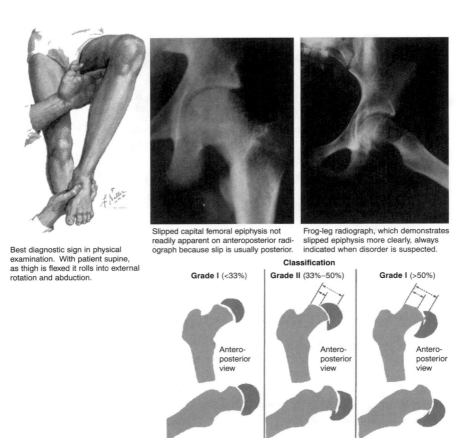

Best diagnostic sign in physical examination. With patient supine, as thigh is flexed it rolls into external rotation and abduction.

Slipped capital femoral epiphysis not readily apparent on anteroposterior radiograph because slip is usually posterior.

Frog-leg radiograph, which demonstrates slipped epiphysis more clearly, always indicated when disorder is suspected.

**Classification**

Grade I (<33%)    Grade II (33%–50%)    Grade I (>50%)

Antero-posterior view    Antero-posterior view    Antero-posterior view

Frog-leg view    Frog-leg view    Frog-leg view

**Figure 2-8** Slipped capital femoral epiphyses. (Reprinted with permission from FH Netter. [1990] *The CIBA Collection of Medical Illustrations, Volume 8: Musculoskeletal System* [p. 70]. West Caldwell, NJ: CIBA-GEIGY Corporation.)

- Forcible reduction is never used.
- The subacute slip is treated in hospital with traction in extension and gradual internal rotation.
- Once the hip can be rotated to neutral internal rotation, and radiographs show that the femoral head is close to a normal relationship with the femoral neck, then closure of the epiphyses with a threaded pin is performed.
- More severe slips need to be treated by proximal femur osteotomy.

- Postoperative physical therapy after SCFE stabilization involves teaching partial or touchdown weightbearing, gentle hip ROM exercises, and submaximal isometrics.

### Complications

- AVN. AVN can occur following surgery to fix SCFE. It occurs more frequently after intra-articular osteotomies.
- Chondrolysis. Chondrolysis is a pathologic process that results in matrix breakdown of articular cartilage. It is represented on x-rays as extraordinarily decreased joint space. Chondrolysis presents clinically as a painful and unusually stiff joint. It can occur independent of surgical intervention and is more common in women. Anti-inflammatory drug use and limited weightbearing can provide some recovery.
- Osteoarthritis. Long-term follow-up in SCFE patients is largely uncharted; however, available evidence suggests that these patients are more likely to develop hip osteoarthritis by the fifth decade. Indeed, many patients thought to have primary OA may, if studied closely with radiographs, show signs of an old, mild SCFE.

### HIP TIPS

- A red flag is the adolescent child (tall and thin or short and obese) with hip pain. He or she should be referred for radiographic evaluation.
- Prognosis for surgical fixation of a minor slip is much better than for the more advanced SCFE; therefore, the importance of early diagnosis cannot be overstated.

## Legg-Calvé-Perthes Disease

### Definition

LCP is a disorder in which there is AVN of the femoral head in a growing child. It is also known as *coxa plana* and *juvenile osteochondrosis*.

### Epidemiology

- LCP affects children 3–12 years in age, with 4 or 5 years being the most common age at onset.
- Boys are involved slightly more often than girls.
- Whites are affected much more than blacks.
- Bilateral involvement is present in 15% of patients.

### Etiology

- LCP is a self-limiting syndrome that can involve all or part of the femoral head.
- Occasionally, onset of the condition is preceded by one or more episodes of transient synovitis.
- The initial stage in LCP is avascularity of the femoral head.
- The cause of LCP is not fully understood.
- Skeletal maturity is often delayed by 1–2 years, but no other abnormalities have been identified.

### Clinical Presentation

- Presentation is similar to transient synovitis, with hip pain, limp, and referred pain to the superior knee joint.
- Decreased abduction, limited rotation, and flexion contracture are usually seen.

### Radiologic Features

- Early radiographs may show capsular swelling or widening of the hip joint. The ossific nucleus becomes dense during the avascular stage. A subchondral fracture or crescent sign may be seen later in the course. The disease process takes from 2 to 8 years to run its course.
- To aid diagnosis and prognosis, five radiographic "head-at-risk" signs have been described (Gruebel Lee 1983): (1) increased inferior-medial joint space indicative of lateral subluxation; (2) abnormal angle of the growth plates; (3) Gage sign, which is an osteoporotic (translucent) region at the lateral end of the growth plate; (4) calcification lateral to the growth plate, indicating collapse of the femoral head; and (5) irregularity of the epiphysis indicative of metaphyseal reaction (the "sagging rope" sign). Presence of three or more "head-at-risk" signs suggests poor prognosis and need for surgery.

### Diagnostic Classification

There are three primary systems for classification of LCP disease:

- Waldenstrom classification: chronological phase
- Catterall classification: extent of disease
- Salter-Thompson classification: extent of disease

The following are two radiographic classifications used in research:

- Mose measurements of concentric circles
- Stulberg classification

The lack of conformity in these classification systems could be a reason for the confusion that often exists in treatment of the problem.

### Management

- The goal of treatment in LCP disease is to minimize hip-joint deformity and delay OA changes later in life.
- Treatment is minimal, and prognosis is excellent for younger children who have involvement of only the anterior part of the epiphyses and not the weightbearing region.
- For older children and those with complete involvement of the femoral head, treatment involves avoiding full weightbearing and increasing coverage of the acetabulum by surgery or bracing in abduction and flexion.
- Currently, there is no evidence to suggest advantage of surgery over bracing. Containment of the femoral head within the acetabulum can be achieved by either method; however, surgery allows sooner return to normal activity and less active cooperation by the child.
- Five common treatment methods for LCP are (1) Scottish Rite orthosis, (2) nonweightbearing and exercises, (3) Petrie cast, (4) varus osteotomy, and (5) Salter osteotomy (Wang et al. 1995).
- Physical therapy. ROM exercises with a physical therapist are important, because loss of ROM leads to poorer results. At first, gait training with crutches is prescribed. After the cast or brace is removed, the physical therapist should work on ROM of ankle, knee, and hip.

### Prognostic Factors

- Age at diagnosis. A younger age at diagnosis indicates a more favorable outcome.
- Extent of femoral head involvement. Less involvement leads to a better outcome.
- Radiographic at-risk signs. The presence of three or more femoral head-at-risk signs indicates a poor prognosis.

### HIP TIPS

- Work closely with the orthopedist and patient's family.

- Maintain ROM and function in prescribed orthotic device.

## Congenital Coxa Vara

### Definition

*Coxa* is Latin for the hip region. *Vara* indicates that there is a reduced angle between the neck of the femur and the shaft. *Valga* indicates an increased neck-shaft angle. Congenital coxa vara is an affliction that becomes apparent once a child starts to walk. It is caused by a neck-shaft angle of less than 120 degrees. At birth, the angle of inclination of the femoral neck is approximately 150 degrees; it decreases to 125 degrees by adulthood, and in the elderly is further reduced to about 120 degrees.

### Etiology

- Acquired coxa vara results from a number of conditions (many of which are described in this chapter) including LCP, SCFE, rickets, osteomalacia, and hip fracture.
- Congenital coxa vara results from malformation of the proximal femur. The infantile form is considered a distinct entity characterized by a triangular defect in the distal part of the femoral neck metaphysis. It is frequently bilateral but is not usually associated with other developmental defects. Familial history is suggestive of a genetic agent in transmission.
- Other forms of coxa vara include children with a congenitally short femur, which is also known as *proximal focal femoral deficiency*.

### Clinical Features

- Congenital coxa vara is not usually identified until the child starts to walk with a painless limp.
- Trendelenburg sign is positive.
- Bilateral involvement results in a duck-waddle gait in which the body sways from side to side.
- Abduction and internal rotation of the affected hip are usually limited.
- A shortened leg is also common.
- There is often an increased lumbar lordosis.

### Radiographic Features

- A decreased neck-shaft angle
- A triangular defect in the inferior aspect of the femoral neck

### Management

- Mild deformities in which the neck-shaft angle is greater than 100 degrees are treated conservatively with a shoe lift and exercises to stretch out contractures. Follow-up exams are necessary to check for deformity progression.
- Varus deformities in which the angle of inclination is less than 100 degrees and is progressively worsening with functional impairment should be treated surgically with a valgus osteotomy. The goal of surgery is to create a normal position for the proximal femoral growth plate at right angles to the resultant weightbearing force across the hip joint. This, in turn, improves abductor muscle function and leg length discrepancy.
- After osteotomy, a hip spica cast is worn for 6 weeks, and then gentle active-assisted activities are initiated. Weightbearing is allowed after union is determined radiographically.

### HIP TIP

A child with a painless limp with decreased hip-abduction range and strength (positive Trendelenburg sign) should be referred for x-rays.

## *Acute Transient Synovitis*

### Definition

Acute transient synovitis is a self-limiting condition of the hip, seen in children 2–10 years of age. It is often seen a couple of weeks after an upper respiratory tract infection. It is also known as *toxic synovitis*, *irritable hip syndrome*, or *observation hip*.

### Epidemiology

- Acute transient synovitis occurs in children from 2 to 10 years of age.
- There are usually no other health problems.
- It is often preceded by an upper respiratory tract infection.
- Up to 5% of children with acute transient synovitis develop AVN or LCP.

### Etiology

The etiology is unknown, but it may be related to infection or minor trauma.

### Clinical Features

- The child experiences hip pain.
- The child walks with a limp.

- The child may refuse to walk.
- The child experiences decreased hip ROM (especially internal rotation).
- Fever may be associated with severe pain.
- Work-up should include erythrocyte sedimentation rate and white blood cell count.

### Radiologic Features

- X-rays should be performed to rule out other problems.
- Bone scan may be positive for a hip problem.

Radiologic tests should be performed to rule out the following:

- LCP
- Juvenile rheumatoid arthritis
- Osteomyelitis
- Tumor

### Management

- Bed rest is the primary treatment.
- Sometimes traction and bed rest in hospital is indicated.
- Partial weightbearing with crutches is indicated for 2–3 weeks in older children.
- Heat and massage are advocated by some.
- Follow-up radiographs are recommended for a few years after the synovitis.
- Aspiration of the joint may be necessary.

HIP TIPS
The following are red flags for acute transient synovitis:

- Child with hip pain and limp. He or she should be referred to an orthopedist for a work-up.
- Previous diagnosis of transient synovitis warrants follow-up with an orthopedist to ensure that LCP is not developing and to instigate early management if it is.

## Conclusion

A comprehensive summation of the primary diseases and disorders that affect the hip is presented in this chapter. Knowledge of these problems is powerful weaponry for enabling the clinician to accurately diagnose and appropriately direct treatment for those who have hip pain and dysfunction. Referral of the patient to an orthopedic surgeon is essential when a serious problem is suspected. Radiologic imaging and other studies (e.g., blood tests) are required to *accurately* diagnose skeletal conditions affecting the hip. Although the clinician should not rely on signs and symptoms alone, skilled history taking and physical examination as presented in Chapter 3 are essential components of the diagnostic process. Subtle diagnostic clues are often the tip that an experienced investigator needs to solve a difficult case. Careful attention to the contents of this chapter provide many such clues.

# 3

# Evaluation of the Hip

Scott L. Jones

Health care professionals face enormous pressure to provide quality service while simultaneously reducing cost. A shift in practice patterns is required for the physical therapist to succeed in this environment. To be efficient yet thorough in the evaluation of a patient requires the use of a systematic and analytic approach. Such a method is employed in this chapter. It is anticipated that this method will be a valuable resource for all physical therapy clinicians (beginning to advanced) with clinical management of this patient population.

## Examination Process

Because the hip joint is deeply situated, it can present numerous problems in evaluation and diagnosis. The clinician must be mindful of the possible effects and influences of other adjacent segments in the trunk and lower quarter of the body and effectively rule out their contribution to the clinical presentation of signs and symptoms.

### *Lower Quarter Segments*

- Inferior thoracic spine (from approximately the tenth thoracic vertebra [T10])*
- Lumbar spine
- Sacrum
- Pelvis

---

*The inferior thoracic spine from T10 is included due to its neurologic sensory contribution to the lumbopelvic region and its facet joint alignment, which permits it to function like an extension of the lumbar spine.

- Femur
- Tibia
- Ankle and foot complex

Physical therapists do not use the full technological means (e.g., x-ray, magnetic resonance imaging [MRI], computed tomography scan) to make a diagnosis across the spectrum of possible hip disorders; however, they need to function as team members with other medical specialists to ensure a complete and accurate diagnosis. It is also crucial that physical therapists are able to identify findings that do not support the presence of a musculoskeletal disorder and require physician referral to determine if a medical condition is present (Table 3-1).

The three primary purposes of the musculoskeletal examination (Figure 3-1) are as follows:

- To determine the etiology of the patient's chief complaint
- To specify the involved structures and tissues and assess their integrity
- To determine the patient's functional status with daily, occupational, and recreational activities

The essential aspects of the musculoskeletal examination consist of two parts: subjective assessment and objective assessment. Although these parts are separated for recording purposes, they are intertwined throughout the examination process. It is common for the patient to share pertinent subjective information with the clinician while the objective assessment is in progress.

### Subjective Assessment

The examination begins with defining the patient's problem through an interview process. The interview is an opportunity to establish a list of provisional diagnoses, from which a logical physical examination can be developed. It should also provide the clinician with an indication of the severity, irritability, and nature of the condition (Maitland 1991).

The clinician must acquire skill in guiding an interview so that contradictory or vague information can be clarified. This can be done effectively by using the following basic interviewing techniques:

- Open-ended questions (e.g., "What positions and activities make your symptoms better or worse?")
- Closed-ended questions (e.g., "Are your symptoms worse with prolonged sitting?")
- Follow-up questions (e.g., "If yes, how long does it take for your symptoms to appear with prolonged sitting?")

**Table 3-1** Diseases and Disorders Causing Hip Pain That Require
Physician Referral

Suspected fractures

Iliopsoas abscess

Lumbar herniated disc with neurologic involvement

Appendicitis

Cauda equina syndrome

Pelvic inflammatory disease

Signs or symptoms of suspected cancer

Crohn's disease

Osteoid osteoma

Femoral hernia

Chondroblastoma

Ureteral colic

Chondrosarcoma

Reiter's syndrome

Giant cell tumor

Ankylosing spondylitis

Ewing's sarcoma

Tuberculosis

Sickle cell anemia

Hemophilia

Osteoporosis

Arterial insufficiency

Source: Adapted from CG Goodman, TEK Snyder. (1990) *Differential Diagnosis in
Physical Therapy*. Philadelphia: Saunders, 566.

- Paraphrasing (e.g., "You have told me that your symptoms are worse
  with sitting. What other positions aggravate your symptoms?")

It is important that the clinician remain objective during the interview
to avoid bias toward any particular diagnosis. Positive and negative findings
should be noted in both subjective and objective assessments to correlate
information when making any initial provisional diagnoses. The objective
assessment either supports or weakens the possible diagnoses until one is
identified as the primary etiology.

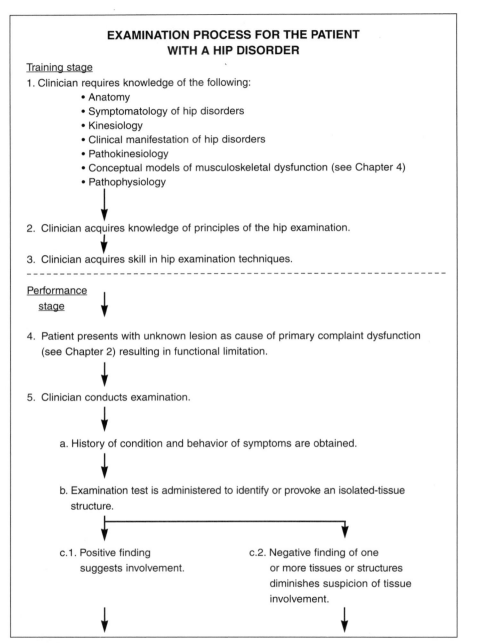

**Figure 3-1** Examination process for the patient with hip dysfunction. (Adapted from DA Dyrek. [1994] Assessment and Treatment Planning Strategies for Musculoskeletal Deficits. In SB Sullivan, TJ Schmitz [eds], *Physical Rehabilitation: Assessment and Treatment* [3rd ed] [p. 63]. Philadelphia: Davis.)

d.1. Clinician administers further tests to isolate a specific tissue.

d.2. Clinician administers further tests to provoke tissue to ensure no involvement.

e. Lesion is identified. Etiology of primary complaint is known.

f. Clinician evaluates the effect of lesion on the functional status of tissues (e.g., range of motion, strength, soft tissue flexibility, joint mobility).

g. Clinician evaluates the functional ability of the patient.

6. Assessment is obtained by correlating information.

7. Goals are identified.

8. Treatment plan is initiated.

9. Clinician monitors effect of treatment (by repeating steps 5–8).

The basic components of the interview are current status, past history, general health, and previous tests and treatment (including effectiveness of prior treatment). Using a patient history form (Figure 3-2) ensures that all appropriate information is gathered. The patient completes the form before the scheduled appointment. The clinician then reviews the information with the patient during the interview to further clarify responses. In a busy clinical environment, this method increases the available time to conduct the patient evaluation.

### Current Status

The chief complaint of a patient with hip dysfunction is typically pain (Grieve 1983). However, I have experienced several instances in which diminished function, in the form of decreased motion, strength, or gait quality, brought the patient to the clinic.

Please provide us with the following information so that we may better serve you. Your physical therapist will review this form with you. If you do not know the information requested or if you need assistance filling out the form, your physical therapist will help you. This information is confidential and will be part of your medical record.

Family and Personal History

Name: _____ Gender: _____

DOB: _____ Age: _____ Date: _____

Occupation: _____

Referred by: _____

Family physician: _____

Diagnosis: _____

Next scheduled physician's appointment for this problem: _____

Date of onset: _____ Onset: (circle)     Gradual          Sudden

Work related? ☐ Yes ☐ No     Under litigation? ☐ Yes ☐ No

Past Medical History

Have you or any immediate family member ever been told you have: (✔ all that apply)

| ✔ | Condition | For the therapist (Do NOT complete) | | |
|---|-----------|---------|---------------|--------|
|   |           | Relation | Date of onset | Status |
|   | Allergies |  |  |  |
|   | Anemia |  |  |  |
|   | Angina or chest pain |  |  |  |
|   | Arthritis or gout |  |  |  |
|   | Asthma or hay fever |  |  |  |
|   | Bladder problems |  |  |  |
|   | Bowel problems |  |  |  |
|   | Cancer |  |  |  |
|   | Cirrhosis or liver disease |  |  |  |
|   | Chronic bronchitis |  |  |  |
|   | Diabetes |  |  |  |
|   | Emphysema |  |  |  |
|   | Hepatitis or jaundice |  |  |  |
|   | High blood pressure or hypertension |  |  |  |
|   | Heart disease |  |  |  |
|   | Hypoglycemia |  |  |  |
|   | Kidney disease or kidney stones |  |  |  |
|   | Migraine headaches |  |  |  |

Figure 3-2 Physical therapy patient history form.

| ✔ | Condition | For the therapist (Do NOT complete) | | |
|---|-----------|----------|---------------|--------|
| | | Relation | Date of onset | Status |
| | Pneumonia | | | |
| | Polio | | | |
| | Rheumatic or scarlet fever | | | |
| | Shortness of breath | | | |
| | Stroke | | | |
| | Tuberculosis | | | |
| | Ulcers or stomach problems | | | |
| | Unusual menstrual problems | | | |
| | Urinary tract infection | | | |
| | Other (specify) | | | |

General Health

1. Have you had any recent illnesses or hospitalizations?  □ Yes □ No
   If yes, please describe the problem. _____
2. Have you had any unexplained weight loss or gain in the last month? □ Yes □ No
3. Do you smoke or chew tobacco?  □ Yes □ No
   If yes, how many packs per day?_____ For how many months or years?_____
4. How much alcohol do you drink during a week?_____
5. How much caffeine do you consume daily (including soft drinks, coffee, tea, or chocolate)?_____
6. Have you noticed any lumps or thickening of skin or muscle anywhere on your body? □ Yes □ No  If yes, where?_____
7. Do you have any sores that have not healed or any changes in size, shape, or color of a wart or mole?  □ Yes □ No
8. Are you on any special diet prescribed by a physician?  □ Yes □ No
9. What hobbies do you enjoy?_____
10. Do you exercise?  □ Yes □ No
    If yes, what do you do, how often, and for how long?_____
11. What type of person do you consider yourself?  □ Calm □ Stressed
                                                      □ Somewhere in between

Special Questions for Women

1. Last pap smear: _____
2. Last breast examination: _____

3. Do you perform a monthly breast self-examination? ☐ Yes ☐ No
4. Do you take birth control pills or use an intrauterine device (IUD)? ☐ Yes ☐ No

Special Questions for Men

1. Do you ever have difficulty with urination (e.g., difficulty in starting or continuing flow or a very slow flow of urine)? ☐ Yes ☐ No
2. Do you ever have blood in your urine? ☐ Yes ☐ No
3. Do you ever have pain on urination? ☐ Yes ☐ No

Work Environment

1. Does your job involve:
   ____Prolonged sitting (e.g., desk, driving)
   ____Prolonged standing (e.g., sales clerk, equipment operator)
   ____Prolonged walking (e.g., delivery person, mill worker)
   ____Use of large or small equipment (e.g., computer, cash register, fork lift, drill press)
   ____Lifting, bending, twisting, climbing, or turning
   ____Exposure to chemicals or gas
   ____Other. Please describe: _____
2. Do you use any special supports?
   ____Back or neck cushion
   ____Back brace or corset
   ____Other kind of brace or support for any body part

Previous Tests and Treatments

1. Do you take medications? ☐ Yes ☐ No
   If yes, please list all your medications (prescribed and over-the-counter):

| Type | Dosage | Frequency | Effect |
|------|--------|-----------|--------|
|      |        |           |        |
|      |        |           |        |

2. Have you had any diagnostic tests for this problem, such as x-rays, sonograms, computer tomography (CT) scans, magnetic resonance imaging (MRI), electromyogram (EMG), or myelogram? If yes, please specify: which? when? results?_____
3. Have you had previous treatment for this problem, such as physical therapy, occupational therapy, or chiropractic treatment? ☐ Yes ☐ No
   If yes, please specify: which? when? type of treatments? results?_____

**Figure 3-2** *Continued*

4. Please list any operations that you have ever had and the date(s) of surgery:

| Surgery | Date |
|---|---|
|  |  |
|  |  |
|  |  |

Present Symptoms

1. How did your problem begin?_____

2. Do you have pain? ☐ Yes ☐ No
   If yes, where is the pain located?_____

3. Do your symptoms seem to be getting: ☐ Better ☐ Worse ☐ Same ☐ Fluctuating

4. When are your symptoms worse? ☐ Morning ☐ Afternoon ☐ Evening
   ☐ Night/Sleeping

5. When are your symptoms better? ☐ Morning ☐ Afternoon ☐ Evening
   ☐ Night/Sleeping

6. Would you describe your pain as: ☐ Sharp ☐ Aching ☐ Burning ☐ Throbbing
   ☐ Shooting ☐ Tingling ☐ Other: _____

7. Do your symptoms disturb your sleep? ☐ Yes ☐ No

8. In what position do you sleep? ☐ Back ☐ Stomach ☐ Left side ☐ Right side
   ☐ Sitting up in a chair

9. How many hours do you sleep?_____

10. How do the following activities affect your symptoms? (✔ appropriate column)

| Activity | My symptoms | | |
|---|---|---|---|
|  | Increase | Decrease | Unchanged |
| Sitting longer than 30 mins |  |  |  |
| Sitting less than 30 mins |  |  |  |
| Sit to stand |  |  |  |
| Driving |  |  |  |
| Bending |  |  |  |
| Leaning backwards |  |  |  |
| Standing |  |  |  |
| Lying down |  |  |  |
| Walking |  |  |  |
| Stairs |  |  |  |
| Twisting |  |  |  |
| Activity in general |  |  |  |
| Work activities |  |  |  |

11. Make a mark (X) along the lines a and b between the given extremes that you think represent your current symptoms in your major area of injury.

a. _____

No pain at all                              Pain as bad as it could be

b. _____

No difficulty performing tasks                    Completely disabling

12. Have you had any of the following symptoms associated with this problem? (Mark all those that apply.)

|   |                                            |
|---|--------------------------------------------|
|   | Stomach ache                               |
|   | Weakness                                   |
|   | Chills                                     |
|   | Dizziness                                  |
|   | Fever                                      |
|   | Hoarseness                                 |
|   | Numbness                                   |
|   | Skin rash                                  |
|   | Persistent cough                           |
|   | Difficulty with breathing                  |
|   | Heart palpitations                         |
|   | Changes in bowel or bladder functions      |
|   | Difficulty with swallowing                 |
|   | Problems with vision                       |
|   | Headaches                                  |
|   | Nausea or vomiting                         |
|   | Unexplained sweating or night sweats       |

13. Finally, what would you like to achieve from therapy? (Goals)_____

_____

_____

_____

_____

**Figure 3-2** *Continued*

Because the hip joint is derived by multiple segments of the mesoderm (primarily the third lumbar vertebra [L3]), there are likely to be several possible pain patterns. Wroblewski (1978) compiled a list of 89 patients (65 men and 26 women with a mean age of 60.3 years) with primary hip osteoarthritis and summarized their various pain distributions (Table 3-2). All patients

**Table 3-2** Pain Patterns in 89 Patients with Osteoarthritis of the Hip Joint

| Area of pain | Number of patients |
| --- | --- |
| Greater trochanter | 71 |
| Medial buttock | 40 |
| Groin | 47 |
| Anterior thigh | 63 |
| Knee | 70 |
| Shin | 40 |

Source: Adapted from BM Wroblewski. (1978) Pain in osteoarthrosis of the hip. *Practitioner* 1315, 140.

presented with multiple sites of pain. This observation, along with the possibility of referred pain from nonhip structures, highlights the challenge of differential diagnosis at the hip.

There are many possible reasons for pain and many types of pain (e.g., radicular, chronic). Usually, a careful assessment of pain behavior is invaluable in determining the nature and extent of the underlying pathology (Figure 3-3). "Failure to listen to a complaint of pain may lead to serious errors in treatment." (Parsons 1945, p. 73)

To elicit a more complete description of symptoms from the patient, the clinician may wish to use a term other than *pain* (e.g., referring to the patient's *symptoms* or using descriptors such as *hurt* or *ache*). This point is especially true when interviewing and eventually treating the prolonged pain sufferer to move the focus away from pain and toward improvement of functional abilities. Furthermore, because physical therapists spend a considerable amount of time investigating pain, it is easy to remain focused exclusively on this symptom when patients may otherwise bring to the forefront other important problems.

### Past Medical History

A careful review of the personal and family medical history is necessary if the current status relates to a past medical problem. This review should include physiologic- and functional-level data, psychosocial factors, and health promotion and disease prevention behaviors.

Several disorders of the hip are related to the patient's age, gender, race, activity level, or mechanism of injury. For example, certain hip problems are seen only in children or only during certain age periods (see Table 2-1). Information about pediatric hip conditions can be found in Chapter 2.

Check any words that describe your pain. If more than one word applies in a category, check *only* the most appropriate. You do not have to check a word in every category; only if it describes your pain.

| | | | | |
|---|---|---|---|---|
| 1. Flicking | ( ) | 13. Fearful | ( ) | |
|   Quivering | ( ) |   Frightful | ( ) | |
|   Pulsing | ( ) |   Terrifying | ( ) | |
|   Throbbing | ( ) | 14. Punishing | ( ) | |
|   Beating | ( ) |   Grueling | ( ) | |
|   Pounding | ( ) |   Cruel | ( ) | |
| 2. Jumping | ( ) |   Vicious | ( ) | |
|   Flashing | ( ) |   Killing | ( ) | |
|   Shooting | ( ) | 15. Wretched | ( ) | |
| 3. Pricking | ( ) |   Blinding | ( ) | |
|   Boring | ( ) | 16. Annoying | ( ) | |
|   Drilling | ( ) |   Troublesome | ( ) | |
|   Stabbing | ( ) |   Miserable | ( ) | |
|   Lancinating | ( ) |   Intense | ( ) | |
| 4. Sharp | ( ) |   Unbearable | ( ) | |
|   Cutting | ( ) | 17. Spreading | ( ) | |
|   Lacerating | ( ) |   Radiating | ( ) | |
| 5. Pinching | ( ) |   Penetrating | ( ) | |
|   Pressing | ( ) |   Piercing | ( ) | |
|   Gnawing | ( ) | 18. Tight | ( ) | |
|   Cramping | ( ) |   Numb | ( ) | |
|   Crushing | ( ) |   Drawing | ( ) | |
| 6. Tugging | ( ) |   Squeezing | ( ) | |
|   Pulling | ( ) |   Tearing | ( ) | |
|   Wrenching | ( ) | 19. Cool | ( ) | |
| 7. Hot | ( ) |   Cold | ( ) | |
|   Burning | ( ) |   Freezing | ( ) | |
|   Scalding | ( ) | 20. Nagging | ( ) | |
|   Searing | ( ) |   Nauseating | ( ) | |
| 8. Tingling | ( ) |   Agonizing | ( ) | |
|   Itchy | ( ) |   Dreadful | ( ) | |
|   Smarting | ( ) |   Torturing | ( ) | |
|   Stinging | ( ) | | | |

| | | | |
|---|---|---|---|
| 9. Dull | ( ) | Key: (for therapist only) | |
|   Sore | ( ) | Group 1 | Suggests vascular disorder |
|   Hurting | ( ) | Groups 2–8 | Suggests neurogenic disorder |
|   Aching | ( ) | Group 9 | Suggests musculoskeletal disorder |
|   Heavy | ( ) | Groups 10–20 | Suggests emotional lability |
| 10. Tender | ( ) | Scoring: Add up total number of checks. | |
|   Taut | ( ) | Patients who mark | |
|   Rasping | ( ) |   4–8 = are within normal limits (WNL). | |
|   Splitting | ( ) |   ≥ 6 = may be getting a "little into pain." | |
| 11. Tiring | ( ) |   ≥ 10 = may be helped more by a clinical psycholo- | |
|   Exhausting | ( ) |       gist than by physical therapy. | |
| 12. Sickening | ( ) |   ≥ 16 = are unlikely to respond to therapy procedures. | |
|   Suffocating | ( ) | | |

**Figure 3-3** Modified McGill-Melzack pain questionnaire. (Adapted from SL Wolf. [1985] Clinical Decision Making in Physical Therapy. In S Paris [ed], *Clinical Decision Making: Orthopedic Physical Therapy* [p. 125]. Philadelphia: Davis.)

*General Health*

Recent colds, influenza, or upper respiratory infections can be an extension of a chronic health pattern of systemic illness. Emotional stress and altered sleep patterns resulting in deprivation can be indicators of underlying physiologic and psychological disease.

The effects of emotional stress can be increased by physiologic changes brought on by the use of medication or poor diet and health habits (e.g., tobacco, alcohol, or drug use). These chemical substances can impair the ability to exercise or alter the perception of pain. Emotions, such as fear and anxiety, are common reactions to illness, and treatment can increase the patient's awareness of pain and symptoms. Furthermore, these emotions can cause autonomic distress and symptoms such as pallor, muscular tension, perspiration, restlessness, stomach pain, diarrhea, constipation, and headache.

Other information in the general health history (e.g., unexplained weight loss) can help to screen for early cancer detection. Weight loss significant for neoplasm would be 10–15 lb in 10–15 days separate from any intentional diet program or fasting (Goodman and Snyder 1990).

*Prior Tests and Treatments*

The clinician should obtain the results of diagnostic tests and know the medications prescribed for the patient. If feasible, the clinician should examine and discuss the available test results either with a radiologist or with the patient's physician. Familiarity with the results of these tests, combined with an understanding of the patient's clinical presentation, can assist the clinician in knowing what to look for clinically with patients in the future. Furthermore, the clinician can offer some guidelines for knowing when to suggest or recommend additional testing for patients who have not had a radiologic work-up or other potentially appropriate medical testing. For further information regarding the various radiologic procedures performed at the hip, refer to Chapter 7.

The following are common questions in regards to the patient's prior medical treatment:

- What home remedies were tried, and what was their effect?
- Have other forms of therapy been tried, and what was their effect?
- Will treatment by other disciplines be administered while undergoing physical therapy?

The potential positive and negative interactions of concurrent treatments should be considered when a patient is receiving care from multiple disciplines. This includes realizing that medications can mask signs and symptoms or produce those that are seemingly unrelated to the patient's current medical problems. The clinician is advised to refer to a reference source, such as the *Physician's Desk Reference* (Barnhart 1989), to check the potential side effects of all prescribed medications.

The clinician should remember that the purpose of the subjective assessment is to gain information about the problem from the patient's perspective. By taking a thorough history, considerable time can be saved with the physical examination, and more valid judgments can be made about objective findings. The clinician should not underestimate the importance of a good history, because the patient can often relate in minutes what might take hours to discover or confirm with various tests and treatment trials.

Before proceeding with the physical examination, the clinician should take a moment to do the following:

- Identify relevant, consistent, and accurate information
- Review data and obtain additional information if needed
- Identify chief and secondary symptoms
- Assess the patient's needs, expectations, and motivation
- Analyze and interpret data to develop a provisional diagnosis of the patient's condition including
  Nature and extent of the symptoms
  Probable etiology of the symptoms
  Anatomic structures involved
  Stage of the condition
  Possible contraindications to physical therapy examination and treatment
- Plan physical examination including
  Comprehensive examination techniques that have a high probability of contributing to the development and refinement of the provisional diagnoses
  Determination of the extent and rigor of the exam consistent with the severity, irritability, nature, and stage of the condition
  Selection of areas to be examined
  Selection of movements, functional activities, or both to be examined
  Selection of examination procedures
  Selection of examination sequence

### Objective Assessment: Physical Examination

The purpose of the objective assessment is to examine for abnormal findings of the neuromusculoskeletal system. It should consist of reproducible, measurable, and reliable data relating to the present disorder. The physical examination of the patient with a hip disorder of unknown etiology begins with a lower quarter screening examination (Figure 3-4), which can be done concurrently with some elements of the specific hip examination (Figure 3-5). The clinician must effectively rule out regions above and below the hip as the source of symptoms. Following this, the clinician proceeds to a specific examination of the hip.

In considering the examination itself, several methods or strategies have been proposed (Cyriax 1982; Hoppenfeld 1976; Maitland 1991; Reid 1992; Saunders 1985; Woerman 1994). Most of the schemes discussed in these sources are adequate, and it is incumbent on the clinician to become familiar enough with a particular method so that the process is systematic, comprehensive, and comfortable. This ensures that the clinician is less likely to miss an important clinical finding that can result in an incorrect diagnosis.

As with any examination, the clinician should compare one side of the body with the other. The comparison is necessary because of the individual differences among normal people. It is particularly pertinent, in the case of an irritable hip disorder, that the patient be subjected to as little movement as possible to diagnose the condition. Therefore, an objective examination is best organized by patient position (Table 3-3). Although this method is proposed, this chapter describes the kind of information that needs to be gathered, not necessarily the order in which it must be gathered.

## *Lower Quarter Screening Examination*

The screening examination is comprised of the following:

- Vital signs (if indicated)
- Functional observation, including gait
- General observation
- Palpation
- Peripheral "joint clearing" tests
- Neurologic assessment (if indicated)

### Vital Signs

Assessment of baseline vital signs should be part of the initial data collected if an active systemic process is suspected.

The following are vital signs with normative range values:

- Resting heart rate (pulse): 60–100 beats per minute (bpm)
- Blood pressure: From 90/60 mm Hg to 140/90 mm Hg for the young adult; less than or equal to 160/100 mm Hg for elderly men; less than or equal to 170/90 mm Hg for elderly women
- Respiratory rate: 12–18 breaths per minute
- Temperature: 97.0–99.4°F (average 98.6°F)

**Vital Signs**
Resting pulse rate:_____beats/min
Resting respiratory rate:_____breaths/min
Oral temperature:_____°F
Blood pressure: first reading ___/___ mm Hg; second reading ___/___ mm Hg
           Extremity:                  Position:

**Functional Observation:**   (+ = Present; − = Not present.)
Gait pattern: Normal__ Antalgic__ Gluteus medius (Trendelenburg)__
               Gluteus maximus__ Psoas__ Other__
Comments:_____
Transfers: Independent___ Assisted___ Assistance required___ Pain___
Assistive device:_____Weightbearing status:_____
Aids:_____
Comments:_____

**General Observation:**   (+ = Present; − = Not present.)
Head: Forward___ Tilted___
Shoulders: Level___ High L___ R___; Protracted L___ R___
Thoracic: Kyphosis___ Decreased curve ___ Scoliosis___
(Convex thoracic L___ R___; Convex lumbar L___ R___)
Lumbar: Lordosis___ Decreased curve___ Lateral shift L___ R___
Pelvic landmarks: IC High L___ R___; PSIS High L___ R___; ASIS High L___ R___
Leg length: L___ R___
Skin: Color___ Condition___ Lesions___ Scars___
Digital-scale weightbearing: L _____lb R _____lb
Comments:_____

**Palpation:**   (+ = Tender; − = Not tender.)
Thoracic: L___ R___ Midline___
Lumbar: L___ R___ Midline___
L5–S1: L___ R___
Sacrococcygeal joint: L___ R___
SIJ: L___ R___ Midline ___
Hip: L___ R___
Thigh: L___ R___
Sacrotuberous ligament: L___ R___
Iliolumbar ligament: L___ R___
Sacrospinous ligament: L___ R___
Piriformis: L___ R___

**Figure 3-4** Lower quarter screen. (ASIS = anterior superior iliac spine; L = left; R = right; IC = iliac crest; PSIS = posterior superior iliac spine; SIJ = sacroiliac joint; SLR = straight leg raise.)

Knee: L___ R___
Calf: L___ R___
Ankle: L___ R___
Foot: L___ R___
Comments:_____

**Joint Clearing Tests**     C = Completes task;
                             D = Completes task with difficulty or discomfort;
                             N = Does not complete task.
___Bending forward from sitting to tie shoes
___Crossing the legs
___Squatting
___Ascending stairs
___Descending stairs (one step, then two steps at a time)
___One-legged standing test: L ____secs R _____secs
___Running straight ahead
___Running and twisting
___Jumping

+ = Symptoms reproduced; – = No reproduction.
SIJ: Compression L___ R___; Distraction L___ R___
Hip: Patrick test (fabere sign) L___ R___
Knee: Varus L___ R___
Valgus L___ R___
Bounce home: L___ R___
Trunk quadrant testing: physiologic forward bending L___ R___; physiologic back-
                        ward bending L___ R___; nonphysiologic forward bending
                        L___ R___; nonphysiologic backward bending L___ R___
Range of motion (ROM): + = Symptoms reproduced; – = No reproduction
Trunk flexion:  Normal ___ Abnormal (degrees of ROM) ___/___ Repeated motion ___
Extension:      Normal ___ Abnormal (degrees of ROM) ___/___ Repeated motion ___
L sidebend:     Normal ___ Abnormal (degrees of ROM) ___/___ Repeated motion ___
R sidebend:     Normal ___ Abnormal (degrees of ROM) ___/___ Repeated motion ___
L rotation:     Normal ___ Abnormal (degrees of ROM) ___/___ Repeated motion ___
R rotation:     Normal ___ Abnormal (degrees of ROM) ___/___ Repeated motion ___
Overpressure: Flexion ___ Extension ___ L sidebend ___ R sidebend ___
              L rotation___ R rotation___
Hip motion: L___ R___ Knee motion: L___ R___ Ankle motion: L___ R___
Comments: _____

**Neurologic**
  Motor: (5 = Normal; 4 = Good; 3 = Fair; 2 = Poor; 1 = Trace; 0 = Absent. + and
  − symbols can be used to provide finer discrimination.)
  Hip flexion (L1–L2):      L___ R___
  Knee extension (L3):      L___ R___
  Dorsiflexion (L4):         L___ R___
  Toe extension (L5):        L___ R___
  Eversion (S1):             L___ R___
  Plantar flexion (S1):      L___ R___
  Knee flexion (S1–S2): L___ R___
  Motor control:  Spastic___ Flaccid___ Rigid___ Clonic___
  Sensation: (Lacking: A = Light touch sensation; B = Sharp-dull discrimination; C =
  Temperature discrimination; D = Proprioception [passive motion and static position].)

  Reflexes: (0 = No response; 1 = Minimum response; 2 = Moderate response; 3 =
  Brisk response; 4 = Clonus.)
  Patellar (L3–L4):          L___ R___
  Achilles (S1):             L___ R___
  Medial hamstrings (L5): L___ R___
  Lateral hamstrings (S1): L___ R___
  Babinski sign:             L___ R___
  Neural tension provocation tests: (− = Normal; + = Abnormal.)
  SLR supine:                L___ R___ (degrees L___ R___)
  Lasègue sign:              L___ R___
  Flip sign:                 L___ R___
  Kernig sign:               L___ R___
  Hoover sign:               L___ R___
  Slump test:                L___ R___

**Figure 3-4** *Continued*

A pulse increase of more than 20 bpm lasting more than 3 minutes after rest or changing positions or a persistent fall or rise of blood pressure should be a warning to alert the clinician to the need for medical follow-up or intervention (Muthe 1981).

Temperature should be assessed for any patient who has night sweats, pain, or symptoms of unknown etiology and for patients who have not previously been medically screened by a physician. Fever in a patient with hip pain, especially if he or she has a prosthetic hip component and no other possible cause for increased temperature (e.g., upper respiratory tract, atelectasis, deep venous thrombosis, urinary tract infection), should be referred due to the red flag of infection.

**Inspection and Palpation:** (+ = Abnormal; – normal.) Involved side: L___ R ___

Body Area or Test

| | L | R | | L | R | | L | R | | L | R |
|---|---|---|---|---|---|---|---|---|---|---|---|
| Iliac crest | | | ASIS | | | PSIS | | | Ischial tuberosity | | |
| Greater trochanter | | | Pubic tuberosity | | | Adductor tuberosity | | | Baer's point | | |
| McBurney's point | | | Femoral triangle | | | Gluteus medius | | | Gluteus maximus | | |
| Adductors | | | TFL | | | Rectus femoris | | | Sciatic nerve | | |
| Cluneal nerves | | | Sciatic | | | Hamstrings | | | | | |

Deformities: (Perform appropriate tests and measures.)
Comments:_____

**Selective Tissue Tension Testing:** (Add * if painful.)

Physiologic movement

| Hip Motion | Active | | Passive | | Resistive |
|---|---|---|---|---|---|
| | ROM L/R | Symptoms | ROM L/R | End-feel | Strength |
| Flexion | | | | | |
| Extension | | | | | |
| Abduction | | | | | |
| Adduction | | | | | |
| Internal rotation (in extension) | | | | | |
| External rotation (in extension) | | | | | |
| Internal rotation (in flexion) | | | | | |
| External rotation (in flexion) | | | | | |

**Accessory Movement**

Hypomobility
(0 = no movement [ankylosis]; 1 = considerable lack of movement;
2 = slight decreased movement.)
Normal (3 = normal.)
Hypermobility
(4 = slight increased movement; 5 = considerable increased movement; 6 =
complete instability.)

| Glide Direction | Mobility | Symptoms |
|---|---|---|
| Lateral distraction | | |
| Compression | | |
| Caudal glide (long-axis traction) | | |
| Anterior glide | | |
| Posterior glide | | |

**Figure 3-5** Physical therapy hip examination. (ASIS = anterior superior iliac spine;
L = left; R = right; TFL = tensor fasciae latae; PSIS = posterior superior iliac spine;
ROM = range of motion; SLR = straight leg raise.)

**Static Arthrokinematic Stability:**     (+ = Positive; − = Negative.)

|  | Left | Right |  | Left | Right |  | Left | Right |
|---|---|---|---|---|---|---|---|---|
| Torque test |  |  | Iliofemoral (inferior band) |  |  | Iliofemoral (iliotrochanteric band) |  |  |
| Pubofemoral |  |  | Ishiofemoral |  |  |  |  |  |

Special Tests
(+ = Positive; − = Negative.)

|  | L | R |  | L | R |  | L | R |
|---|---|---|---|---|---|---|---|---|
| Thomas test |  |  | Rectus femoris stretch test |  |  | Ely test |  |  |
| Adduction flexibility test |  |  | Ober test |  |  | 90–90 degrees SLR |  |  |
| Tripod sign |  |  | Piriformis test |  |  | Patrick test |  |  |
| Grind test |  |  | Flexion and adduction test |  |  | Scour test |  |  |
| Sign of the buttock test |  |  | Trendelenburg test |  |  |  |  |  |

Comments:_____
    (Note: This document includes tests primarily specific to the hip. Tests of the
    sacroiliac joints and lumbar spine may also be warranted in certain cases.)

**Assessment and Diagnosis**

**Prognosis:**

**Goals:**

| Short-term | Time | Long-term | Time |
|---|---|---|---|
| 1. |  |  |  |
| 2. |  |  |  |
| 3. |  |  |  |
| 4. |  |  |  |
| 5. |  |  |  |

**Plan:**
Frequency (circle) 1 2 3 4 5 times per week
Other: _____
Duration (circle) 1 2 3 4 5 6 7 8 weeks
Other: _____
Treatment: _____
Instructions given: _____
_____

**Figure 3-5** *Continued*

**Table 3-3** Hip Examination Sequence

Standing

Observation

Posture
Transfers
Gait

Examination

Specific palpation of anatomic landmarks
Repetitive toe raises (if indicated)
Balance
Digital-scale weightbearing
One-leg standing test
Trendelenburg test
Trunk AROM
Squatting
Q-angle
Leg length (iliac crest heights)

Sitting

Observation

Posture
Transfers

Examination

Vital signs (if indicated)
Ability to bend forward and tie shoes
Ability to cross leg over opposite thigh
Trunk AROM: rotation and quadrant tests (if indicated)
Active and resistive knee extension and ankle dorsiflexion, inversion,
eversion, and toe extension (if indicated)
Active, passive, and resisted hip internal and external rotation
Active and resistive hip flexion
Patellar DTR (if indicated)
Slump test (if indicated)
Tripod sign

Supine

Examination

Palpation of anterior aspect
Passive knee flexion and extension and all ankle motions
Active, passive, and resisted hip flexion, abduction, and adduction
Sensory testing (if indicated)
Pathologic reflexes (if indicated)
SIJ compression and distraction
Knee bounce home test
Knee varus and valgus stress tests
Static arthrokinematic and ligamentous testing

**Table 3-3** *Continued*

> Neural tension provocation tests (if indicated)
> Deformity assessment and measurement (if indicated)
> Accessory motion testing
> Thomas test
> Rectus femoris stretch test
> Adduction flexibility test
> 90 degree–90 degree SLR
> Piriformis test
> Patrick test
> Grind test (if indicated)
> Flexion and adduction test (if indicated)
> Scour test (if indicated)
> Sign of the buttock test

Side-lying

> Examination

>> Palpation of lateral and posterior aspects
>> Active, passive, and resisted hip extension, abduction, flexion, and adduction
>> Ober test

Prone

> Examination

>> Palpation of posterior aspect
>> Active, passive, and resisted hip extension; internal and external rotation; and knee flexion
>> Hip accessory motion testing of anterior glide
>> Ely test
>> Sensory testing (if indicated)
>> Achilles and hamstring DTRs (if indicated)

Other testing (if indicated)

> Functional activity

>> Up and down stairs
>> Running straight ahead
>> Running and twisting
>> Jumping

AROM = active range of motion; DTR = deep tendon reflex; Q-angle = quadriceps muscle-tendon angle; SIJ = sacroiliac joint; SLR = straight leg raise.
Source: Adapted from DC Reid. (1992) *Sports Injury Assessment and Rehabilitation.* Edinburgh, UK: Churchill Livingstone.

## Functional Observation

The clinician should observe how the patient sits in the waiting area, how he or she moves from sitting to standing and vice versa, and how he or she ambulates. In vivo research demonstrating high acetabular contact pressures during the sit-to-stand maneuver (Fagerson et al. 1995) helps to explain the difficulty and pain that patients with severe hip dysfunction often report when rising from a chair. As the patient ambulates into the treatment area, particular attention should be paid to the gait pattern.

The clinical gait evaluation should note the following:

- Stride-length difference
- Cadence
- Equal versus unequal timing
- Abnormal pelvic movements (e.g., shifting, listing, or rotation)
- Abnormal hip or trunk movements (e.g., circumduction or lurch)
- Distance walked before fatigue
- Loading response and progression angles of the knees and feet
- Description of aids, assistive devices, and weightbearing status required by patient
- Type of gait pattern

Common gait patterns seen with hip pathology are the following:

- Antalgic gait
- Trendelenburg gait
- Compensated Trendelenburg gait or gluteus medius lurch
- Waddling gait
- Gluteus maximus or hip extensor gait
- Scissor gait
- Psoas gait
- Short-leg gait
- Stiff-hip gait

Refer to Chapter 1 for a more detailed description of each pathologic gait pattern.

Abnormal gait patterns are the result of pain, weakness, contractures, or limitations in range (Table 3-4). An understanding of the mechanisms of normal gait is needed to understand pathologic disturbances. Observing gait with a trained eye can give helpful clues as to possible diagnoses.

### General Observation

With the adult patient adequately exposed, the clinician observes static standing posture from head to toe for evidence of asymmetry. A triplanar assessment is conducted for all body segments, joints, and bone shafts. *Triplanar assessment* refers to visual inspection of body parts in the sagittal, coronal, and transverse planes. Inspection should be performed from anterior, posterior, and lateral views. A plumb line or postural grid is useful for establishing a standard reference point.

**Table 3-4** Causes of Gait Deviations at the Hip

| Diagnosis | Inadequate flexion | Excessive flexion | Inadequate extension | Excessive extension | Excessive abduction | Excessive adduction | Excessive rotation |
|---|---|---|---|---|---|---|---|
| Flexion contracture | X | X | — | — | — | — | — |
| ITB contracture | X | X | — | — | I | C | — |
| Abduction contracture | — | — | — | — | I | C | — |
| Adduction contracture | — | — | — | — | C | I | — |
| Arthrodesis | X | X | X | X | X | X | X |
| Flexor spasticity | X | X | — | — | — | — | — |
| Pelvic obliquity | — | — | — | — | I/C | I/C | — |
| Hip anteversion | — | — | — | — | — | — | X |
| Muscle overactivity | — | — | — | — | — | — | X |
| Abductor weakness | — | — | — | — | C | I | — |
| Pain | X | X | — | — | — | — | — |
| Voluntary muscle overactivity | X | X | X | — | I | — | X |

ITB = iliotibial band; C = contralateral; I = ipsilateral; I/C = ipsilateral and contralateral; X = not side oriented.

Source: Adapted from J Perry. (1992) *Gait Analysis: Normal and Pathological Function* (p. 250). Thorofare, NJ: Slack.

Visual inspection should include the following:

- Observation of equal weight on both limbs
- Observation and measurement of atrophy, hypertrophy, or swelling (i.e., edema, effusion) of the following areas:
    Lumbopelvic region
    Thigh
    Leg
- Observation of pelvis, trunk, and limb alignment
- Observation of the overall skin quality and appearance, including visual description of the following areas:
    Birth marks
    Discoloration
    Abrasions
    Erythema
    Sinus tracts
    Previous surgical incisions
- Observation of muscle spasm, guarding, and protective splinting
- Observation of general body movement

A digital scale reading can indicate asymmetry in weightbearing, which is diminished on the painful side. In the absence of a digital scale, two bathroom scales can be used. The presence or absence of pelvic obliquity is noted as a clue to leg length discrepancy or contracture around the hip joint. The clinician should determine if both knees are in full extension and both feet are flat on the floor. A patient with a painful hip may tend to hold the hip in the resting position (i.e., flexion, abduction, and external rotation) to accommodate joint effusion.

The depth of the hip joint renders it difficult to inspect for changes in shape; however, clinical indications of anteversion or retroversion exist (see "Bony Disorder Techniques"). This point reinforces the importance of using hip radiographs and other diagnostic studies in diagnosis. The same is true for swelling. Swelling in the hip joint itself (effusion) is virtually impossible to detect by observation alone. Special testing and diagnostic testing, such as radiographs, help to confirm its presence. (Refer to Chapter 7 for details.)

### Palpation

Palpation of bony prominences and soft tissue can be accomplished during the general observation portion of the examination. I suggest performing bony and soft tissue palpation concurrently, while separating the patient anteriorly, medially, laterally, and posteriorly for reasons previously mentioned in "Objective Assessment: Physical Examination."

Careful palpation identifies the following:

- Asymmetry
- Tenderness
- Flexibility
- Density
- Nodules
- Masses
- Swelling
- Texture
- Temperature

The clinician's palpatory examination should begin with light touching over the area under observation. This allows somewhat of a scanning examination of the area and reveals the presence of any large abnormalities in the superficial or deep layers of tissue. The clinician can then identify structures as palpatory tissue deformation increases. The clinician should apply forces parallel and perpendicular to the long axis of structures first to identify them and then under conditions of resting length, passive stretch, and active contraction to determine the extent of a possible lesion. The palpatory examination takes time and concentration, and errors in reception result from excessive pressure or movement of the palpatory fingertips.

### Peripheral Joint Clearing Tests

The emphasis with peripheral joint clearing tests should be assessing functional activities involving the use of the hip. The clinician can use a series of functional activities to see if increased intensity of activity produces pain or other symptoms at or from the lumbar spine, sacroiliac joint, knee, or hip. With all the active tests, the clinician is trying to "clear" adjacent joints of pathology and attempting to reproduce symptoms from the hip. The functional clearing activities must be geared to the individual patient. Older individuals should not be expected to perform the last four activities listed in Table 3-3, unless they have been performing them in the recent past.

Other nonfunctional joint clearing tests include the following:

- Thoracolumbar spine active movements (backward bending, lateral side bending, and rotation)
- Quadrant testing of the thoracolumbar spine
- Sacroiliac compression and distraction
- Knee varus and valgus stress and bounce home tests

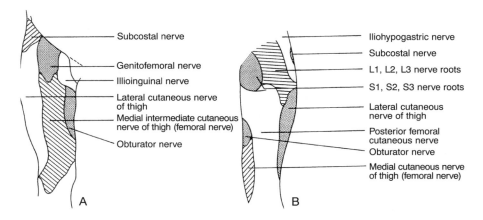

**Figure 3-6** Sensory distribution of peripheral nerves about the hip. A. Anterior view. B. Posterior view. (L = lumbar, S = sacral.) (Reprinted with permission from DJ Magee. [1992] *Orthopaedic Physical Assessment* [p. 358]. Philadelphia: Saunders.)

With these tests, along with peripheral neural tension, selective tissue tension, and specific hip tests, the clinician applies an external force while palpating and observing the response of the tissue. The external force can be modified by altering the following (Dyrek 1994):

- Magnitude of the force
- Duration of force application
- Velocity of application
- Frequency of application
- Location of force application and the degree of pretest tension in the tissue
- Direction of force application

*Each of these variables can by manipulated by the clinician to thoroughly assess a specific tissue.*

### Neurologic Testing

If a neurologic deficit is suspected, it is appropriate to perform sensory, motor, reflex, and proprioceptive tests involving the nerve root levels from L1 to the fourth sacral level (S4).

- Sensation. The clinician should be aware of the dermatomal nerve root as well as the peripheral nerve supplies (Figures 3-6 and 3-7). The following sensations should be assessed:

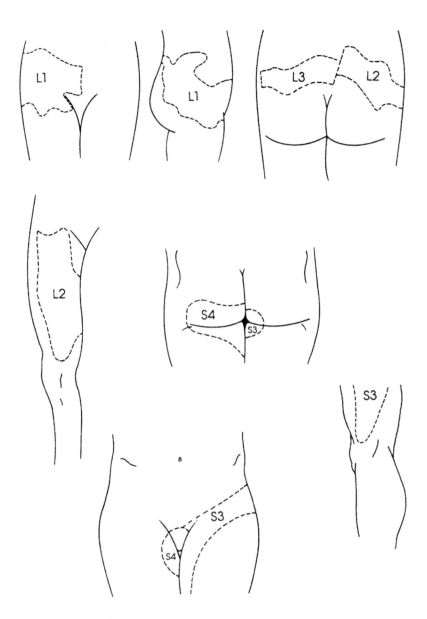

**Figure 3-7** Dermatomes about the hip. One side only is illustrated. (L = lumbar, S = sacral.) (Reprinted with permission from DJ Magee. [1992] *Orthopaedic Physical Assessment* [p. 357]. Philadelphia: Saunders.)

Superficial tactile sensation (with light touch or brush)
Superficial pain (with pin prick or pin-wheel)
Temperature (with hot and cold test tubes)
Vibration (with tuning fork)

- Motor. The clinician should conduct a lower quarter myotomal assessment. A positive finding of weakness can indicate involvement of a specific nerve level.
- Deep tendon reflexes
- Pathologic reflexes. The clinician should test for upper motor neuron disease or lesions of the corticospinal tracts (e.g., Babinski reflex).
- Proprioception
  Passive motion sense
  Static position sense
- Neural tension provocation*

## Specific Hip Examination

With other potential causes of hip pain ruled out, the clinician proceeds to further examine the hip region. Included in this exam, the clinician assesses the following:

- The appearance of the hip area
- The hip joint and adjacent soft tissues
- Tension tolerance of soft tissue via selective tissue tension testing
- Differential (special) testing
- Relevant radiology of the hip

### Inspection and Palpation

Hoppenfeld (1976) suggested an approach to inspection and palpation that is organized by region, separating bony from soft tissue palpation. Even though Hoppenfeld separated bony from soft tissue palpation, the two should be done concurrently in each region to improve efficiency for the clinician and minimize changes in position for the patient.

---

*Peripheral neural tension provocation or passive neural mobility testing assesses the mobility of the neural elements (e.g., nerve, neural sheath, dura mater) under externally applied passive tensile loading. It also determines whether this tissue is a source of pain, neurologic symptoms, or both. Neural elements are subjected to progressive tensile loading via osteokinematic movements of body parts with the patient in a position of maximum relaxation either sitting (slump test), supine (straight leg raising test), or prone (Ely or prone knee-bend test).

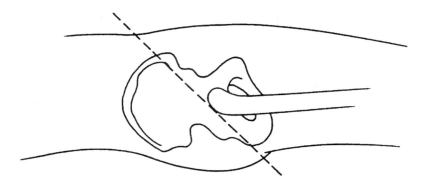

**Figure 3-8** Nélaton line. (Reprinted with permission from DJ Magee. [1992] *Orthopaedic Physical Assessment* [p. 346]. Philadelphia: Saunders.)

Most of the muscles that are superficial and cross the hip region can be palpated. A method to palpate these is to divide them into their respective groups by function: the flexor group, the adductor group, the abductor group, external rotator group, and the extensor group. Since selective tissue tension is also part of the examination, it is suggested to perform the muscle palpation portion concurrently with portions of the selective tissue tension testing. This method promotes not only efficiency but also effectiveness in differentiating muscles within the same group.

**Deformity Assessment**

*Bony Disorder Techniques*
The following are clinical techniques to inspect for changes in shape or alignment of the hip joint:

- Allis sign: Visual inspection of relaxation of the soft tissue between the crest of the ilium and the greater trochanter implicating a femoral neck fracture.
- Desault sign: Visual inspection of any deviation of the arc described by rotation of the greater trochanter, which normally describes the segment of a circle, but in a displaced intracapsular fracture rotates only at the apex of the femur as it rotates about its own axis.
- Langoria sign: Visual inspection of relaxation of the hip extensor muscles, implicating intracapsular fracture.
- Nélaton line (Figure 3-8): Visual inspection by forming a line from the anterior superior iliac spine (ASIS) to the ischial tuberosity, which normally touches the tip of the greater trochanter. If trochanter is superior to line, hip dislocation is suspected.

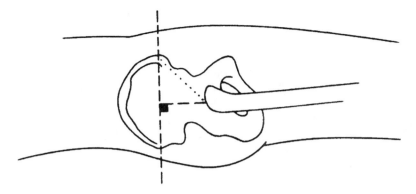

**Figure 3-9** Bryant's triangle (area within dashed and dotted lines). (Reprinted with permission from DJ Magee. [1992] *Orthopaedic Physical Assessment* [p. 346]. Philadelphia: Saunders.)

- Bryant's triangle (Figure 3-9): Visual inspection of a triangle formed by a perpendicular down from the ASIS in a supine patient. The base of the triangle is a line extending from the tip of the greater trochanter to this perpendicular, while the hypotenuse is represented by the line joining the ASIS and the tip of the greater trochanter. The base of the triangle is shortened if fracture is present, allowing upward displacement of the greater trochanter.
- Schoemaker line: Visual inspection of a line from the tip of the greater trochanter through the ASIS and extended toward the midline. The continuation of the line meets the midline of the body below the umbilicus when the trochanter is upwardly displaced.
- Rotational deformity signs: Visual inspection of the lower limbs via the reference point of the patellae with the patient supine. If the patellae face inward ("squinting" patellae), it is an indication of medial rotation of the femur or tibia. If the patellae face outward away from each other ("frogs eye" or "grasshopper eye" patellae), it is an indication of lateral rotation of the femur or tibia. If the tibia is affected, the feet face inward ("pigeon toe") for medial rotation and face out more than 10 degrees for excessive lateral rotation of the tibia (Magee 1992).
- Trochanteric prominence test: Maneuver in which the knee of a prone patient is flexed to 90 degrees. The patient's hip is rotated medially until the clinician palpates that the greater trochanter is most prominent and subsequently parallel to the table top. The angle formed between the tibia and the vertical when the greater trochanter is most laterally prominent is the angle of anteversion. This test is most commonly

known as the *Craig test* by physical therapists (Magee 1992). Ruwe et al. (1992) found that this clinical method of assessing anteversion was superior to radiologic techniques in children who have not had hip surgery.

- Medial femoral torsion: An alternative method for assessing the angle of anteversion (i.e., medial femoral torsion) is to compare the amount of hip medial rotation to lateral rotation. This is best done with the patient prone and knees flexed 90 degrees. Staheli et al. (1985) graded the severity of medial femoral torsion as follows:

   Mild: Medial rotation is between 70 and 80 degrees and lateral rotation is between 10 and 20 degrees (two or three standard deviations from the mean).

   Moderate: Medial rotation is between 80 and 90 degrees and lateral rotation is between 0 and 10 degrees (three or four standard deviations from the mean).

   Severe: Medial rotation is greater than 90 degrees and no lateral rotation is possible (more than four standard deviations from the mean).

- Q-angle (quadriceps or patellofemoral angle): The clinician marks the ASIS, center of the patella, and tibial tuberosity preferably with a skin pencil. The patient stands with feet under the hips. A modified, extended goniometer is aligned with the markings. The axis of the goniometer is placed over the center of the patella. The extended arm is in line with the ASIS, and the other arm is in line with the tibial tuberosity. Normal Q-angle is 13 degrees for men and 18 degrees for women with the knee straight (Magee 1992).

- True leg length: Before measurement, the clinician must level the pelvis in relationship to the lower extremities via active bridging, followed by passive longitudinal distraction of the patient's lower extremities. This should allow both ASIS to form a straight line with the lower extremities perpendicular to that line. The clinician should avoid fluctuations in soft tissue girth. It is recommended that the clinician measure from ASIS to ipsilateral lateral malleolus (or medial malleolus). Firm manual fixation of the tape measure should be applied to each bony prominence. A slight difference (1.0–1.5 cm) is considered within normal limits but can still cause symptoms (Magee 1992). If one leg is shorter than the other, the clinician can determine where the difference is by measuring

   from the most superior portion of the iliac crest to the greater trochanter for coxa vara;

   from the greater trochanter to the lateral knee joint line for femoral shaft shortening; and

   from the medial knee joint line to the medial malleolus for tibial shaft shortening.

- Apparent leg length: Apparent or functional shortening of the leg can exist if the patient has altered pelvic obliquity. The clinician measures the distance from the tip of the xiphisternum or umbilicus to the medial malleolus.

### Soft Tissue Disorder Techniques

The following are clinical techniques to inspect for changes in adjacent soft tissue to the hip joint. (See Table A-1 in Appendix for detailed descriptions of special tests.)

- Gill sign. If the hip region has swelling, it feels thicker than the contralateral side. Swelling is assessed bilaterally by placing the thumbs over the femoral artery where it crosses the inguinal ligament, while the other four fingers are placed posteriorly over the buttock opposite the position of the thumb.
- Bursitis. Refer to "Soft Tissue Disorders" in Chapter 2.

Bony and soft tissue techniques have inherent errors in correctly and consistently palpating landmarks and making reliable and valid conclusions. The conventional radiograph is to bony alignment, as the MRI is to soft tissue—gold standards for reliable measurement.

### Selective Tissue Tension Testing

Selective tissue is the assessment of soft tissue's (contractile and noncontractile) tensile capabilities and pain response under active and passive loading conditions.

Selective tissue tension consists of the following:

- Active range of motion (ROM)
- Passive ROM
- Physiologic
- Accessory
- Active and passive motion combinations
- Resistive movements
- Static arthrokinematic stability
- Passive neural mobility (which is included secondary to external force manipulation variables)

Active and passive ROM testing of the hip joint should include flexion and extension with the femur in neutral rotation, abduction and adduction in extension, and internal and external rotation in both extension and flexion. The clinician should test and measure bilaterally with a goniometer and

**Table 3-5** Anatomic Structures Limiting Hip Motion

| Hip motion | Anatomic structure |
|---|---|
| Flexion | Anterior soft tissues |
| | Posterior capsule |
| Extension | Iliofemoral ligament |
| | Pubofemoral ligament |
| | Ischiofemoral ligament |
| Abduction | Adductor muscles |
| | Pubofemoral ligament |
| | Ischiofemoral ligament |
| Adduction | Abductor muscles |
| | Iliofemoral ligament |
| External rotation | Iliofemoral ligament |
| | Pubofemoral ligament |
| Internal rotation | Ischiofemoral ligament |
| | External rotator muscles |

Source: Adapted from SP Hicklin, MC DePretis. (1995) Lower Extremity: Hip. In RS Myers (ed), *Saunders Manual of Physical Therapy Practice* (p. 960). Philadelphia: Saunders.

note and measure any pain during or following each movement. This should be compared with the uninvolved side and normal values.

The capsular ligaments define and limit normal hip motion except flexion (Table 3-5). There is considerable variation in range, based on inherent laxity, age, and training. Flexion of the normal hip is limited primarily by soft tissues of the thigh and abdomen when the knee is flexed and by hamstring tension when the knee is extended. Caillet (1988) used the term *lumbar-pelvic rhythm* to describe the phenomenon in the hip joint, pelvis, and lumbar spine in which coordinated activity of the segments produce a larger ROM than is available to one segment alone. This phenomenon should be kept in mind and controlled for by the clinician through proper patient positioning and concurrent inspection and palpation to ensure isolated movement patterns.

With all movements, the clinician assesses and notes capsular versus noncapsular patterns of restricted motion. Furthermore, the clinician should assess the end-feel pain and tissue response and any crepitus during passive physiologic and accessory joint motions. Several different end-feels are possible. Both physiologic and pathologic end-feels exist in the hip joint.

The following are normal end-feels of the hip joint and anatomic limitation to motion (Norkin and Levangie 1992):

- Soft: Soft tissue approximation (i.e., flexion)
- Firm:
    Joint capsule (i.e., internal and external rotation)
    Muscle (i.e., hip flexion with knee extension)
    Ligaments (i.e., extension)
    Abduction and adduction are limited by muscle or ligament, or both.

The following are abnormal end-feels of the hip joint (Cyriax 1982; Kaltenborn 1989):

- Muscle spasm: Abrupt stop with mild "rebounding" sensation
- Boggy: "Mushy" resistance (e.g., effusion)
- Springy: "Rubbery" rebound with firm unyielding resistance (e.g., fragment of cartilage [loose body])
- Empty: No resistance due to severe pain (e.g., bursitis)
- Capsular: Firm yet resilient with maintained force; occurs prematurely in the range if abnormal (e.g., adhesive capsulitis)
- Bony block: Sudden, abrupt limitation with no resiliency with maintained force (e.g., osteophyte)
- Laxity: Excessive mobility beyond normal anatomic ROM

### Active Range of Motion

The osteokinematic active movements are done in such a way that the movements most likely to be painful are done last. The clinician should note not only the joint ROM but also the patient's willingness to move. Specific techniques for measuring hip joint movement can be found in standard texts. Values for active ROM of the hip are presented in Chapter 1, and normative data on hip active ROM are presented in Chapter 4 (see Table 4-3). Pain during active movement implicates both contractile and noncontractile tissue pathology: Passive testing needs to be performed to differentiate between the two.

### Passive Range of Motion

*Physiologic*

Physiologic passive movement tests provide the clinician with information about full available joint motion and the end-feel response of the tissue when overpressure is applied.

The pattern of pain accompanying resistance during passive ROM yields valuable diagnostic and prognostic information. Cyriax (1982) described three patterns that can occur:

1. Pain before resistance. Pain occurs before reaching the extreme of available motion. This pattern is suggestive of an acute inflammatory lesion of either extra-articular or articular origin.
2. Pain simultaneous with resistance. Pain that occurs simultaneously with resistance is suggestive of a subacute inflammatory process.
3. Resistance before pain. Pain is not elicited at the point of resistance, rather, overpressure must be applied to elicit pain (i.e., a greater force to passively stretch the tissues beyond the physiologic range). This pattern is indicative of a mild or chronic lesion that could tolerate aggressive treatment.

Thorough assessment of a joint requires that the pattern of pain and resistance be correlated with the point at which the normal resistance to motion is expected to occur. Crepitus, snapping, and any other abnormal joint sounds should be noted during this portion of the evaluation. Pain during passive movement is more likely due to inert tissue pathology. If passive movements are pain-free and active movements are painful, then two possibilities exist: (1) the problem involves the contractile tissues, or (2) greater stress is required to reproduce the symptoms.

### Accessory
The arthrokinematics, or accessory motions, of the hip joint are equally assessed for the quantity and quality of movement and the irritability of the hip joint structures. Normal arthrokinematics are necessary for normal osteokinematics. Given this condition, if arthrokinematic testing reveals decreased mobility concurrently with decreased osteokinematic function, an articular restriction is confirmed.

The following are accessory motions of the hip joint:

- Caudal glide (long-axis distraction)
- Lateral distraction (short-axis distraction)
- Compression
- Anterior glide
- Posterior glide

The joint play movements are performed with the patient in the supine and prone positions. Due to strong ligamentous support and large soft tissue bulk, these motions can be quite difficult to assess. Achieving optimal patient-clinician positioning for force application, with or without the use of mobilizing belts, greatly enhances assessment and treatment. Joint play movements should be assessed bilaterally. Kaltenborn's scale for grading arthrokinematic movements is useful for quantifying findings (Kaltenborn 1989). (This is provided in the "Accessory Movement" section of Figure 3-5.)

### Active and Passive Motion Combinations

Two specific patterns of active and passive motions exist to identify further the type of tissue responsible for the symptoms:

1. Active and passive ROM are restricted, painful, or both in the same direction. This pattern is indicative of a capsular or arthrogenic lesion.
2. Active and passive ROM are restricted, painful, or both in opposite directions. This pattern is indicative of a contractile tissue lesion. Resistive motion is indicated to further incriminate the tissue.

### Resisted Muscle Testing

Resisted muscle testing assesses the contractile tissues for the following:

- Torque production
- Source of pain
- Ability to perform a specific function in a coordinated manner during a movement task

With the patient sitting, supine, or prone, and the hip joint held in midrange, the clinician resists maximal isometric contractions of muscles controlling all major hip movements. It is imperative that no motion is allowed at the joint as this "muddies the waters" as to whether contractile or noncontractile structures are the source of pain.

The following are the isometric movement tests:

- Hip flexion
- Hip extension
- Hip abduction
- Hip adduction
- Hip external rotation
- Hip internal rotation
- Knee flexion
- Knee extension

Strength should be graded for clinical recording purposes. Specific positions are used to isolate individual muscles for testing (Daniels and Worthingham 1986).

### Static Arthrokinematic Stability (Stress) Testing

Static arthrokinematic tests of hip joint stability should be normal in a patient with joint hypomobility; however, proprioception and dynamic stability are often impaired due to altered neurophysiology (Lee 1989).

To test the integrity of the hip extra-articular ligaments, the clinician must stress the ligaments to their maximal available end range, while again manipulating the external force variables. To accomplish this, the patient is supine while the clinician takes the involved extremity passively to a point of maximum elongation for the ligament under investigation and notes any pain response. Once again, a thorough knowledge of anatomy guides the clinician as to correct position for force application.

Static arthrokinematic stress tests of the hip include those presented in Figure 3-5. The torque test is a global provocation test that is performed first to stretch all extra-articular ligaments of the hip. If this test is positive, then the clinician can proceed to further differential ligamentous testing.

### Passive Neural Mobility

See "Neurologic Testing."

### Strength Assessment

The following is a numerical grading system for strength assessment (Daniels and Worthingham 1986):

0   There is no palpable or observable contraction.
1   Trace muscle contraction is palpable.
2   Full ROM is present with gravity eliminated or minimal ROM is present against gravity.
3   Full ROM is present against gravity.
4   Full ROM is present against gravity with considerable resistance to motion provided by the clinician.
5   Full ROM is present against gravity with strong resistance to motion provided by the clinician.

*Note:* + and – symbols can be used to provide finer discrimination among the criteria.

Following a gross strength assessment, the clinician can test for strength under various conditions (e.g., using combinations of muscles, effect of testing at different lengths) to more adequately assess the contractile tissue function, especially when the goal is to determine the source of pain.

The following are variables that may be altered to further assess strength:

- Hip ROM
- Velocity of resistance
- Duration of resistance
- Amount of repetitions

Advanced strength assessment, with or without the use of equipment, such as an isokinetic dynamometer, permits testing of these variables under concentric, isometric, and eccentric loading conditions. Normative values for isokinetic strength are presented in Chapter 4 (see Tables 4-5 and 4-6).

Resisted motion is used to aid in the assessment of tissue reactivity. As would have been discerned from active movements, the clinician should test the most painful movements last.

The following are four patterns of pain and strength to assess tissue reactivity (Cyriax 1982):

1. Strong and painless indicates normal function.
2. Strong and painful indicates a minor lesion (e.g., tendinitis).
3. Weak and painful indicates a major lesion (e.g., fracture).
4. Weak and painless indicates a neurogenic lesion or total rupture of myotendinous unit.

In addition to routine ROM and strength testing, several *special tests* that have noncontractile and contractile implications can be performed at the hip joint. These help to further differentiate structures and tissues, aiding the clinician to arrive at a primary diagnosis (see Table A-1 in the chapter appendix).

## Assessment

The examination process is completed with the formulation of a diagnosis (Table A-2 in the chapter appendix) and a list of the problems to be addressed with treatment. Chapter 4 also discusses the issue of diagnosis.

A thorough assessment dictates the goals and plan of care. Included in the assessment are the following (Dyrek 1994):

- Mechanism of onset of symptoms
- Diagnosis
- Stage of symptoms
- Contributing factors to etiology
- Physical therapy prognosis
- Frequency and duration for treatment

The physical therapist, with the patient's participation, formulates treatment goals and a plan of care based on the results of the evaluation.

The physical therapist explains the risks and benefits of the proposed treatment, outlines the alternative treatments available, explains the risks of foregoing treatment, and obtains the patient's consent before proceeding with treatment.

## Conclusion

This chapter provides an extensive framework of methods and techniques for comprehensive and effective evaluation of the adult outpatient with hip dysfunction. Careful history taking and systematic tissue differentiation ensure that all relevant information is gathered and analyzed, so that an accurate diagnosis can be made.

# Appendix

**Table A-1** Differential (Special) Tests of the Hip Joint

| Test | Purpose | Key indications | Technique | Findings |
|------|---------|-----------------|-----------|----------|
| Thomas test | To assess for hip flexion contracture | History of compensatory lumbar lordosis, c/o lumbar pain, or both<br><br>Presence of anky-losed or contrac-tured hip gait | Patient is supine with the thighs midway over the edge of the plinth. Both knees are flexed toward the chest to reduce the lumbar lordosis. The patient holds one leg against the chest, and the leg to be tested is extended toward the plinth. The clinician should palpate the lumbar spine during this maneuver to ensure that the patient maintains a posterior pelvic tilt. The position of the tested leg is then observed.<br>If the tested hip does not reach 0 degrees of extension, then a hip flexion contracture is sus-pected, and the amount of hip flexion is measured and recorded. If the addition of hip abduction allows the hip to reach 0 degrees, shortening from the TFL may be the cause.<br>The test is repeated for the oppo-site leg, beginning again with the knees-to-chest position. | Classically, this test is used as an assessment of iliopsoas length. However, shortening of other structures can be involved (i.e., rectus femoris, hip capsule, TFL, adductors, sartorius), or there may be pelvic hypomobility, derangement, or contracture. It is important to differentiate the extent of involvement that is achieved through selective loading of each of these structures and thus the findings of a cluster of tests. |

| Test | Purpose | Key indications | Technique | Findings |
|---|---|---|---|---|
| Rectus femoris stretch test | To assess the flexibility of the two-joint hip flexor: rectus femoris | Same as Thomas test (see above) | Same as Thomas test (see above), with the emphasis on the amount of observable knee flexion of the leg in extension at the hip | The angle of knee flexion should be approximately 80 degrees with the leg hanging relaxed. If not, the clinician should attempt to passively flex the knee to 80 degrees or greater. If the knee does not flex beyond 80 degrees in this position of hip extension, then shortened length of rectus femoris is suspected. The clinician should always palpate for tissue resistance when performing any contracture test. If there is no palpable resistance, the probable cause of limitation is contracture of intra-articular structures (i.e., the capsulo-ligamentous complex of the hip). |
| Ely test or prone knee-bending test | To assess the length of the rectus femoris muscle and neural tension or irritation of the femoral nerve | c/o pain in the lateral or anterior thigh or neurologic signs involving L1–L3 nerve-root distribution<br><br>An anterior pelvic tilt or an ipsilateral short leg resulting in postural deviations, gait deviations, or both can be associated with | The patient is prone. The clinician passively flexes the patient's knee to 90 degrees or greater. Limitation in knee flexion, symptom production, or both is noted. Then, while maintaining knee flexion at 90 degrees, the examiner passively extends the hip while also stabilizing the pelvis. Limitation in hip extension, symptom production or both is noted. | Before the test with the patient lying prone with knees extended on the firm examination table, the clinician should note if the hip is slightly flexed: This can indicate an iliopsoas contracture. Such a finding should be confirmed using the Thomas test. During the Ely test, if passive knee flexion provokes a compensatory increase in hip flexion and hyperlordosis of the lumbar spine, then the rectus femoris muscle is likely shortened. When hip extension ROM is limited, the clinician should differentiate a capsulo-ligamentous source by performing hip extension with the knee extended rather than flexed. If hip extension is equally limited with the knee extended, as when flexed, then hip capsular con- |

**Table A-1** *Continued*

| Test | Purpose | Key indications | Technique | Findings |
|---|---|---|---|---|
| | | this condition. | | tracture is likely. Neurologic pain or symptoms along the anterolateral thigh in the distribution of the L1–L3 nerve roots can indicate femoral nerve root involvement. The flexed knee position should be maintained up to 45–60 seconds to provoke symptoms. |
| Adduction flexibility test | To isolate the two-joint hip adductor (i.e., gracilis) from the one-joint hip adductors | c/o pain in the groin inner thigh, or medial thigh with or without concurrent gait deviation | The patient is supine. The clinician abducts the patient's leg with the knee in extension, ensuring isolation of the movement through stabilization of the ipsilateral ASIS of the pelvis. By maintaining knee extension, the gracilis is maximally lengthened. This same maneuver with the knee in flexion places the gracilis on slack, isolating the one-joint hip adductors (i.e., pectineus, adductor longus, adductor brevis, and adductor magnus). | If pain is elicited during the maneuver, the clinician should identify the site of pain, the firmness of end-feel, and any limited motion. An indication of adductor involvement is abduction less than 45 degrees with knee extension and less than 65 degrees with knee flexion. |
| Ober test (modification by | To identify restricted ITB, TFL, and gluteus | c/o pain in buttock, peritrochanteric region, lateral iliac crest area, | Patient is side-lying with the lower hip (untested hip) placed in 45-degrees hip flexion and 90-degrees knee flexion to | Positive test results include reproduction of pain and symptoms, identification of a tissue restriction, or both. The clinician should note type of end-feel tissue |

| Test | Purpose | Key indications | Technique | Findings |
|------|---------|-----------------|-----------|----------|
| Dyrek 1996) | maximus at the proximal or distal site as a source of dysfunction, pain, or both (The assumption is that hip capsule and femoral congenital anomalies have or will be ruled out as a source of tissue impairment or pain.) | ASIS, lateral thigh, distal thigh superior to lateral femoral condyle, anterior knee compartment pain, and superior tibiofibular joint with or without concurrent gait deviations | create a stable base. The pelvis is firmly stabilized to prevent lateral and anterior pelvic tilt. The upper hip is adducted in maximum extension, and then again while progressively more flexion is added in 20- to 30-degree increments until 90 degrees of hip flexion. In each position, while applying an adduction force, the variables of (1) hip internal rotation, (2) hip external rotation, (3) 0-degree knee extension, and (4) 20-degree knee flexion are added. So, in each position of hip flexion, four variables involving hip rotation and the degree of knee flexion are controlled by the clinician. If a restriction is found, the clinician should consider the use of neuromuscular inhibition techniques to further differentiate contractile versus non-contractile tissue as the cause of the lesion. | resistance. |

**Table A-1** *Continued*

| Test | Purpose | Key indications | Technique | Findings |
|---|---|---|---|---|
| Noble compression test | To access ITB friction syndrome at the knee | c/o lateral knee compartment pain with activity (e.g., running) | The patient is supine with the tested extremity in 90-90 degree position (90 degrees of concurrent hip flexion and knee flexion). The patient is asked to slowly extend the knee, while the examiner maintains firm finger pressure on the ITB just proximal to the lateral femoral epicondyle. | A positive test result is sharp pain produced short of approximately –30 degrees knee extension. |
| 90–90 degrees SLR | To assess the flexibility of the hamstrings | c/o pain in the buttock, posterior thigh, or postero-lateral or postero-medial knee compartments<br>Decreased knee extension ROM | The patient is supine. The clinician passively flexes the patient's hip to 90 degrees, with the knee flexed at 90 degrees. The clinician then attempts to fully extend the knee while maintaining the hip at 90-degrees flexion. To avoid error, the pelvis should be maintained in a posterior pelvic tilt. | An angle of 20 degrees from full-knee extension is within normal limits; however, a larger angle is considered indicative of decreased hamstring flexibility.<br>Any motion less than or greater than 20 degrees knee extension is documented. |
| Tripod sign | Alternative test to assess hamstring length | See 90–90 degrees SLR above | The patient is seated upright with both knees flexed to 90 degrees over the edge of the plinth. The clinician passively extends one knee while observing | The test is positive if the pelvis is pulled into a posterior tilt (usually with trunk extension) as the knee is extended. |

| Test | Purpose | Key indications | Technique | Findings |
|---|---|---|---|---|
| Piriformis tests | To assess the flexibility, strength, and pain response to passive and active loading of the piriformis muscle | Buttock pain, sciatic radicular symptoms, firmness of end-feel to hip flexion or adduction, limited hip motions (usually flexion, adduction, and internal rotation), altered sacroiliac arthrokinematics, and toeing-out gait with involved extremity | the pelvis and trunk. Frieberg test: The patient is supine while the clinician performs passive internal rotation of the extended thigh (hip). Pace test: The patient is sitting while the clinician performs resisted hip abduction. Beattie test: The patient is side-lying with the painful side up. The painful hip and knee are flexed, with the knee resting on table. The patient is asked to lift and hold knee several inches from the table. Lee test: The patient is supine. The clinician resists active hip abduction with the hip at 60 degrees flexion (foot resting on table with hip and knee flexed). | A positive result for each test is reproduction of the patient's symptoms from contraction or stretch of the piriformis muscle. Symptoms are usually buttock pain, sciatica, or both. Firmness of end-feel, limited motion, and weakness should be noted, as well as symptom reproduction. Dyrek (1996) suggested an alternative method in which the patient lies prone, and hip internal rotation and external rotation are combined with motion palpation and resting palpation at different lengths of the piriformis. The density, resistance, and quality of piriformis should be noted, as well as pain responses (with and without palpation), flexibility, and contractile strength. |
| Patrick test (also known as *fabere test* and | A provocation test to the hip joint articular surfaces via externally applied | Serves as a gross clearing test History of crepitus; locking; instability; or pain in the hip, buttock, or groin | The patient is supine. The clinician passively takes the tested lower extremity and places the ankle on top of the contralateral knee. The tested hip should now lie in flexion, abduction, and external rotation. | Positive test results include pain (identify site), crepitus, click, firmness of end-feel, and limited motion. |

**Table A-1** *Continued*

| Test | Purpose | Key indications | Technique | Findings |
| --- | --- | --- | --- | --- |
| *figure 4 test)* | compression forces to rule out joint pathology Also stresses sacroiliac joint, pubic symphysis, adductors, lumbar spine, and inguinal ligament | | The clinician applies a dorsally directed pressure through the tested LE (knee), while stabilizing the contralateral ilium. Oscillations can be used to spring the hip joint. | |
| Hip grind test | To assess joint surface integrity of acetabulum and femur | Suspect joint degeneration by history. Pain (deep ache) in hip, buttock, thigh, groin, or knee Crepitus, click, locking, or instability | Patient is supine. The clinician passively places the tested hip in the loose-packed position (i.e., ideally 55 degrees abduction, 55 degrees flexion, and 5 degrees external rotation, but probably less than this will be possible due to pain, capsular contracture, or degenerative change) to avoid stress on non-joint surface tissue. The clinician cradles the tested LE to his or her chest and applies a compressive force through the long axis of the femur. While main- | Positive findings include pain, crepitus, click, and intermittent lock. |

| Test | Purpose | Key indications | Technique | Findings |
|------|---------|-----------------|-----------|----------|
| | | | taining a compressive load, the tested hip is passively moved into flexion and then extension. Small internal and external rotation oscillations are applied during these movements. The clinician can perform long and short axis distraction as opposite testing forces and compare the findings. | |
| Hip flexion and adduction test | To test for synovial-capsular impingement in the antero-inferior hip region | c/o sharp groin pain c/o pain with movement while sitting and with sit-stand and stand-sit maneuvers | The patient is supine. The clinician firmly stabilizes the pelvis and passively flexes the hip to 95–100 degrees. Next he or she adds an adduction force and oscillates between hip flexion of 75 degrees and 100 degrees. To differentiate if capsule is involved, the clinician brings the hip out of adduction while maintaining the hip flexion and asks for a few submaximal isometric iliopsoas contractions. He or she then repeats test. If retest is negative, then the likely cause is a cap- | A positive finding is sharp groin pain that immediately resolves after test. The clinician should monitor for sacroiliac or lumbar origin of pain. |

**Table A-1** *Continued*

| Test | Purpose | Key indications | Technique | Findings |
|---|---|---|---|---|
| | | | sular impingement. Contraction of iliopsoas can free an impinged anterior capsule because it attaches to the muscle. | |
| Scour or quadrant test | Gross clearing test to assess for pain, limitation of ROM, and end-feel of hip joint at expense of capsular flexibility and joint motion This test should not be done with the irritable or surgical hip. | c/o hip pain, snapping psoas tendon, impingement symptoms, crepitus, click, or any combination of these | The patient is supine. The clinician passively circumducts the tested extremity through extremes of motion, while applying overpressure. The four quadrants in the manuever can be broken down into the following arcs of movement: (1) flexion-abduction–external rotation to extension-abduction–external rotation; (2) flexion-adduction–external rotation to extension-adduction–external rotation; (3) flexion-abduction–internal rotation to extension-abduction–internal rotation; and (4) flexion-adduction–internal rotation to extension-adduction–internal rotation. At two positions in test, either Patrick or flexion and adduction test | Positive findings include pain (ache to sharp), intermittent locking, impingement, crepitus, click, premature limitation of ROM, and snapping tendon. The clinician should monitor for lumbar spine and sacroiliac joint as pain source. |

| Test | Purpose | Key indications | Technique | Findings |
|---|---|---|---|---|
| | | | are duplicated. | |
| Sign of the buttock test | To assess disease in the buttock region (e.g., septic bursa, tumor, abscess) | Pain in the buttock region with or without gait deviation | The patient is supine. The clinician performs a passive unilateral SLR. If there is unilateral restriction, the clinician then flexes the knee to assess whether hip flexion increases. | If the problem involves a lumbar nerve root, hip flexion increases. This finding indicates a negative test. If hip flexion does not increase when the knee is flexed, it is a positive sign and can indicate osteomyelitis, septic SI arthritis, ischiorectal abscess, neoplasm, rheumatic fever with bursitis, septic bursitis, or a fractured sacrum. The patient may also exhibit a noncapsular pattern of the hip. |
| Trendelenburg test or sign | To assess the strength and functional ability of the ipsilateral hip abductors (especially the gluteus medius) to maintain stability of the contralateral pelvis | Trendelenburg or compensated Trendelenburg gait pattern | The patient is standing and is asked to stand on one leg and then the other. The patient should flex the nonweight-bearing hip not more than 30-degrees flexion. While the patient is balancing on one leg, the clinician observes the angle between the pelvis (a line joining the iliac crests) and the ground. Movement of the trunk to the weightbearing side should be noted and then warned against for repeat of the test. If the patient is unable to balance on one leg, the exam- | Negative Trendelenburg: The pelvis should remain level or rise slightly on the contralateral side. Neutral Trendelenburg: The pelvis remains level with the ground, but the patient is unable to hike the contralateral pelvis maximally when asked to do so (compare with other side if normal). Positive Trendelenburg: Pelvis drops on the contralateral side to the stance leg. Compensated Trendelenburg: Excessive lateral trunk lean toward the same side (compare with effect on other side if normal). A positive or compensated Trendelenburg test indicates weak hip abductors. There may be an inability to control the abductors due to neural problems, pain inhibition, or mechanical factors (e.g., short abductor lever arm after hip |

**Table A-1** *Continued*

| Test | Purpose | Key indi-cations | Technique | Findings |
|---|---|---|---|---|
| | | | iner can provide minimal support to the patient's *ipsilateral* hand (a cane can be used) or support the patient's shoulders. The patient should hold the one-leg stance for 30 seconds, while the examiner observes for any delayed response of lateral pelvic tilt. | replacement) (Hardcastle and Nade 1985). |

ASIS = anterior superior iliac spine; c/o = complains of; ITB = iliotibial band; L1–L3 = first through third lumbar nerve root levels; LE = lower extremity; ROM = range of motion; SLR = straight leg raising; SI = sacroiliac; TFL = tensor fasciae latae.

**Table A-2** Differential Diagnosis of Common Hip Disorders (Refer also to Chapter 2)

| Disorder | Chief complaint | Etiology | Symptoms | Static physical signs | Dynamic physical signs | Special tests |
|---|---|---|---|---|---|---|
| **Osteoarthritis (OA) or degenerative joint disease** | Early stages: Pain with weightbearing at the end of the day or with fatigue Occasional radicular pain along L3 dermatome Advanced stages: Constant aching with morning stiffness Sleep difficulty secondary to pain Difficulty with functional activity secondary to decreased ROM in a capsular pattern and pain | Primary OA: Idiopathic with no known predisposing cause Secondary OA See Chapter 2 | Insidious, gradual onset of pain in groin, anterior thigh, and knee that increases with prolonged activity Joint stiffness after rest Crepitus, including squeaking, creaking, and grating | Atrophy of adjacent hip musculature, especially gluteals and abductors Flexion contracture, compensated by lumbar lordosis, and subsequent shortening of the affected leg Moderate effusion Tenderness possible, occurring over the site of capsular inflammation | Early stages: Mild limitation at end range of internal rotation, abduction, and extension associated with pain Advanced stages: Difficulty with functional activities such as stair climbing, squatting, and dressing Trendelenburg or antalgic gait Possible use of assistive device Motion limited in capsular pattern Decreased strength, especially of gluteals and abductors Hypomobility of all joint play movements | Patrick test Grind test Scour test Trendelenburg test |

**Table A-2** Continued

| Disorder | Chief complaint | Etiology | Symptoms | Static physical signs | Dynamic physical signs | Special tests |
|---|---|---|---|---|---|---|
| **Stress fracture** Femoral neck Pelvic | Local tenderness to pressure over (1) inguinal or anterior groin or (2) pubic rami (inferior) | Related to repetitive weightbearing activity (e.g., long-distance running or aerobics) with osteoporosis being a contributing factor | Local pain and tenderness Night pain if fracture progresses | Pain at end ranges of hip motion | Equilibrium and balance impairment Usually antalgic gait pattern | Anvil test (progressive striking to heel of supine patient) |
| **Osteo-myelitis** | Local tenderness to pressure over proximal femur | Usually due to entry of infective organisms (*staphylococcus aureus*) through the bloodstream | Local extreme pain and tenderness | Local swelling and erythema with increased skin temperature | Decreased and painful joint ROM in all directions with empty end-feels Antalgic gait pattern | Sign of the buttock test |
| **Contusion (hip pointer)** | Local tenderness to pressure to the iliac crest | Usually the result of athletic activity resulting in direct impact to the iliac crest | Local pain and tenderness Antalgic gait pattern Occasionally, numbness of lateral buttock and hip | Local ecchymosis, edema, or both | Symptoms increased with coughing, active trunk flexion or rotation, and active hip flexion | None |
| **Nerve entrapment syndromes** | Tingling, numbness, weakness, and burning pain in nerve | | | | | |

| Disorder | Chief complaint | Etiology | Symptoms | Static physical signs | Dynamic physical signs | Special tests |
|---|---|---|---|---|---|---|
| Lateral femoral cutaneous nerve (meralgia paresthetica) | Anterior and lateral aspect of thigh distribution | Sudden weight gain<br>Direct trauma<br>Pregnancy<br>Overuse of abdominal musculature<br>Restricted athletic garments<br>Leg length discrepancy<br>Short leg opposite of symptoms | Pressure pain over the ASIS<br>Tingling and numbness in nerve distribution | Postural alteration (e.g., increased anterior pelvic tilt or ipsilateral short leg) | Pain<br>Symptom magnification at end range of passive abduction or extension | Adductor and flexibility test |
| Superior gluteal nerve | Gluteal region | Overuse syndrome involving the piriformis muscle and pelvic obliquity, or both | Pressure pain just lateral to the edge of the greater sciatic notch | Increased anterior pelvic tilt with possibility of atrophy of iliopsoas and sartorius | Pain<br>Symptom magnification at end range of passive internal rotation with possible weakness of hip abductors. If severe, increased lumbar lordosis with Trendelenburg gait pattern | Trendelenburg test |
| Femoral nerve | Anteromedial thigh to the medial surface of the foot | Direct trauma<br>Hematoma | Pressure pain in the groin | Possibility of atrophy of iliopsoas, sartorius, pect- | Pain<br>Symptom magnification at end range of passive hip | Femoral nerve stretch test |

**Table A-2** *Continued*

| Disorder | Chief complaint | Etiology | Symptoms | Static physical signs | Dynamic physical signs | Special tests |
|---|---|---|---|---|---|---|
| | | | | ineus, and quadriceps | extension with knee flexion Possible weakness of iliopsoas, sartorius, pectineus, and quadriceps If severe, antalgic or psoas gait | |
| Sciatic nerve | Posterolateral thigh to the plantar and dorsal aspects of the foot | Overuse syndrome involving the piriformis muscle Hematoma Direct trauma (rare) | Pressure pain at greater sciatic notch, with sensory impairment along nerve distribution possible | Possibility of atrophy of the hamstrings, adductor magnus, and all musculature distal to knee | Pain Symptom magnification with SLR or SLR derivative Weakness in myotomal distribution with antalgic gait pattern | SLR, SLR derivatives, or both |
| Obturator nerve | Medial thigh from the groin | Obturator hernia Osteitis pubis | Increased pain in nerve distribution with Valsalva maneuver and unrelieved with rest | Possibility of atrophy of the adductors | Pain Symptom magnification with active or passive hip abduction Weakness in myotomal distribution with waddling gait | Adduction flexibility test |
| Ilio- | Groin | Direct trauma | Pressure pain | No visible | Symptom magni- | None |

| Disorder | Chief complaint | Etiology | Symptoms | Static physical signs | Dynamic physical signs | Special tests |
|---|---|---|---|---|---|---|
| inguinal nerve | Scrotum | Hematoma | medial to the ASIS | changes | fication with active trunk flexion, standing erect, or with active and passive hip motion (especially extension) Probable antalgic gait pattern | |
| **Acetabular labrum tear** | Intermittent sharp pain with weightbearing activity (e.g., subjective report of hip instability when walking) | Most likely due to strong rotatory forces at the hip | Same as chief complaint | None | Palpable click with probable pain elicited by passively adducting and internally rotating the hip while it is maintained in extension Antalgic gait pattern | Flexion and adduction test Grind test Scour test |
| **Loose body in the hip joint** | See acetabular labrum tear above | A piece of articular cartilage can flake off secondary to trauma or consequence of OA changes (Cyriax 1982). | Same as acetabular labrum tear, especially with high contact pressures (e.g, rising from chair, ascending stairs) | None | Painful Springy end-feel on passive ROM in a set of movements in the noncapsular pattern | Grind test Scour test |
| **Bursitis** | Local tenderness to pressure over: | | Local pain and tenderness with occasional radiating | | Symptoms increased by: | |

**Table A-2** *Continued*

| Disorder | Chief complaint | Etiology | Symptoms | Static physical signs | Dynamic physical signs | Special tests |
|---|---|---|---|---|---|---|
| Ilio-pectineal (psoas) | Anterior hip or inguinal region | Can develop from hip joint inflammation, limited iliopsoas muscle flexibility, or chronic poor posture | pain into: L2–L3 dermatomes | Local swelling | Combined passive hip flexion and adduction Resisted hip flexion and passive extension | Femoral nerve stretch test, Flexion/adduction test, Scour test if others negative |
| Ischio-gluteal (ischial) | Ischial tuberosity | Related to irritating activity such as prolonged sitting, or repetitive motions or hip flexion with external rotation Direct trauma secondary to fall | Pain at ischial tuberosity with hamstring contraction Pain with sitting | Local swelling | Active forward trunk flexion Walking Ascending stairs Sitting | None |
| Superficial and deep trochanteric (gluteal) | Greater trochanter | Can develop from hip abductor or adductor imbalance, poor posture, increased Q-angle, inadequate running shoes or surface, or leg length discrepancy | L5 dermatome or proximally referred into lumbosacral region | Local swelling | Passive internal and external rotation, adduction, or resisted abduction Activities such as crossing legs, walking, and ascending stairs | Ober test |

| Disorder | Chief complaint | Etiology | Symptoms | Static physical signs | Dynamic physical signs | Special tests |
|---|---|---|---|---|---|---|
| **Muscle strain** | | | | | | |
| Hip adductors (particularly adductor longus) | Local tenderness to pressure over medial thigh, usually proximally at the musculotendinous junction | Can develop insidiously from overuse. Can develop traumatically by forced extension of the lower extremity as the hip is actively being flexed | Local pain and tenderness. Progressive stiffness | Hip usually held in flexion, adduction, and external rotation | Progressive ambulation. Resisted hip flexion. Limited hip extension | Thomas test. Ely test. Adductor length test |
| Gluteus medius | Sharp pain with prolonged running | Usually caused by overuse with long-distance running. Can develop due to surrounding pelvic muscle weakness | Local pain and tenderness over the region of the greater trochanter with resisted hip abduction | None | Symptoms increased with the following: Prolonged running. Resisted hip abduction. Limited hip adduction | Trendelenburg test. Ober test |
| Hamstring | Local tenderness to pressure either proximally at the ischial origin or more distally in the muscle belly or insertion at the knee | Can develop insidiously from poor posture, fatigue, or pelvic muscle imbalance. More likely to develop traumatically due to decreased flexibility, inappropriate quadriceps-to-hamstring ratios, comparative | Local pain and tenderness | Local ecchymosis and hemorrhage. In severe cases, palpable muscle defect. Increased stiffness | Symptoms increased by the following: Walking or running acceleration. Resisted hip extension, knee flexion, or both | 90–90 degrees. SLR. Tripod sign |

**Table A-2** Continued

| Disorder | Chief complaint | Etiology | Symptoms | Static physical signs | Dynamic physical signs | Special tests |
|---|---|---|---|---|---|---|
| | | limb-strength deficits, or forced hip flexion with the knee extended | | | | |
| Rectus femoris | Tenderness to pressure at the proximal AIIS origin, muscle belly, or distal patellar tendon insertion | Usually develops traumatically due to decreased flexibility, inappropriate quadriceps-to-hamstring ratios, comparative limb-strength deficits, or forced hip extension with the knee flexed | Local pain and tenderness | Local ecchymosis and hemorrhage. Possible palpable muscle defect and increased stiffness in severe cases | Symptoms increased by the following: Walking or running accelerations; Resisted hip flexion, knee extension, or both; Maintained hip extension with resisted knee extension | Ely test |
| **Snapping hip syndrome** | Crepitus or sensation of clicking, usually with associated pain: | | Sensation and possibly pain and tenderness: | | | |
| Internal (deep tissue; articular) | Anteriorly | Iliofemoral ligament over femoral head; Iliopsoas tendon over iliopectineal eminence; Iliopsoas tendon over AIIS; Femoral head in relationship to acetabulum | Anteriorly or anteromedially | None | Possibly an antalgic gait pattern | Thomas test; Adduction or flexibility test; Ober test; Grind test; Scour test |

| Disorder | Chief complaint | Etiology | Symptoms | Static physical signs | Dynamic physical signs | Special tests |
|---|---|---|---|---|---|---|
| | | (subluxation) | | | | |
| External (superficial tissue; nonarticular) | Laterally | ITB over greater trochanter Gluteus maximus tendon over greater trochanter Contributing factors include decreased flexibility of ITB; narrow biliac width; unbalanced flexibility; and muscle imbalance | Laterally | Decreased flexibility, strength, or both of adjacent soft tissue | Same as internal | Same as internal |
| **Myofascial pain syndromes** | Referred pain and tenderness over: | | | | | |
| Tensor fasciae latae | Greater trochanter | Acute or chronic overload to muscle Emotional stress Visceral disease OA | Hyperirritable foci or trigger points with referred pain patterns | Possible increased soft tissue density in area of involved tissue with altered bony alignment or posture (i.e., pelvic obliquity) | Pain worse with resisted abduction and passive adduction Prolonged sitting if hip flexed greater than 90 degrees | Ober test |
| Quadratus lum- | Iliac crest Greater trochanter | Same as tensor fasciae latae | Same as tensor fasciae latae | Same as tensor fasciae latae | Pain worse in upright position | Leg length assessment |

**Table A-2** *Continued*

| Disorder | Chief complaint | Etiology | Symptoms | Static physical signs | Dynamic physical signs | Special tests |
|---|---|---|---|---|---|---|
| borum | SIJ<br>Lower buttocks | | | | Limited passive and active forward trunk bending, lateral side bending away from involved side, and rotation secondary to pain | |
| Piriformis muscle | SIJ<br>Buttock<br>Posterior hip | Same as tensor fasciae latae | Same as tensor fasciae latae | Same as tensor fasciae latae | Pain worse with sitting; occasionally squatting and rising from chair; lateral rotation of hip; or trunk rotation with occasional numbness and tingling along sciatic nerve distribution | Piriformis test |
| Gluteus medius | Posterior iliac crest and SIJ<br>Center of iliac crest and caudally to mid-gluteal region<br>Lower lumbar and sacrum | Same as tensor fasciae latae | Same as tensor fasciae latae | Same as tensor fasciae latae | Pain worse with walking (antalgic gait pattern) | Trendelenburg test |

| Disorder | Chief complaint | Etiology | Symptoms | Static physical signs | Dynamic physical signs | Special tests |
|---|---|---|---|---|---|---|
| Gluteus minimus | Anterior fibers: Lower lateral buttocks Lateral thigh Caudally into perineal region Posterior fibers: Greater portion of buttocks Posterior thigh and calf | Same as tensor fasciae latae | Same as tensor fasciae latae | Same as tensor fasciae latae | Antalgic gait pattern secondary to constant pain, worse with rising from chair | Trendelenburg test |

AIIS = anterior inferior iliac spine; ASIS = anterior superior iliac spine; ITB = iliotibial band; L2–L3 = second and third lumbar nerve roots; L5 = fifth lumbar nerve root; ROM = range of motion; SIJ = sacroiliac joint; SLR = straight leg raising.

# 4

# Physical Therapy Treatment of Hip Dysfunction

Timothy L. Fagerson

> Physical therapy is a health profession whose primary purpose is the promotion of optimal health and function through the application of scientific principles to prevent, identify, assess, correct, or alleviate acute or prolonged movement dysfunction. (American Physical Therapy Association 1989, p. 26)

Information regarding physical therapy treatment for the hip is sparse. Most orthopedic physical therapy texts have chapters on evaluation of the hip, but very few deal with physical therapy treatment. Equally sparse is research on physical therapy for the hip (Cibulka and Delitto 1993; Smidt 1997).

The purpose of this chapter is to provide a framework for physical therapy intervention and management of hip dysfunction, as well as to present a broad selection of treatment options. A framework for intervention and basic principles behind treatment techniques are provided because the reasoning and planning behind use of any technique is seen as prerequisite to its application. Being able to explain why is essential to physical therapy autonomy. Thus, problem solving as a scientist and performing treatment as an artist go hand in hand.

To most effectively apply the information in this chapter, the following should be known:

- The diagnosis and list of impairments (see Chapters 2 and 3)
- The natural history of the disorder (see Chapter 2)
- A good understanding of anatomy and biomechanics of the problem (see Chapter 1)
- The limitations of a particular surgery (see Chapter 5)
- The special needs of individual population groups
- The goals and expectations of the individual patient

On deciding to use a particular treatment, it is each practitioner's ethical responsibility to base that decision on a thoughtful review of the theoretical foundation of the approach and its scientific basis (Harris 1996). The patient should then be informed of the diagnosis, prognosis, treatment plan, and preventative measures.

## Diagnosis: A Prerequisite for Physical Therapy Treatment

> *Diagnosis* is the term that names the primary dysfunction toward which the physical therapist directs treatment. The dysfunction is identified by the physical therapist based on information obtained from the history, signs, symptoms, examination, and tests the therapist performs or requests. (Sahrmann 1988, p. 1705)

The issue of diagnosis continues to be debated in the physical therapy literature, and a consensus has yet to be reached as to accepted "physical therapy diagnoses." The primary purpose of diagnosis by a physical therapist is to identify the primary impairment or functional limitation toward which the clinician will direct his or her treatment. Physical therapy interventions for a given condition cannot be shown to be effective unless there is a clear statement as to what that condition is (Guccione 1991).

Why a physical therapy diagnosis?

1. Medical diagnoses based on disease do not adequately direct physical therapy intervention. Physical therapy treatment is better directed by diagnosis of movement system dysfunction.
2. A diagnosis provides an effective and efficient means of communication with colleagues and consumers.
3. A diagnosis provides a classification by which research can be directed and a means by which research findings can in turn direct treatment and determine prognosis (Sahrmann 1988).

The two models most frequently proposed as a framework for physical therapy diagnosis and classification are the Nagi model (Nagi 1965) (Figure 4-1) and the World Health Organization's taxonomy, *International Classification of Impairments, Disabilities, and Handicaps* (World Health Organization 1980). These models are simple hierarchies and have been adapted by Guccione (1991) (see Figure 4-1) and the National Center for Medical Rehabilitation Research (Figure 4-2) to more accurately express the complex interrelated dimensions of dysfunction.

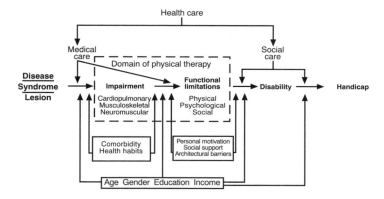

**Figure 4-1** Working expansion of Nagi's model of the process of disablement to account for the influence of service delivery and personal factors. (Reprinted with permission from AA Guccione. [1991] Physical therapy diagnosis and the relationship between impairments and function. *Physical Therapy* 71, 502.)

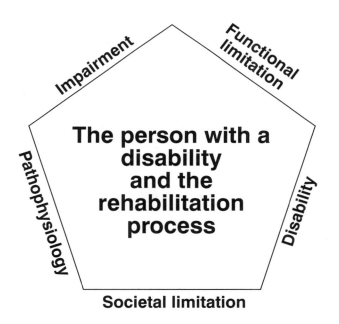

**Figure 4-2** Interrelated dimensions of disability. (Reprinted with permission from National Institutes of Health. [1993] *Research Plan for the National Center for Medical Rehabilitation Research* [p. 34]. NIH Publication no. 93-3509. Bethesda, MD: National Institutes of Health.)

When planning rehabilitation of the hip patient, each of the dimensions in Figure 4-2 should be considered. Managing disability and societal limitation requires an interdisciplinary approach. In physical therapy, a common assumption is that by intervening at the impairment level, resolution of functional limitations can be achieved. Such a simplistic view is often inaccurate and ineffective. A useful model of orthopedic dysfunction developed by Harris and Dyrek (1989) offers an understanding of pathophysiologic and pathokinesiologic processes to explain the cause and effects of orthopedic dysfunction (Figure 4-3). An important message of the model in Figure 4-3 is that impairments identified on examination can and should be related to the internal tissue response. Considering the effects of therapeutic interventions at the tissue and cellular level enables appropriate progression of treatment and prevents unnecessary complications.

Another model, developed by Schenkman and Butler (1989) for neurologic dysfunction also has implications for treating orthopedic dysfunction. Impairments are classified as *direct effects* of the lesion, *indirect effects* of the lesion, or *composite effects*. In the acute phase of an injury, pain, redness, swelling, increased local temperature, and decreased function may be direct effects; indirect effects may be joint contracture and muscular imbalance (which should be preventable with appropriate management); and composite effects may be abnormal gait and decreased balance. Impairments that are composite effects can have multiple underlying causes, which are likely to be a combination of direct and indirect impairments. In focusing treatment, it is important to have an understanding as to which problems are amenable to physical therapy and which are not. Treatment is most effective when it is focused at the source of the problem (i.e., the lesion): This is achieved through accurate diagnosis. When physical therapy is not the best method for treating the lesion, other means should be recommended (e.g., medication, injection, surgery). In such cases, physical therapy is often still warranted to address indirect or composite effects, such as preventing contracture; preventing atrophy and muscular imbalance; and reducing swelling, pain, and muscle spasm. Communication between physical therapist, physician, and patient is an essential ingredient to successful management.

Based on factors derived from the previously stated models (i.e., Harris and Dyrek 1989; Guccione 1991; Nagi 1965; Schenkman and Butler 1989) the physical therapist should determine at the end of the diagnostic process:

- The site of the lesion (i.e., intra-articular, extra-articular, or both)
- The cause of dysfunction
- The internal tissue response
- The stage of the lesion (i.e., acute, subacute, chronic)

- Natural healing versus clinical intervention
- The impairments (i.e., direct, indirect, composite)
- Functional limitations
- Any disability
- Any societal limitations (handicaps)
- Which impairments and functional limitations are amenable to physical therapy
- What morbidity factors need to be considered (e.g., age, disease process)
- An idea of the most effective treatment and its prognosis

The clinician should then define the problem with a diagnostic label that most accurately describes the problem. Ideally, this diagnostic label should have a standardized definition and be widely accepted.

## Diagnostic Categories for the Hip

Sahrmann and Woolsey (1992) suggested the following framework of diagnoses for physical therapists:

I. Diagnoses for physical therapy management. For example, postural or muscular imbalances, soft tissue disorders caused by minor trauma or overuse (e.g., sprains, strains, tendinitis, bursitis, fasciitis, capsulitis), nerve entrapment syndromes (e.g., piriformis syndrome)

II. Conditions needing referral for confirmation by another practitioner. Physical therapy can begin before confirmation. For example, osteoarthritis, rheumatoid arthritis

III. Conditions that need to be referred for medical diagnosis before physical therapy treatment can begin (does not include first-aid treatment). For example, signs and symptoms suggestive of fracture, dislocation, avascular necrosis, infection, neoplasm

An important determinate of groups I and II are the absence of *red flags**
that suggest immediate work-up with imaging studies, laboratory tests for confirmation, or both. A list of red flags is given in Table 3-1.

Most of the non–soft tissue diagnoses listed in Chapter 2 require diagnostic studies that are out of the physical therapist's realm. Any signs and symptoms suggestive of such conditions should prompt referral to a physi-

---

*Red flags* is a jargon term referring to conditions outside the diagnostic scope of physical therapy (e.g., tumors, fractures, disease, infection, or osteonecrosis).

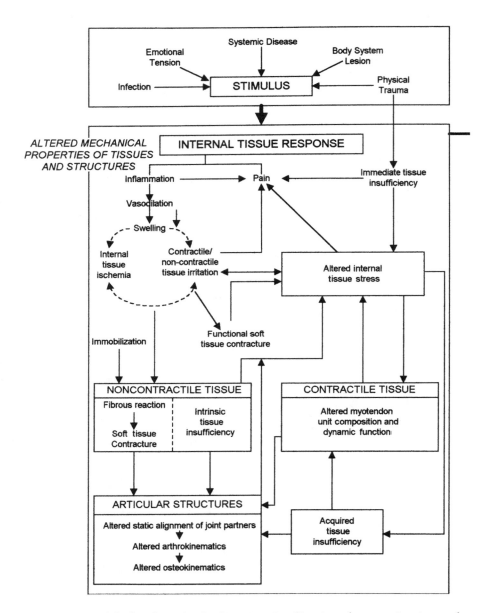

**Figure 4-3** Model of orthopedic dysfunction: Implications for examination and treatment. (Reprinted with permission from BA Harris, DA Dyrek. [1989] A model of orthopaedic dysfunction for clinical decision making in physical therapy practice. *Physical Therapy* 69, 550.)

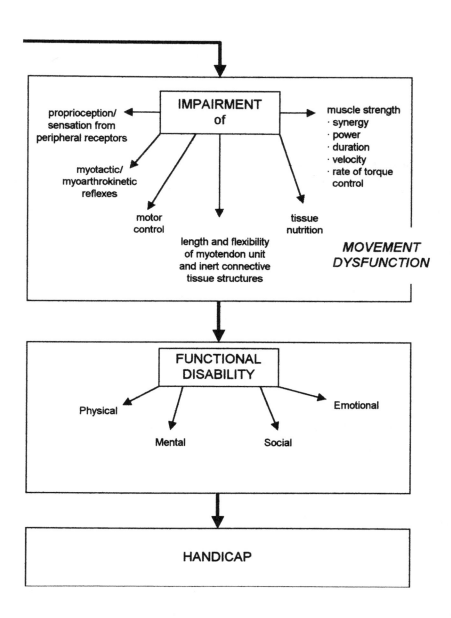

cian. Cyriax (1982) used a test called the sign of the buttock (see Chapter 3) in addition to presenting signs and symptoms to differentiate red flags (i.e., major lesions in the buttock) from non–red flags (i.e., minor lesions). Like Sahrmann and Woolsey's (1992) proposed classification, Cyriax required that major lesions be referred for medical work-up, and minor lesions be treated by injection, physical therapy, or both.

Cyriax's (1982) differential involves determining the following:

- If there is lumbar or sacroiliac involvement
- Capsular pattern versus noncapsular pattern
- Contractile versus noncontractile lesion
- Type of end-feel
- Presence or absence of the sign of the buttock

In essence a diagnosis that a physical therapist can make is one that can be made based on history and physical examination alone without imaging or laboratory studies to confirm. Such a diagnosis is usually an impairment, functional limitation, or recognized cluster of these. In the future, a broad selection of standardized diagnostic classifications should be available for use by physical therapists and other professionals involved with movement system dysfunction.

## Treatment Planning

### Planning the Physical Therapy Intervention

Maitland's (1991) "permeable brick wall" idea, in which the therapist compares clinical findings with theoretical findings, is a very useful intervention planning approach (Table 4-1). Maitland said of the diagnosis issue, "[m]any people consider that treatment should not be administered unless an accurate diagnosis is available. This is true to some extent; it IS necessary to know whether a patient's symptoms are believed to be arising from a musculo-skeletal disorder rather than an active disease, but it is not always necessary to have a precise diagnostic title." (Maitland 1991, p. 3)

Even when a precise diagnostic title is given, a detailed problem list of impairments should also be generated. From this problem list, the therapist must determine which impairments are related to the functional limitation and are also treatable by physical therapy. Then the therapist must determine the order in which to treat the impairments and the type of treatment methods to use. Of foremost importance is determining what *the patient's problems* are and intervening to resolve these problems. Active listening is essential to success in this process along with demonstrating a "positive personal commitment to understand what the patient is enduring." (Maitland 1991, p. 1)

**Table 4-1** Maitland's "Permeable Brick Wall"

| *Theoretical* | *Clinical* | |
|---|---|---|
| Pathology | | History |
| Biomedical engineering | *Diagnosis* | Symptoms |
| Neurophysiology | | Signs |
| Anatomy | | |

Source: Reprinted with permission from GD Maitland. (1991) *Peripheral Manipulation* (3rd ed) (p. 2). Boston: Butterworth–Heinemann.

When hip dysfunction coexists with pelvic dysfunction, lumbar dysfunction, or both, the hip problem should usually be addressed first. The following is a suggested order of treatment for lesions of the lumbopelvic region (Dyrek 1996):

1. Hip
2. Lumbar spine
3. Pelvis
   a. Pubis lesions
   b. Sacral lesions
   c. Ilium lesions

This sequence should be modified, however, to address lesions with greater malalignment, tissue resistance, or both.

Successful rehabilitation of the hip requires a broad knowledge base and understanding, which includes:

- The hip as part of the lumbo-pelvic-hip complex, comprising both hip joints, both sacroiliac joints, the lumbar spine, and the pubic symphysis
- The hip as the proximal end of the lower extremity kinetic chain
- Anatomy and biomechanics of the hip
- The pathophysiology of diseases and disorders of the hip
- Surgical procedures and their implications to rehabilitation

### Goal Setting

Dyrek (1994) has suggested the following generic treatment goals:

1. Promote healing by improving the nutritional status of tissue.
2. Restore or prevent the loss of soft tissue flexibility and length for contractile and noncontractile tissue.

3. Restore or prevent the loss of normal joint alignment.
4. Restore or prevent the loss of normal joint mobility.
5. Promote normal myotactic and myoarthrokinetic reflexes.
6. Promote normal motor control.
7. Resolve pain and associated symptoms.
8. Prevent recurrence of the lesion.
9. Restore the functional ability of the patient.

In summary, goals for treatment of joint dysfunction are to relieve pain and to restore normal alignment, mobility, stability, and function (Figure 4-4).

## Treatment Strategies

When implementing treatment, applying a scientific and rational approach is crucial. Incorporating one treatment variable per session is an approach that achieves this. The adding of one treatment variable at a time is straightforward and logical. If the patient is made worse, it is likely that the last added intervention was the cause. If the patient shows marked improvement, then the latest ingredient may be among the most important factors. The downside of this approach is that progression can be slow. Obviously, when research, experience, or both indicate that a recognized cluster of signs and symptoms respond to a particular approach, then that approach should be used. Since positive treatment effects are often the result of a combination of techniques and advice, physical therapy researchers are starting to compare the effects of treatment combinations and not just one technique versus another technique. This paradigm shift is similar to that seen in the classic pyramid approach to treating rheumatoid arthritis. In this approach, the foundation of the pyramid is comprised of accepted, recognized, and safe methods; added to it are progressively more aggressive and experimental forms of drug therapy. The shift in rheumatology has been toward a reverse pyramid approach, as used in oncology, in which the patient is started on an aggressive medication regimen and gradually medications are removed until the baseline therapy is reached (Williams 1993). In physical therapy, unless indicated by experience or scientific evidence or both, the traditional pyramid approach (see Figure 4-4) is advised for treatment progression because:

1. When uncertain, one intervention at a time can be safely built on;
2. When irritability and severity of symptoms are high, the patient often will not tolerate multiple interventions at the same session; and
3. This approach complements the natural healing process involving progressive increase in loads and the tissues adapting to the imposed demands.

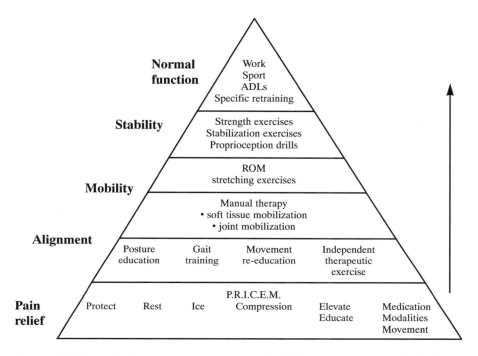

**Figure 4-4** Physical therapy treatment pyramid. (ADLs = activities of daily living; ROM = range of motion.)

Musculoskeletal dysfunction at any synovial joint, including the hip, can exhibit any combination of the following sequelae (Dyrek 1996):

- Pain
    Mechanical
    Chemical
- Contracture, adhesion, restriction
- Instability, tissue insufficiency
- Weakness
    Motor control
    Tissue weakness

Determining which of these sequelae is "driving" the patient's impairment or functional limitation and specifying the anatomic location is, perhaps, a more precise diagnosis than assigning the primary impairment or functional limitation. Such precision is encouraged whenever it can be made with a reasonable level of certainty. Figure 4-5 demonstrates how treatment strategies can be applied to these sequelae of dysfunction.

**1. Soft tissue lesion without a mechanical deficit**

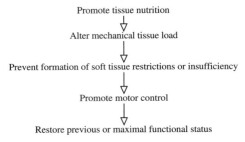

Promote tissue nutrition

↓

Alter mechanical tissue load

↓

Prevent formation of soft tissue restrictions or insufficiency

↓

Promote motor control

↓

Restore previous or maximal functional status

**2. Soft tissue flexibility or length deficit without an articular component**

*The first two steps below are appropriate if soft tissue inflammation is present*

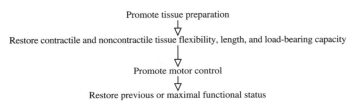

Promote tissue preparation

↓

Restore contractile and noncontractile tissue flexibility, length, and load-bearing capacity

↓

Promote motor control

↓

Restore previous or maximal functional status

**3. Articular deficit with soft tissue lesion, length and flexibility deficit, or both**

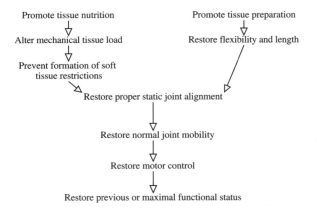

Promote tissue nutrition          Promote tissue preparation

↓                                        ↓

Alter mechanical tissue load          Restore flexibility and length

↓

Prevent formation of soft
tissue restrictions

↘          ↙

Restore proper static joint alignment

↓

Restore normal joint mobility

↓

Restore motor control

↓

Restore previous or maximal functional status

**Figure 4-5** Treatment strategies for musculoskeletal deficits. (Reprinted with permission from DA Dyrek. [1994] Assessment and Treatment Planning Strategies for Musculoskeletal Deficits. In SD Sullivan, TJ Schmitz [eds], *Physical Rehabilitation: Assessment and Treatment* [3rd ed] [p. 79]. Philadelphia: Davis.)

## Treatment Interventions

Throughout this section, helpful assessment and reassessment tips and treatment recommendations are given. In addition, relevant normative data are given by which to target an individual patient's outcome, tempered of course with comparison to preinjury function, opposite limb values, and natural history of the disorder. Continuous analytic assessment is the key to applying the most appropriate treatment intervention and to directing the best possible outcome (Maitland 1991).

### Gait Training

Perhaps the most significant result of hip dysfunction is the effect on gait. Therefore, determining which impairments are responsible for abnormal gait is a sensible first step.

The first aspect to consider in gait training is as follows: What is the permitted weightbearing status? A patient who is status post-surgery, -fracture, or -severe soft tissue injury may be on limited weightbearing. The therapist's first task should be to ensure that the weightbearing status is known and adhered to by the patient. Second, the clinician should teach a normal gait pattern. An abnormal gait pattern can predispose a patient to hip region inflammation and pain. Not to mention the effect that altered mechanics have on the lumbar spine, knee, and foot.

The following are "hip tips" for gait training:

HIP TIPS

- Patients with hip pain, regardless of the source, can benefit from a period of limited weightbearing to decrease the loads on weak and sensitive tissues. Even a cane in the contralateral hand can decrease significantly the loads on the hip (see Chapter 1). The advice of Blount (1956, p. 695), "don't throw away the cane," is always worth considering as an option in management of hip dysfunction.
- Patients with weak hip abductors (i.e., positive Trendelenburg or compensated Trendelenburg sign) are strong candidates for use of a cane in the opposite hand until the abductors are sufficiently strong. This is not only for purposes of a more aesthetic-looking gait but also to normalize lumbo-pelvic-hip mechanics.
- Instructing the patient to sleep and rest with the hip in abduction is important advice to help resolve stretch weakness, which is often a contributory factor in abductor weakness.
- Eccentric strengthening of the abductors is essential, since this is how they are recruited during gait.

- A mirror and parallel bars are useful tools in re-education of a normal gait pattern.
- Encourage symmetry and timing. De-emphasize compensatory mechanisms.
- Recognize component problems and treat them with joint mobilization, stretching, muscle re-education, strengthening, and so on.
- Walking at a faster speed can sometimes allow a patient to overcome a limp due to weak abductors and is good advice to patients on a progressive walking program.
- Pool walking (see the section "Aquatics") is also an excellent method, especially in the early phases of gait re-education.

Refer also to Chapter 6 for additional information on gait re-education.

## Posture and Muscle Imbalance

Gregory Grieve (1983, p. 200) wrote, "[t]he genesis of painful, degenerative joint conditions may frequently lie in regional and major chronic imbalance of functional movement patterns, which place sustained and abnormal stress on joints."

Addressing posture and muscle imbalance is essential for effective rehabilitation of the hip. These variables form the basis around which all treatment is directed.

### Posture

Poor postural and movement habits need to be addressed, as they may be contributory or the cause of the current complaint. This approach requires appreciation of the body as a working whole and does not focus just on the hip joint. Obviously, to make a judgment as to faulty posture requires comparison with a normative standard, ideal posture. For sagittal-plane ideal posture (side view) a plumb-line aligned just anterior to the lateral malleolus should pass through the following reference points (Figure 4-6):

- Slightly anterior to lateral malleolus
- Slightly anterior to axis of knee joint
- Slightly posterior to axis of hip joint (through greater trochanter)
- Bodies of lumbar vertebrae
- Shoulder joint
- Bodies of most of cervical vertebrae
- Ear lobe

Symmetry should also be observed on anterior and posterior viewing of the body, bearing in mind that some normal variation is accepted for hand-

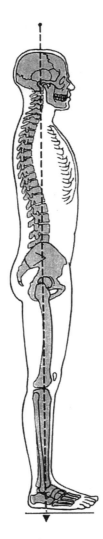

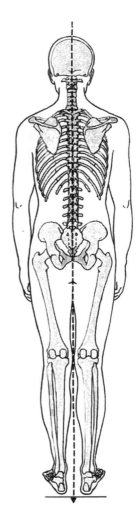

**Figure 4-6** Ideal alignment: Sagittal view. (Modified from FP Kendall, EK McCreary, PG Provance. [1993] *Muscles Testing and Function* [4th ed] [p. 76]. Baltimore: Williams & Wilkins.)

**Figure 4-7** Ideal alignment: Posterior view. (Modified from FP Kendall, EK McCreary, PG Provance. [1993] *Muscles Testing and Function* [4th ed] [p. 88]. Baltimore: Williams & Wilkins.)

edness (i.e., right-handed people tend to have a slightly lower shoulder girdle and higher pelvic girdle on the right, and vice versa for left-handed people). Landmarks for frontal plane (left to right) symmetry include (Figure 4-7):

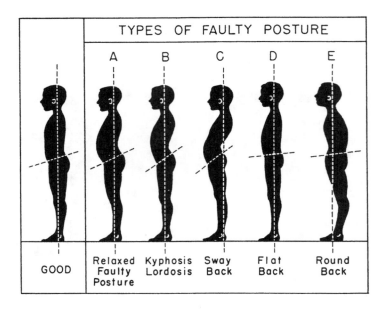

**Figure 4-8** Types of faulty posture. (Reprinted with permission from RO McMorris. [1961] Faulty posture. *Pediatric Clinics of North America* 8, 217.)

- Foot and ankle alignment
- Knee creases
- Buttock creases
- Iliac crest
- Inferior angle of scapulae
- Acromion processes
- External occipital protuberances

Note that a plumb line is a useful tool in a physical therapist's armamentarium. It is far too underused (Kendall et al. 1993).

Five "abnormal" posture types are commonly seen (Figure 4-8):

- Relaxed faulty posture (lordotic)
- Kyphosis-lordosis
- Sway back
- Flat back
- Round back

### Muscle Imbalance

Restoring normal length-tension relationships where realistically possible is the underlying principle for treating muscle imbalance.

Shortened muscles should be lengthened with stretching and soft tissue mobilization. Weak muscles should be strengthened, and their endurance capacity increased. Painful trigger points that are more likely to develop in shortened muscles should be released.

The following are "hip tips" for muscle imbalance:

## HIP TIPS

- Identify the posture type.
- Identify which muscles are elongated and weak.
- Identify which muscles are short and strong.
- Very weak muscles exhibiting stretch weakness should be immobilized in the shortened position (Kendall et al. 1993).
- Isometrically contract weak muscles in shortened range; stop just before fatigue (Kendall et al. 1993).
- Actively work lengthened muscle in shortened range (White and Sahrmann 1994).
- Maintain correct posture and movement habits throughout the day.
- Taping or bracing can be used to facilitate maintenance of correct posture.
- Exercise and work synergists in functional patterns, incorporating eccentric exercise and proprioceptive training.
- Progressively increase loads, time, and required skill.

## *Therapeutic Exercise*

Therapeutic exercise (therex) is a major component of physical therapy. The purpose of exercise includes

- Improve joint mobility
- Increase soft tissue flexibility
- Improve muscle control
- Increase muscle strength
- Improve muscle endurance
- Increase circulation
- Improve joint lubrication and nutrition
- Increase bone density
- Hypertrophy muscle
- Prevent contracture
- Prevent atrophy
- Improve balance
- Improve posture

- Improve gait
- Improve function

Listed above are most of the effects of exercise on the musculoskeletal system. Exercise can also have major effects on the cardiopulmonary and nervous systems.

In the wrong hands, exercise can be harmful. Exercise can increase pain from an injury, can increase wear and degeneration of joints, can cause muscle strain and joint sprain, can cause fracture, can prevent healing of fractures, can cause failure of surgical fixation, can exacerbate arthritis, can cause or increase inflammation of bursitis and tendinitis, and can make an acute problem chronic.

Consistently effective exercise prescription is a skilled task. It requires consideration of the following variables:

- Whole-body exercise or localized body-part exercise
- Passive, active-assisted, active, or resisted
- Isometric, isotonic (concentric or eccentric), or isokinetic
- Static, ballistic, proprioceptive neuromuscular facilitation (PNF)
- Open chain or closed chain
- Supine, prone, hook-lying, sidelying, quadruped, kneeling, sitting, standing
- Nonweightbearing (NWB), touch down weightbearing (TDWB), partial weightbearing (PWB), weightbearing as tolerated (WBAT), full weightbearing (FWB)
- Warm-up
- Use of heat and ice
- Duration
- Intensity
- Frequency
- Repetitions
- Sets
- Resistance
- When to progress and when to modify or stop

A useful reminder for establishing components of an exercise program, especially for athletes, is the *s* principle (Norris 1995):

- Strength
- Stamina
- Suppleness
- Specificity
- Skill

- Speed
- Psychology
- Coordination

## Hip Exercise Portfolio

The list of exercises in Table 4-2 is presented by way of progression from NWB through FWB. It is hoped that this portfolio will provide the clinician with ideas from which to tailor a program for a specific need and as a basis from which to be appropriately creative in exercise prescription. To illustrate and define each exercise is a book or computer program in itself. The intention of this list is to jog the memory and generate ideas. Remember, few exercises (three to five) are better than many, and an individualized program is better than a generic list.

## Manual Therapy: Passive Joint Mobilization

Diane Lee (1989, p. 121) wrote, "[s]light restriction of motion at [the hip] joint can produce dramatic compensatory effects at both the sacroiliac joint and the lumbosacral junction. The subsequent decompensation of the lumbo-pelvic region can only be resolved by restoring the mobility of the hip."

The "classic" capsular pattern for the hip described by Cyriax (1982) is maximum loss of internal rotation, flexion, abduction, and a minimal loss of extension. The two hip-movement restrictions that probably have the most significant functional implications are decreased extension (Ingber 1989) and decreased medial rotation (Ellison et al. 1990). With every gait cycle, increased stresses are imparted to the lumbosacral region, particularly when extension, internal rotation, or both is limited. It has been demonstrated that patients with low back pain frequently display a range of motion (ROM) pattern of hip medial rotation less than lateral rotation, suggesting that this pattern can be a cause, effect, or both of low back pain; however, further research is necessary to fully substantiate this (Ellison et al. 1990).

For determining ROM goals for hip patients, it is worth using a normative standard (Table 4-3) and the patient-specific standard of contralateral side.

### Arthrokinematics

An important premise of passive accessory joint mobilization is to restore normal arthrokinematic motion. Without normal arthrokinematics, there cannot be normal osteokinematics (physiologic movements).

**Table 4-2** Hip Exercise Portfolio

Supine

    Ankle pumps (postoperative circulatory exercise)
    Quadriceps sets
    Gluteal sets
    Hamstring sets
    Terminal knee extension
    Hip and knee flexion (heel slides)
    Straight leg raise (SLR)
    Hip abduction, with suspension and without
    Bilateral hip abduction with hips and knees flexed
    Thomas test stretch (Figure 4-9A)
    Bridging
    Piriformis stretch (Figure 4-9B)
    Hip rotation (internal and external)
    Flexion, abduction, and external rotation
    Hip hiking (hula)
    Pelvic tilt
    Hip adduction stretch with hips at 90-degrees flexion and legs supported
      by a wall
    Rectus femoris stretch with leg over side of bed and ankle held by hand
      (Figure 4-9C)

Sidelying

    Gravity-eliminated hip flexion and extension with suspension
    Against gravity abduction SLR and slow, eccentric lowering (Figure 4-9D)
    Against gravity adduction SLR
    External rotation
    Ober test stretch (Figure 4-9E)

Prone

    Calf raises (postoperative exercise)
    Active hip extension with knee straight
    Active hip extension with knee flexed
    Hip rotation (internal and external) with knees flexed (Figure 4-9F)
    Ely test stretch (Figure 4-9G)
    Opposite arm and leg lifts
    Trunk extension

Quadriped

    Buttocks to heels
    Single limb lifts
    Opposite arm and leg lifts (Figure 4-9H)
    Pelvic tilt

Sitting

    Hip flexion: knee to chest
    Hip flexion: fingers to floor
    Hip flexion, abduction, and external rotation (Figure 4-9I)
    Hip internal and external rotation (feet on floor)

Knee flexion and extension
Thigh slides (moving knee over fixed foot)
Resisted hip flexion (Figure 4-9J)

Long sitting

Hamstring stretch (Figure 4-9K)
Adductor stretch with hips and knees flexed
Piriformis stretch (Figure 4-9B)

Kneeling

Rectus femoris stretch

Standing

Hip and knee flexion
Hip abduction
Hip adduction
Hip extension
Two-joint hip flexor stretch with knee flexed and supported on stool on side to be stretched
Closed-chain hip extension (similar to a runner's calf stretch)
Hip hiking (Figure 4-9L)
The "rhumba" (sidegliding of pelvis)
Groin stretch
Rectus femoris stretch
Hip abductor stretch
Hamstring stretch (Figure 4-9M)
Closed-chain hip rotation (internal and external)
One-leg stance

Dynamic exercises and therapeutic interventions

Walking
Bicycling
Nordic Trak
Pool exercises and activities
Swimming
Yoga
Step exercises
Slide board
Body Blade
Aerobic and calisthenic routines
Thera-Band resistance
Sandbag resistance
Isotonic resistance machines
Isokinetic resistance
Proprioceptive neuromuscular facilitation
Muscle energy techniques
Passive stretching
Joint mobilization
Traction
Re-education ball
Balance board

**Table 4-3** Normative Hip Range of Motion: Percentile Distribution for Hip Active Range of Motion (in Degrees) by Age in the First National Health and Nutrition Examination Survey

| Motion | All ages (n = 1,683) | 25–39 years of age (n = 433) | 40–59 years of age (n = 727) | 60–74 years of age (n = 523) |
|---|---|---|---|---|
| **Hip flexion** | | | | |
| $\bar{x}$ | 121 | 122 | 120 | 118 |
| SD | 13 | 12 | 14 | 13 |
| CI | 120–121 | 121–123 | 119–121 | 117–120 |
| 100% | 160 | 150 | 160 | 150 |
| 75% | 130 | 130 | 130 | 125 |
| 50% | 120 | 120 | 120 | 120 |
| 25% | 110 | 115 | 115 | 110 |
| 0% | 0 | 55 | 0 | 0 |
| **Hip extension** | | | | |
| $\bar{x}$ | 19 | 22 | 18 | 17 |
| SD | 8 | 8 | 7 | 8 |
| CI | 19–20 | 21–23 | 18–19 | 16–17 |
| 100% | 45 | 45 | 40 | 40 |
| 75% | 25 | 25 | 20 | 20 |
| 50% | 20 | 20 | 20 | 15 |
| 25% | 15 | 15 | 15 | 10 |
| 0% | 0 | 0 | 0 | 0 |
| **Hip abduction** | | | | |
| $\bar{x}$ | 42 | 44 | 42 | 39 |
| SD | 11 | 11 | 11 | 12 |
| CI | 42–43 | 43–45 | 41–43 | 38–40 |
| 100% | 90 | 90 | 90 | 90 |
| 75% | 50 | 50 | 50 | 45 |
| 50% | 40 | 45 | 40 | 40 |
| 25% | 35 | 35 | 35 | 30 |
| 0% | 0 | 0 | 0 | 0 |
| **Hip internal rotation** | | | | |
| $\bar{x}$ | 32 | 33 | 31 | 30 |
| SD | 8 | 7 | 8 | 7 |

| Motion | All ages (n = 1,683) | 25–39 years of age (n = 433) | 40–59 years of age (n = 727) | 60–74 years of age (n = 523) |
| --- | --- | --- | --- | --- |
| CI | 31–32 | 32–34 | 31–32 | 29–30 |
| 100% | 60 | 60 | 55 | 50 |
| 75% | 35 | 40 | 35 | 35 |
| 50% | 30 | 30 | 30 | 30 |
| 25% | 25 | 30 | 25 | 25 |
| 0% | 0 | 10 | 0 | 5 |
| **Hip external rotation** | | | | |
| $\bar{x}$ | 32 | 34 | 32 | 29 |
| SD | 9 | 8 | 8 | 9 |
| CI | 32–33 | 33–35 | 32–33 | 29–30 |
| 100% | 65 | 65 | 60 | 55 |
| 75% | 40 | 40 | 40 | 35 |
| 50% | 30 | 35 | 30 | 30 |
| 25% | 25 | 30 | 25 | 25 |
| 0% | 0 | 10 | 0 | 5 |

SD = standard deviation; CI = 95% confidence interval, $\bar{x}$ = mean.
Source: Reprinted with permission from KE Roach, TP Miles. (1991) Normal hip and knee active range of motion: The relationship to age. *Physical Therapy* 71, 659.

Accessory joint mobilization techniques commonly performed at the hip are presented in the following list. The Maitland term for each technique is stated with other terms for the same technique in parentheses. Maitland (1991) used three asterisks in his text to denote most frequently used techniques and no asterisk for least frequently used techniques. The following are some of the more commonly used accessory mobilizations at the hip:

- ***Lateral movement (short-axis or lateral distraction): straps or belts could be used, but remember that what is gained in force is often lost in quality of movement.
- ***Longitudinal movement caudad (long-axis distraction): useful for the very painful hip and as a good general stretch of the capsule (Figure 4-10).
- ***Longitudinal movement cephalad compression: best suited for patient with pain on weightbearing; therefore, needs to be done as a grade III or IV and can be combined with gentle grades of rotation.
- ***Compression medially: useful for the patient with chronic hip pain that prevents lying on the affected side.

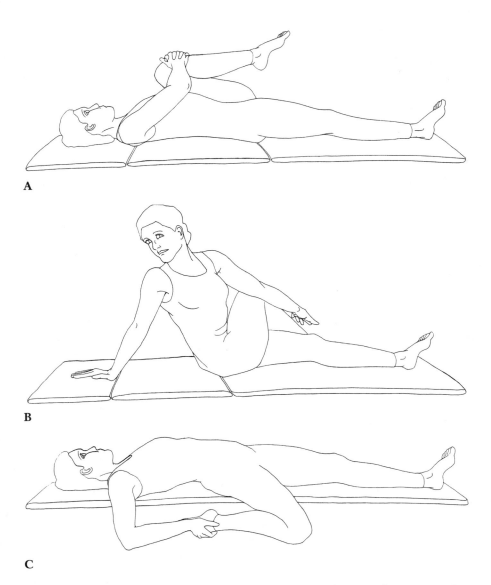

**A**

**B**

**C**

**Figure 4-9** Hip exercise portfolio. A. Thomas test stretch. B. Piriformis stretch. C. Rectus femoris stretch with leg over side of bed and ankle held by hand (posterior pelvic tilt should be maintained, which is not done in this illustration). D. Against gravity abduction straight leg raise with slow, eccentric lowering. E. Ober test stretch. F. Hip rotation (internal) with knees flexed. G. Ely test stretch.

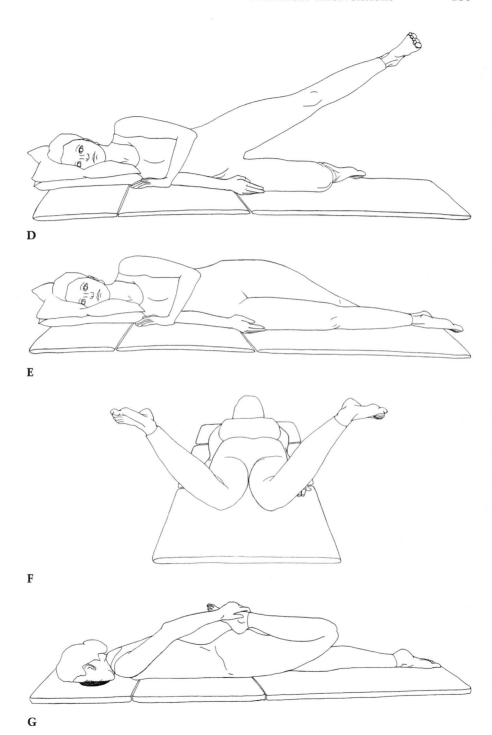

**D**

**E**

**F**

**G**

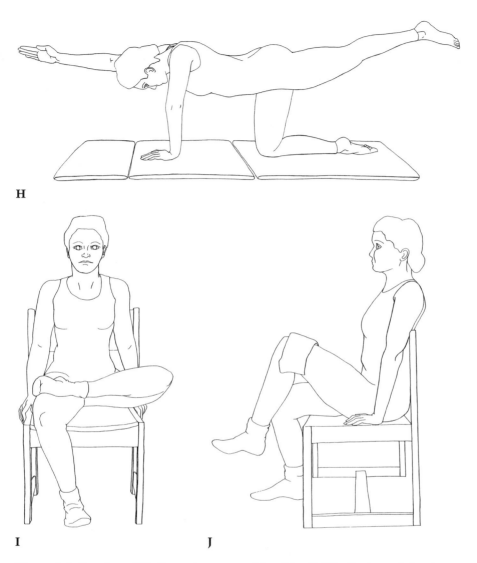

**Figure 4-9** *Continued* H. Opposite arm and leg lifts. I. Hip flexion, abduction, and external rotation. J. Resisted hip flexion. K. Hamstring stretch. L. Hip hiking. M. Hamstring stretch.

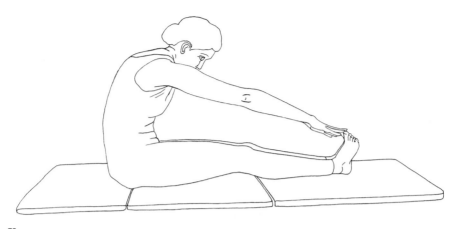

**K**

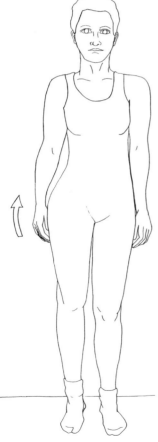

**L**

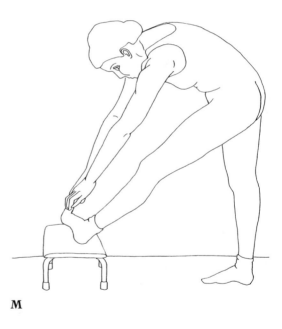

**M**

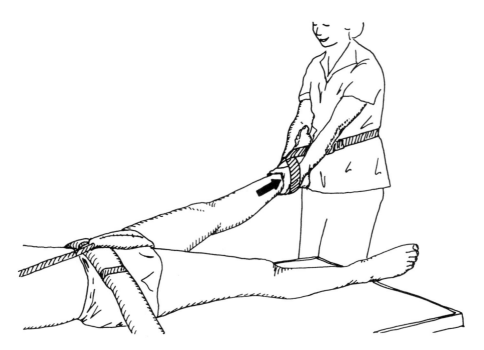

**Figure 4-10** Hip joint long-axis distraction. (Reprinted with permission from C Kisner, LA Colby. [1990] *Therapeutic Exercise: Foundations and Techniques* [p. 198]. Philadelphia: Davis.)

- ***Posteroanterior (posteroanterior glide, ventral glide, anterior glide): can be useful for the painful joint; when used to increase ROM, it should be used at the extreme of the restricted extension range (Figure 4-11).
- Anteroposterior (anteroposterior glide, dorsal glide, posterior glide): the value of this technique performed with the hip near 0 degrees flexion is for a capsular restriction of medial rotation (Figure 4-12).

Applying Kaltenborn's convex-concave rule to mobilization of the hip (Kaltenborn 1989), the femoral head (convex surface) is moved on the acetabulum (concave surface). Because the convex surface is the moving surface, the convex rule applies, which means that the femoral head should be mobilized using joint glides (arthrokinematics) in a direction opposite to the restricted bone movement (osteokinematics). For example, if extension range is limited, then an anterior glide should be used (the femoral head is moving anterior on extension as the femoral shaft moves posterior to the hip axis).

If one considers that the normal acetabulum permits limited joint play of the femoral head (try this with a skeleton), then the importance of taking

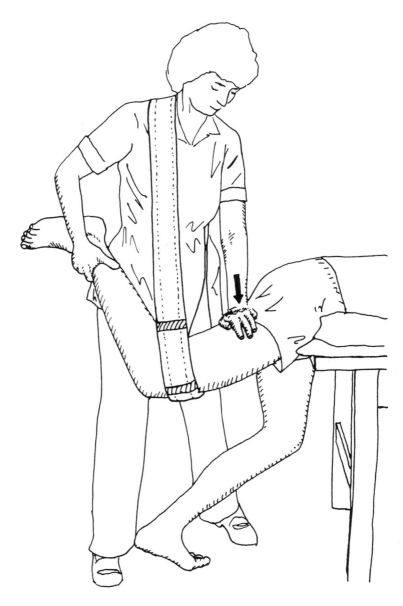

**Figure 4-11** Hip joint anterior glide in prone. (Reprinted with permission from C Kisner, LA Colby. [1990] *Therapeutic Exercise: Foundations and Techniques* [p. 200]. Philadelphia: Davis.)

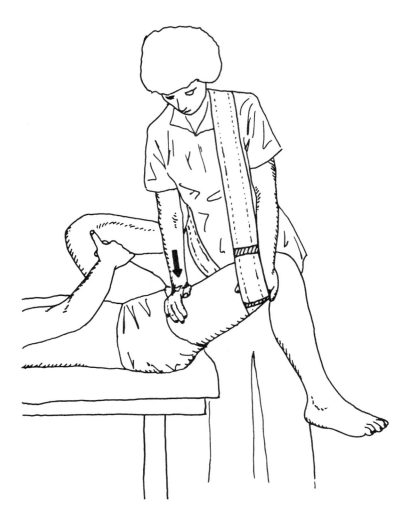

**Figure 4-12** Hip joint posterior glide in supine. (Reprinted with permission from C Kisner, LA Colby. [1990] *Therapeutic Exercise: Foundations and Techniques* [p. 199]. Philadelphia: Davis.)

up as much capsuloligamentous slack as possible before applying accessory movements is crucial to achieving significant changes in capsular flexibility and length. Some authorities state that the only joint-play movement possible at the hip is traction (Mennell 1964; Saunders 1992). However, where motion is limited, the importance of restoring arthrokinematic motion is crucial to the restoration of normal osteokinematics, and many authors advocate use of techniques in addition to traction (Grieve 1983; Kaltenborn 1989; Kisner and Colby 1990; Lee 1989; Maitland 1991; Patta 1989; Wadsworth 1988; Woodman 1993).

The patient's level of tissue reactivity should be monitored closely to ensure that technique vigor is not progressed too soon. Maitland's (1991) mnemonic is helpful:

*Severity*
*Irritability*
*Nature*
*Stage of pathology*

The *SINS* affect the grade of mobilization used (Maitland 1991):

Grade I: small amplitude at the beginning of range
Grade II: large amplitude into middle of range
Grade III: large amplitude to end range
Grade IV: small amplitude at end range

The clinician should document technique, grade, repetitions (or time), sets, response, and effect on range.

## Osteokinematics

Each of the osteokinematic or physiologic movements of flexion and extension, abduction and adduction, and internal rotation and external rotation should be performed passively if active movement is aggravating or end-range stretching is required. Consider moving through PNF patterns instead of cardinal planes for passive, active, and resistive exercise due to the simulation of functional patterns (Table 4-4). The following are useful physiologic mobilizations for the hip (see Maitland 1991 for greater detail):

- ***Flexion and adduction: useful for the moderately painful hip.
- ***Medial rotation: a frequently restricted and painful hip motion that should be tested in both flexion and extension and treated in the position of restriction (Figure 4-13).
- Lateral rotation: limitation of this motion is less common.

## Mobilization with Movement

A manual therapy concept popularized in recent years by Mulligan (1995) is the application of arthrokinematics (mobilization) to osteokinematics (movement) using functional (natural) planes. Terms that are used to

**Table 4-4** Optimal Proprioceptive Neuromuscular Facilitation Patterns for Hip Muscles with Consideration for Action on Two or More Joints

| Patterns | Muscles |
| --- | --- |
| Flexion-adduction-external rotation | Psoas major |
| (Diagonal 1 [D1] flexion) | Psoas minor |
| | Iliacus |
| | Obturator externus |
| | Pectineus |
| | Adductor longus |
| | Adductor brevis |
| With knee flexion | Gracilis |
| | Sartorius |
| Extension-abduction-internal rotation | Gluteus medius |
| (diagonal 1 [D1] extension) | Gluteus minimus |
| Flexion-abduction-internal rotation (diagonal 2 [D2] flexion) | Tensor fascia lata |
| Extension-adduction-external rotation | Gluteus maximus |
| (diagonal 2 [D2] extension) | Piriformis |
| | Obturator internus |
| | Gemellus superior |
| | Gemellus inferior |
| | Quadratus femoris |
| | Adductor magnus |

Source: Modified from DE Voss, MK Ionta, BJ Myers. (1985) *Proprioceptive Neuromuscular Facilitation: Patterns and Techniques* (3rd ed). Philadelphia: Harper & Row.

describe these techniques in treatment of the spine are *NAGS* (natural apophyseal glides) and *SNAGS* (sustained natural apophyseal glides). In the extremity joints, Mulligan refers to mobilization with movement. Whereas in the spine the facet mobilization is usually performed in the direction of the active movement, in the extremity joints the joint glide is often at right angles to the osteokinematic movement (active or passive).

Mulligan (1995) recommended performing passive hip ROM for a restricted movement while at the same time applying lateral distraction with a mobilization belt. Using the example of internal rotation, he stated, "one of the movement losses that inculpates the hip joint is internal rotation, and provided

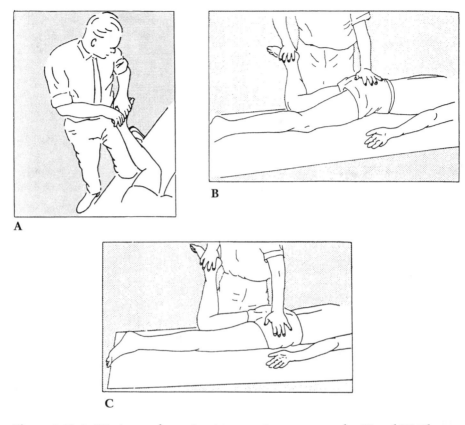

**Figure 4-13** A. Hip internal rotation in extension prone, grades III and IV. The right hip is being mobilized in A. The left hip is being mobilized in B and C. B. At end range of hip (left) internal rotation, the opposite (right) ilium will raise. C. Further range can be gained in left hip internal rotation by holding end-range and applying posteroanterior pressure or oscillations to the raised right ilium. (Reprinted with permission from GD Maitland. [1991] *Peripheral Manipulation* [3rd ed] [p. 226]. Oxford, England: Butterworth–Heinemann.)

the patient does not have too much joint deterioration on x-ray, this mobilization is excellent even if I say so myself." (Mulligan 1995, p. 103)

In addition to mobilization with movement, Mulligan described two pain release phenomenon techniques for the hip:

- Posterior glide in flexion and adduction
- Pressing knee toward plinth while in Patrick test position

When performing the pain release phenomenon, the clinician should reproduce the patient's pain and then hold the joint in that position for 20 seconds. In many cases, the patient reports dramatic relief of symptoms. Pain relief phenomena should not be used for acute conditions; it is recommended that they be used not sooner than 6 weeks after injury.

### Loose-Body Manipulation

Cyriax (1982) believed a cartilage fragment (loose body) to be a potential source of a painful limitation of motion and weightbearing. This loose body is differentiated from osteoarthritis in that it gives rise to a sudden onset of pain, whereas osteoarthritis typically results in a gradual onset of pain. The concept of loose-body manipulation can be likened to having a pebble in your shoe—you shake it around until it sits in a less painful location. Surgical removal of a loose body is only advocated if it has an osseous nucleus and can be visualized on radiograph.

The technique for "reducing" a loose body in the hip involves applying strong traction to the hip while it is in a position of 80-degrees flexion and then lowering the hip to 0-degrees flexion while maintaining the traction and applying several small-amplitude, high-velocity external rotation maneuvers. If this method is unsuccessful, then the clinician should try the same procedure using small thrusts into internal rotation. Another alternative suggested by Cyriax and Russell (1980) entails applying traction to the hip at 90-degrees flexion (with the knee also at 90-degrees flexion), passively moving the hip to the extreme of external rotation, and applying a quick, short overpressure. The effect on pain and function should be dramatic if indeed a mobile loose body is the culprit. The clinician should not persist if not effective after several attempts, but it should be repeated, as needed, if it works.

### Capsular Impingement Reduction

Anterior hip pain reproduced by the flexion and adduction test can be caused by impingement of the iliopsoas bursa or the anterior capsule. Due to the attachment of some iliopsoas fibers to the anterior capsule and the fact that the bursa communicates with the joint in 15% of cases, creating iliopsoas contractions in 90-degrees flexion can pull the impinging capsule, bursa, or both from the joint, thus, resulting in a negative retest. This is not only useful for treatment but also for differential diagnosis.

### Manual Therapy: Soft Tissue Mobilization

Soft tissue techniques can be useful in the treatment of hip dysfunction, especially for myotendon syndromes. To quote Kendall et al. (1993, p. 337), "[m]assage is often underrated and underutilized as a therapeutic measure. When applied correctly, it can be very effective in the management of musculoskeletal conditions."

Effleurage is useful in the acute and subacute stage for swelling, tissue desensitization, and relaxation of muscles. Many massage techniques (traditional and alternative) can be used with good effect in the treatment of hip and buttock pain syndromes. A common mistake in application of techniques to this region is inadequate access to the involved tissues(s). Helpful hints in this situation include (1) draping appropriately with towels and (2) having another person in the room and clearly explaining the reason for exposing the skin over the involved tissue(s). Caution: some societies and cultures deem the use of massage techniques in this region inappropriate, especially if the patient and therapist are of the opposite sex from one another.

Cyriax and Russell (1980) indicated deep friction massage (DFM) for treatment of tendinitis, tenosynovitis, strained muscle bellies, and sprained ligaments. The rationale for DFM is to "break up" scar tissue and eliminate a stress-riser source. In a chronic injury, it can also create an inflammatory response that improves local blood supply, thus accelerating healing. The chronic condition should be treated for 6–20 minutes with DFM every other day for 6–12 treatments. In the subacute phase, gentle friction massage performed for 5 minutes daily can be used to prevent excessive formation of actin-myosin crossbridges in the collagen scar. Combined with a graduated program of stretching and strengthening exercises, a strong and mobile scar should develop.

The following are important principles of DFM:

- Treatment should be directed at the precise site of the lesion.
- The massage should occur perpendicular to the tissue fibers.
- Transverse friction, not pressure, is paramount.
- The patient should be positioned to render the lesion accessible to the surface and in the appropriate amount of tension. For optimal success (1) a muscle belly lesion should be put on slack, and (2) a tendon with a sheath should be put on stretch.

Hip lesions that are commonly treated with DFM are muscle-tendon lesions of distal psoas, proximal rectus femoris, adductors, and hamstrings.

### Friction Massage Versus Steroid Injection

An alternative to deep friction massage is corticosteroid injection. Cyriax and Russell (1980) stated that steroid injection works well for tenoperiosteal lesions and bursitis, but DFM is better for musculotendinous lesions. Corticosteroid injection has the advantage of giving dramatic relief (sometimes after a couple days of soreness); however, it has a smaller mar-

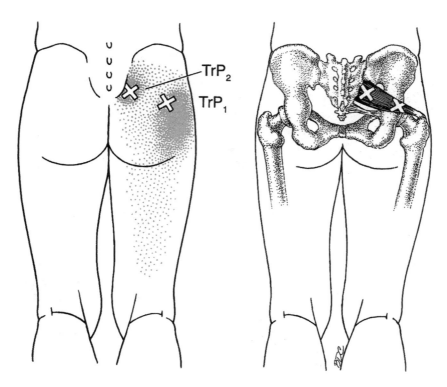

**Figure 4-14** Piriformis trigger points (TrPs) (Xs) and referral pattern. (Reprinted with permission from JG Travell, DG Simons. [1992] *Myofascial Pain and Dysfunction. The Trigger Point Manual, Volume 2, The Lower Extremities* [p. 188]. Baltimore: Williams & Wilkins.)

gin for error than DFM, and it removes the inflammation but not always the cause, which are the adhesions (Cyriax and Russell 1980). Due to the possible complications of corticosteroid injection, additional injections to the same location are spaced at least 1 month apart and limited to three in a year (Butcher et al. 1996).

### Trigger Point

Travell and Simons (1992) have added a new dimension to the understanding of myofascial syndromes. Figure 4-14 illustrates the piriformis trigger points and typical referral pattern. Trigger points are associated with myofascial syndromes and tender points with fibromyalgia (Buschbacher 1994). Trigger points can be treated with procaine injection, ischemic compression, ultrasound with electrical stimulation, strain and counterstrain, and spray and stretch (i.e., stretching preceded with a brief application of ice or Vapo coolant spray). A dry-needle technique to an iliopsoas trigger point (located in the femoral triangle, two finger breadths lateral to the femoral artery and one finger breadth below the inguinal ligament) has been described for successful treatment of "failed" low-back syndrome (Ingber 1989).

## Muscle Re-Education and Strengthening

Movement and stability go hand in hand. Mobility has been dealt with before stabilization (muscle strengthening) in this chapter based on the rationale that restoring motion needs to occur early to prevent contracture. However, regaining strength and control needs to follow soon after (e.g., a patient with an anterior pelvic tilt needs to rapidly regain abdominal strength because stretching hip flexors alone [notably rectus femoris] are not enough to correct the abnormal posture).

### Proprioceptive Neuromuscular Facilitation

PNF techniques can be used for movement re-education and muscle strengthening (slow reversals), active joint stabilization (rhythmic stabilization), and increasing flexibility (hold relax and contract relax). Although PNF methods are often labor intensive, they are useful in early stage re-education and give the therapist good feedback as to the patient's progress throughout the rehab process. PNF can be an effective technique in hamstring and quadriceps stretching, and its superior value has been demonstrated in a number of studies (Markos 1979; Prentice 1983). Incorporating rotational and oblique (functional) patterns into independent exercise programs is, in effect, applying PNF principles to active exercise.

### Normative Hip Strength

Normative values for isokinetic hip strength provide a useful target for strength training (Table 4-5). The hierarchy of hip muscle strength (regardless of age and gender) in descending order is as follows (Cahalan et al. 1989):

1. Extensors
2. Flexors
3. Adductors
4. Abductors
5. Rotators (no significant difference between internal and external rotation)

**Table 4-5** Normative Strength: Isokinetic Averages (N*m) Measured at 30, 90, 150, and 210 Degrees Per Second

| | Men | | Women | |
|---|---|---|---|---|
| Variable | Younger (20–39 years) | Older (40–81 years) | Younger (20–39 years) | Older (40–64 years) |
| Flexion | | | | |
| 30 degrees | 152 ± 50 | 113 ± 21 | 91 ± 24 | 67 ± 21 |
| 90 degrees | 126 ± 50 | 84 ± 21 | 70 ± 26 | 46 ± 17 |
| 150 degrees | 102 ± 47 | 68 ± 17 | 57 ± 17 | 37 ± 13 |
| 210 degrees | 91 ± 50 | 57 ± 20 | 46 ± 16 | 27 ± 12 |
| Extension | | | | |
| 30 degrees | 177 ± 42 | 157 ± 22 | 110 ± 22 | 101 ± 27 |
| 90 degrees | 163 ± 49 | 132 ± 32 | 97 ± 41 | 70 ± 26 |
| 150 degrees | 142 ± 49 | 122 ± 34 | 85 ± 34 | 60 ± 22 |
| 210 degrees | 125 ± 52 | 111 ± 44 | 77 ± 34 | 45 ± 21 |
| Abduction | | | | |
| 30 degrees | 103 ± 26 | 75 ± 18 | 66 ± 19 | 48 ± 14 |
| 90 degrees | 79 ± 20 | 63 ± 19 | 54 ± 20 | 38 ± 13 |
| 150 degrees | 57 ± 20 | 46 ± 15 | 43 ± 21 | 23 ± 9 |
| 210 degrees | 45 ± 20 | 32 ± 23 | 32 ± 19 | 11 ± 9 |
| Adduction | | | | |
| 30 degrees | 121 ± 26 | 99 ± 18 | 82 ± 26 | 63 ± 17 |
| 90 degrees | 103 ± 32 | 83 ± 28 | 62 ± 32 | 44 ± 19 |
| 150 degrees | 85 ± 32 | 55 ± 25 | 50 ± 25 | 25 ± 14 |
| 210 degrees | 66 ± 39 | 33 ± 26 | 39 ± 22 | 17 ± 15 |
| External rotation | | | | |
| 30 degrees | 65 ± 24 | 50 ± 15 | 43 ± 13 | 32 ± 11 |
| 90 degrees | 49 ± 24 | 38 ± 12 | 31 ± 12 | 21 ± 8 |
| 150 degrees | 43 ± 20 | 30 ± 9 | 25 ± 9 | 15 ± 5 |
| 210 degrees | 36 ± 18 | 23 ± 10 | 20 ± 7 | 12 ± 5 |
| Internal rotation | | | | |
| 30 degrees | 72 ± 17 | 61 ± 17 | 47 ± 13 | 34 ± 9 |
| 90 degrees | 53 ± 19 | 41 ± 16 | 36 ± 14 | 22 ± 7 |
| 150 degrees | 42 ± 15 | 32 ± 14 | 25 ± 9 | 15 ± 6 |
| 210 degrees | 34 ± 14 | 27 ± 14 | 22 ± 9 | 12 ± 5 |

N*m = Newton meters.

Source: Reprinted with permission from TD Cahalan, ME Johnson, S Liu, EYS Chao. (1989) Quantitative measurements of hip strength in different age groups. *Clinical Orthopaedics and Related Research* 246, 142.

Demographically, younger men produce the greatest torques, and older women produce the lowest.

The strength values of older men and younger women are similar (Tables 4-5 and 4-6). In the older elderly (older than 75 years of age), increasing age has been shown to be the most significant factor for explaining decreasing strength (Rice et al. 1989).

### Eccentric Exercise

Most functional use of hip musculature is by eccentric contraction, and a primary mechanism in chronic tendinitis is repetitive eccentric loading (Stanish et al. 1986). Therefore, it is not surprising that the three most common soft tissue disorders of the hip are gluteus medius tendinitis, trochanteric bursitis, and hamstring strain (Lloyd-Smith et al. 1985). All three injuries have been associated with eccentric muscle contractions.

The use of progressive eccentric exercise programs has been advocated as vital to successful rehabilitation (Stanish et al. 1986; Stanton and Purdam 1989). Transforming the cause (repetitive eccentric stress) into the cure (progressive repetitive eccentric loads) is the challenge of treating overuse injuries. The injured tissue must be developed into one that can successfully handle the stresses and strains of the imposed demands.

Curwin and Stanish (1984) suggested an eccentric exercise protocol that consists of the following:

- Static stretching of the involved tissue (15- to 30-second hold, repeated three to five times) performed before and after eccentric strengthening
- Eccentric exercise of involved muscle (three sets of 10 repetitions daily), with speed of contraction and resistance to contraction increased progressively as tolerated
- Ice application (crushed ice pack or ice massage) for 5–10 minutes after exercise

It is important not to exacerbate pain when implementing this program, and the therapist should consider the stage of the lesion (i.e., acute, subacute, chronic) when it is prescribed. This approach may not be appropriate for an acute lesion.

### Balance Re-Education

Human balance is maintained through a complex process that involves integration of sensory, neuromuscular, and biomechanical factors. Nashner (1990, p. 5) stated that, "the basic task of balance is to position the center of gravity (COG) over some portion of the support base (i.e., the feet while standing or the buttocks while seated)."

**Table 4-6** Normative Strength: Isometric Data (N*m)

| | Men | | Women | |
| --- | --- | --- | --- | --- |
| Variable | Younger (20–39 years) | Older (40–81 years) | Younger (20–39 years) | Older (40–64 years) |
| Flexion | | | | |
| 10 degrees | 167 ± 30 | 166 ± 37 | 105 ± 26 | 86 ± 24 |
| 45 degrees | 108 ± 23 | 89 ± 23 | 66 ± 16 | 51 ± 18 |
| Extension | | | | |
| 45 degrees | 160 ± 42 | 156 ± 65 | 95 ± 35 | 82 ± 27 |
| 90 degrees | 204 ± 50 | 203 ± 70 | 126 ± 45 | 110 ± 34 |
| Abduction | | | | |
| 10 degrees | 120 ± 23 | 108 ± 26 | 81 ± 19 | 69 ± 20 |
| 0 degrees | 108 ± 19 | 90 ± 19 | 72 ± 17 | 55 ± 20 |
| 10 degrees | 89 ± 18 | 73 ± 22 | 55 ± 15 | 46 ± 22 |
| Adduction | | | | |
| 0 degrees | 83 ± 27 | 77 ± 26 | 58 ± 19 | 49 ± 17 |
| 10 degrees | 111 ± 26 | 104 ± 29 | 70 ± 26 | 59 ± 17 |
| 20 degrees | 129 ± 29 | 107 ± 33 | 79 ± 30 | 62 ± 19 |
| External rotation | | | | |
| 10 degrees internal rotation | 67 ± 21 | 65 ± 20 | 47 ± 13 | 36 ± 8 |
| 0 degrees | 62 ± 21 | 54 ± 14 | 38 ± 9 | 31 ± 7 |
| Internal rotation | | | | |
| 10 degrees external rotation | 85 ± 25 | 75 ± 24 | 58 ± 13 | 45 ± 12 |
| 0 degrees | 68 ± 22 | 62 ± 18 | 46 ± 13 | 34 ± 11 |

N*m = Newton meters.
Source: Reprinted with permission from TD Cahalan, ME Johnson, S Liu, EYS Chao. (1989) Quantitative measurements of hip strength in different age groups. *Clinical Orthopaedics and Related Research* 246, 142.

Motor control research has identified three equilibrium strategies for standing balance control (Nashner 1990):

- Ankle strategy: large, slow movements of the COG occurring about the ankle joints
- Hip strategy: small, quick movements of the COG occurring at the hips
- Stepping strategy: when the COG moves to the limit of the support base or beyond, there comes a point when neither the hip nor ankle strategy is able to maintain balance and a step or stumble is required to set a new reference of support and prevent a fall (Figure 4-15).

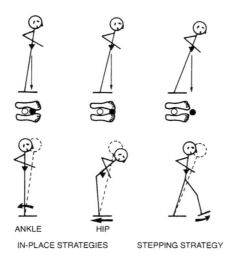

ANKLE               HIP

IN-PLACE STRATEGIES        STEPPING STRATEGY

**Figure 4-15** Strategies for regaining equilibrium. Triangles reflect center of gravity position. Dashed-line figures represent positions after a perturbation. Solid figures represent equilibrium positions after corrective movements. When the center of gravity remains over the base of support, the ankle or hip strategies can be used to return the body to vertical without moving the feet. For larger displacement of the center of gravity, a stepping or stumbling strategy is necessary to restore equilibrium. (Reprinted with permission from LM Nashner. [1990] Sensory, Neuromuscular, and Biomechanical Contributions to Human Balance. In PW Duncan [ed], *Balance: Proceedings of the APTA Forum, Nashville, June, 1989* [p. 6]. Alexandria, VA: American Physical Therapy Association.)

One-leg stance is the most frequently occurring posture in humans, based on the fact that during gait (our most frequent activity) humans are in one-leg stance on the right and left legs for 60–85% of the time. Muscles that maintain this posture are, therefore, true postural muscles (Janda 1983). Testing one-leg stance is not only useful for testing and training of balance but also a crucial functional test (Trendelenburg test) and training method for abductor strength. To measure the posture of one-leg stance, a plumb line or postural grid is recommended to measure deviation from midline and as training feedback together with a mirror. A positive test for hip abductor weakness is termed either *compensated* or *noncompensated Trendelenburg*. (See Chapter 3 for more information on the Trendelenburg test.) A positive test for single-leg balance (younger than the age of 50 years) is the inability to stand unsupported on one leg for longer than 30 seconds.

Bohannon et al. (1984) provided the following age-related normative data for timed one-leg stance (for men and women):

50–59 years: 29.4 seconds (standard deviation [SD] 2.9)
60–69 years: 22.5 seconds (SD 8.6)
70–70 years: 14.2 seconds (SD 9.3)

Balance re-education should be performed when single-leg balance is below these values. Tinetti (1986) defines abnormal one-leg stance in the elderly as the inability to balance on one leg longer than 5 seconds. Along with other performance-oriented findings, she proposed that this is an indicator for intervention. A person younger than 50 years of age with single-leg balance less than 30 seconds should probably also undergo balance training, especially if there is a marked difference between right and left sides.

Balance drills include

- One-leg standing time
- Heel-to-toe stepping
- Side-stepping
- Backward walking
- Rhythmic stabilization in double stance
- Throwing and catching a ball (Patient should be required to reach progressively further outside base.)
- Resisted hip movements while standing on involved and noninvolved limbs (This enables eccentric as well as concentric training and closed chain as well as open chain rehabilitation.)
- Resisted one-third knee bends with elastic tubing (e.g., sports cord), progressing from double stance to single-leg stance
- One-leg stance with vibration of Body Blade in front and to the side for as long as the client is able (an excellent balance challenge)

The progression of these balance drills is as follows:

- Eyes open to eyes closed
- Firm surface to soft surface (e.g., pillow)
- Stationary surface to moving surface (e.g., balance board)

Current motor control research suggests that there is limited carryover of practice of gait components to gait itself (Winstein 1990). This implies that gait itself should be rehearsed, not only the component parts. However, one need only look to the arts and sports to see that practice of component parts is still necessary. What great musician did not practice scales? What great athlete trains by only playing his or her sport?

Enthusiasm for use of the eccentric, closed-chain, functional one-leg stance should, however, be balanced with the understanding that single-leg standing exercises are among the most stressful activities to the human hip (Tackson 1996). Moderation is therefore key.

### Aquatics

Aquatics is also referred to as *pool therapy*, *hydrotherapy*, and *water therapy*. Water is an excellent medium for rehabilitation of hip patients, namely for its load-reducing capabilities. Pool therapy has the following general benefits:

- Reducing joint-compression forces
- Improving mobility due to relaxation and decreased pain
- Allowing finely graded progressive resisted exercise using water to assist or resist movement
- Improving coordination and balance due to a different challenge than dry land
- Cardiovascular benefits without the joint stresses of land exercise
- Positive effect on mood
- Excellent medium for rehabilitation when pain, weakness, weightbearing status, or any combination of these is a limiting factor to land therapy

The following are disadvantages of pool therapy:

- Stabilization of body parts is more difficult in water than on dry land.
- Contraindications and precautions include open wounds, infection, cardiac conditions and high blood pressure, chronic obstructive pulmonary disease, fear of water, fever, and seizure disorder.
- The cost of building and maintaining a pool is high.
- A high ratio of staff to patients is usually required.

Therapy in the water should not be considered a rarity or left to complicated cases that are not responding to therapy on land. It should always be considered as a therapeutic option, particularly in rehabilitation of the hip due to the negation of ground reaction load. Figure 4-16 illustrates the effect that different levels of immersion have on weightbearing status. Walking and running in water are especially popular (Awbrey 1995). Swimming itself has many benefits and is encouraged whenever tolerated (Thomas 1989).

The physical properties of water that are used in aquatics are as follows:

1. Buoyancy. *Buoyancy* is an upward force acting in the opposite direction to gravity. It is based on Archimedes' principle, which states that

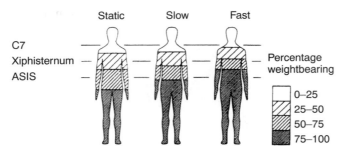

**Figure 4-16** Partial weightbearing at different levels of immersion. (ASIS = anterior superior iliac spine.) (Reprinted with permission from RA Harrison, M Hillman, S Bulstrode. [1992] Loading the lower limb when walking partially submersed: Implications for clinical practice. *Physiotherapy* 78, 166.)

a partially or fully immersed body will experience an upward thrust equal to the weight of the fluid it displaces. The buoyancy of each body part is not equal as a result of varying specific gravity values. For example, the chest area tends to float due to the decreased specific gravity caused by air in the lungs. Likewise, the higher specific gravity of the pelvis and lower extremities requires the use of flotation devices to keep the body horizontal. *Specific gravity* (or relative density) is the ratio of an object's mass to water's mass. Using equipment, such as floats, the effect of buoyancy can be adjusted to make an exercise more or less challenging. Thus, patients can perform buoyancy-supported, buoyancy-assisted, and buoyancy-resisted exercises.

2. Hydrostatic pressure. *Hydrostatic pressure* is based on Pascal's law, which states that the pressure of a fluid is exerted on an object equally at a given depth; this pressure increases with the density of a fluid and with its depth. Exercising in water can thus help to prevent venous pooling and control dependent edema.

3. Viscosity. *Viscosity* is a fluid's resistance to the adjacent fluid layers sliding by one another, which occurs only with motion. The basis for aquatic strengthening programs is that water is more viscous than air; therefore, there is more resistance to movement in water than on land. The resistance to movement can be increased by increasing the speed of movement in water.

4. Hydrodynamic forces. *Hydrodynamic forces* are different types of resistive force that can be created in water (see Figure 4-16). By increasing the velocity (the effect of laminar flow), the surface area (effect of frontal resistance or turbulent flow), or both of the body

part being moved through water, the resistance to movement can be increased. Pressure differentials created by turbulent flow result in drag, which can be used to assist or resist movement (more tapered structures have less drag).

The following is useful equipment for pool therapy:

- Rescue tubes
- Inner tubes
- Swim bars
- Arm floats
- Neck floats
- Wet vest
- Hand paddles
- Pull buoys
- Paddles
- Kick boards
- Fins
- Plastic milk jugs
- Balls
- Resisted tubing

Because humans live on the land, function in water is only as good as it translates to function on land (McLaughlin 1996). Therefore, aquatics should be an adjunct in rehabilitation and not the only intervention.

### Lumbo-Pelvic-Hip

Understanding that the hip is part of a six-joint complex consisting of two hip joints, two sacroiliac joints, the lumbosacral junction, and the pubic symphysis is a crucial concept to grasp and incorporate into evaluation and management. This is a complex issue, and, although the scope of this book only allows for it to be touched on briefly, the reader is strongly encouraged to view the hip joint as a part of the lumbopelvic complex. Much like the glenohumeral articulation is viewed as part of the shoulder complex.

### Get Hip!

Several articles entitled "Get hip!" have appeared in lay magazines, namely *Skiing* (Larsson 1991, 1994) and *Golf* (Prichard 1993). The hip region is of fundamental importance not only for golf and skiing but also for skating, gymnastics, ballet, hammer throwing, pole vaulting, and weight lifting, to name a few.

*Skiing: Hip Counterrotation*

Hip counterrotation is also known as *hip angulation* or *reverse shoulder*. Larsson (1991, 1994) provided a series of exercises and drills for teaching and improving hip counterrotation in skiing. Although Larsson referred to the technique as *hip counterrotation*, it is in fact the ability to dissociate movement of the upper half from the lower half of the body (i.e., lumbo-pelvic-hip control). Control of the lumbo-pelvic-hip area is crucial for effective skiing. Reasons for the hip region being crucial to effective skiing are (Larsson 1991, 1994):

- This area is the junction between what should be independent upper and lower body movements.
- The hip region is near the center of mass for the body and is thus important for balance.
- The powerful muscles about the hip can make edging the skis much more effective.
- Use of the hips for edging lessens the stresses on the knees and can decrease knee injuries.

*Golf: Internal Hip Rotation*

Prichard (1993, p. 78) reported the findings of sports (golf) mechanics and flexibility research, stating that "how you swing is largely determined by 20 ranges of motion in your body. Key among the ranges is internal hip rotation [IHR]. Increase IHR and you'll hit the ball longer and eliminate a major cause of back problems."

**Body Mechanics**

An important component in rehabilitation of the hip is training correct body mechanics. Recent research suggests that the classic mechanical advice taught for back injury prevention (i.e., bend the knees, create a wide base with the feet, and keep the back straight) creates greater hip pressures than lifting with the back (i.e., spare the back and spoil the hip [Luepongsak et al. 1997]). It may be that the answer lies in the little known concept proposed by Vasey and Crozier (1977, 1982) that was developed in response to an increase in industrial back injuries despite body mechanics education. This concept is based on neurophysiologic (reflexive) principles, in addition to mechanical principles. Vasey and Crozier identified two basic whole-body movement patterns defined by the initial movement:

- Top-heavy movement. The trunk and arms move first, while the legs stay straight and stiff

- Base movement. (1) The initial movement is one of relaxation of the knees (lowering the center of gravity), followed by (2) moving a foot in the direction the body would fall if equilibrium were lost (widening the base of support), followed by (3) bending of the back (to get close to the object to be lifted). Then (4) a palmar hold (i.e., from below) is taken on the object (preventing a stiffening reaction through the arms into the neck caused by gripping from above), and, (5) as the lift is executed, unwinding occurs with movement of the head first (a neurodevelopmental response that also relieves tension on the low back by shortening one end of the spinal column).

Base movement should occur as a dynamic functional pattern incorporating momentum to decrease strain on the body parts. Integral to success is conditioning the individual from a top-heavy–movement reflex to a base-movement reflex. Incorporating such principles should spare the back *and* the hip.

Obviously, advice such as "don't lift anything too heavy," "test the load before you lift," and "ask for help if needed" should also be incorporated.

### Orthotics

Orthotic devices used for hip patients include a hip-abduction brace as prevention against hip dislocation, shoe raise, heel insert, medial heel wedge, and an arch support for pronating feet. Pronating feet allows for excessive hip internal rotation during gait.

A new type of orthotic device for hip fracture prevention is hip-protection padding. Such pads have been shown to decrease the rate of hip fracture from falls in nursing home residents (Lauritzen et al. 1993).

### Biofeedback

The role of biofeedback in hip rehabilitation is as an adjunct to motor learning and muscle re-education. For example, a patient with weak hip abductors can have electromyogram electrodes applied over the gluteus medius to encourage normal recruitment of this muscle during gait and exercise. Attaching another set of electrodes on the normal side provides the patient with a normative comparison. Where abductors are affected bilaterally, a demonstration of normal muscle response can be done on a nonaffected individual. In patients who overuse tensor fascia lata, biofeedback can be used to facilitate recruitment of gluteus medius fibers. Use of biofeedback in hip rehabilitation is certainly an area for future research.

A limb-load monitor is a biofeedback device that can be used for weight-bearing re-education (Betts and Watson 1992). This is described in Chapter 6.

**Electrical and Physical Modalities**

Modalities can be useful adjunctive interventions and, if used appropriately, can greatly enhance the therapeutic effect. Described here are frequently used methods in the treatment of hip dysfunction.

*Cold*

Ice packs are recommended in the acute phase after an injury or surgery. As with other body parts, 20–30 minutes of ice repeated every 2 hours can relieve pain and spasm and minimize swelling. Alternatively, maintaining a constant cool environment with commercially available temperature-controlled blankets is effective (Cohn et al. 1989). Cold application can also be used at other phases in rehabilitation and can be most appropriate after a vigorous exercise session.

*Heat*

Conductive methods of heat application are popular with the arthritis population. Moist heat in the form of hydrocolator pads for 20 minutes can be soothing and is often used as a preliminary (warm-up) to exercise with irritable conditions. Use of heat is not advised until at least 72 hours after an injury.

*Ultrasound*

Although touted as the best modality for treatment of hip ligaments and capsule due to the deep penetration at 1 MHz frequency, there is little in vivo research to support this. For the effects of ultrasound to reach the hip capsuloligamentous complex, obviously a 1 MHz frequency should be used as it is capable of heating tissues 2.5–5.0 cm deep. A frequency of 3 MHz should be employed for tissues less than 2.5 cm from the skin (Draper et al. 1995). Recent research suggests that there is a critical window of opportunity after ultrasound of about 3 minutes, during which the tissues remain sufficiently warm and therefore capable of the stretching gains attributed to increased temperature (Draper and Ricard 1995). This "stretching window" can be expanded by starting mobilization (soft tissue, joint, or both) during the last few minutes of ultrasound application. Also of note is that the loss of heat in the deeper tissues (1 MHz) is about twice as slow as in the superficial tissues (3 MHz), so that the stretching window for hip capsule, ligaments, and deep muscles after continuous ultrasound at 1 MHz is about 6 minutes (Rose et al 1996).

*Phonophoresis*

Phonophoresis is the technique in which ultrasound energy is used to drive anti-inflammatory drugs and local analgesics through the skin into the underlying tissue. Most frequently, 10% hydrocortisone cream is used. Phonophoresis is used for treatment of localized inflammation (e.g., trochanteric bursitis).

### Iontophoresis

Iontophoresis is the technique of transmitting ions into the tissues using a continuous low-voltage direct current. It has the advantage over injection in that it is noninvasive, is less painful, and does not result in tissue damage as overuse of steroid injection can. It is most applicable at the hip for localized and superficial inflammation associated with trochanteric bursitis and gluteus medius tendinitis.

### Electrical Stimulation

Electrical stimulation is best used when a voluntary contraction of a muscle cannot be achieved. Electrical stimulation about the hip is not used as frequently as it is for quadriceps weakness at the knee.

### Interferential Therapy

Interferential therapy uses two medium-frequency alternating currents that, at their point of intersection, produce a low-frequency therapeutic effect in the tissues. Its use is indicated for any combination of pain, muscle spasm, swelling, and trigger points. A text on interferential therapy states that, "treatment of the osteoarthritic hip is particularly rewarding." (Savage 1984, p. 76) The protocol suggested by Savage (1984) suggests placing the patient in sidelying and using vacuum electrodes if available, because they are easier to secure around the hip. The recommended treatment duration and frequency are as follows: treat for 7 minutes at a constant sedative frequency of 100 Hz or 130 Hz, followed by 7 minutes of 10–100 Hz sweep, followed by moving the electrodes to treat the lumbosacral spine with a 10–100 Hz sweep (Figure 4-17). Treatment should precede exercise, as pain is less after treatment, which enables gains in ROM. Treatment two to three times per week for 12 treatments is recommended. No research evidence was provided to support these claims. An expert in the field of electrotherapy has noted, however, that interferential therapy is no more than glorified transcutaneous electrical nerve stimulation (TENS) (Alon 1995).

### Transcutaneous Electrical Nerve Stimulation

The advantage of TENS over other modalities is the portable nature of the device. As with other modalities, TENS should not be considered a cure-all, but it can be a useful adjunctive intervention and gives many patients significant relief.

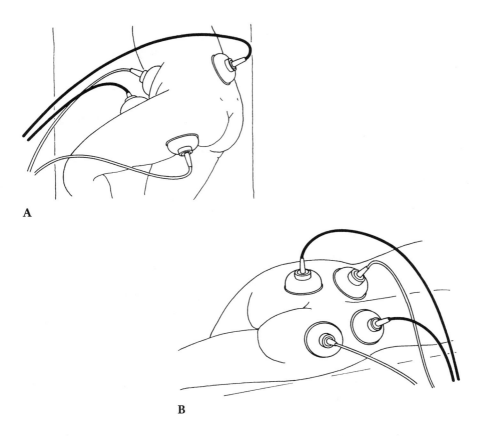

**Figure 4-17** A. Osteoarthritic hip treated using vacuum electrodes. B. Osteo-arthritic hip: treating the lumbar spine as an adjunct to the hip treatment. (Reprinted with permission from B Savage. [1984] *Interferential Therapy* [p. 77]. London: Faber & Faber.)

*Mind-Body Effect*

The placebo effect is frequently found to explain more than the often quoted one-third of treatment effectiveness (Turner et al. 1994). The patient's belief in the treatment, the healer, or both is seen as the vital factor. If a patient or physical therapist (ideally both) have a strong belief in a form of treatment, then it is more likely to be effective. The master clinician no doubt wields placebo to its greatest effect! A most engaging and strongly recommended reading on the mind-body subject is *Timeless Healing: The Power of Biology and Belief* by Benson and Stark (1996).

**Advice and Education**

Involving the patient as an active partner in the rehabilitation process is crucial to long-term success. Clinicians must teach patients how to help themselves. This requires that the clinician act more as a coach and less as a healer. Patient education tips include

- Educate patients as to the nature of their condition and what can reasonably be expected from physical therapy.
- Adapt your approach to different patient populations and levels of understanding of physical therapy procedures.
- Avoid teaching too much too soon, three to five exercises performed correctly is better than a dozen that the patient does not perform at all or does with poor form.
- Tailor exercises to the patient's specific needs not just a generic list.
- Involve the patient in the setting of goals and planning a home program.
- Give written instructions—patients forget.
- Gain the patient's confidence and cooperation with your knowledge and handling of their case, as well as their limbs.

## Conclusion

This chapter has provided an overview of common methods used in rehabilitation of the hip in the outpatient setting. Accurately diagnosing the dysfunction, planning a logical intervention, skillfully carrying out the treatment measures, and frequently reassessing effect are the hallmarks of effective rehabilitation.

Although frequency and duration of treatment has not been addressed in this chapter, given the natural history of many disorders, settling, for example, for physical therapy two or three times per week for 6 weeks as may be dictated by an insurance company may not only be inappropriate but also wasteful. Following some patients for 8–12 visits over 6 months or even 1 year may be a much more rational approach. Faulty posture, muscle imbalances, and movement disorders rarely resolve in 6 weeks. These are habits, and habits are hard to change (Kendall et al. 1993; Snyder-Mackler 1996).

# 5

# Surgeries of the Hip: The Approaches and the Basics

Andrew A. Shinar

This chapter covers details of the most common surgeries performed about the hip, focusing on the surgical approaches involved and their relation to postoperative physical therapy. As hip surgery is complex and replete with controversy, I have attempted to meld the views of most hip surgeons with mine. I do not intend this text to be fully complete or dogmatic. A scholarly dissertation would not be as helpful to a physical therapist in my opinion as is this summary view of how most hip surgeons work.

## Total Hip Arthroplasty

Modern hip replacements were developed in the late 1950s and have since evolved in surgical approaches, implants, and postoperative care. Consequently, surgeons use a wide variety of methods today to implant more than 120,000 total hip prostheses in the United States per year (National Institutes of Health 1994). The basic technique of total hip arthroplasty (THA), a synonym for total hip replacement (THR), has been present since the late 1950s. Surgeons have benefited from the decades of experience and now understand the procedure well. THA is most often performed for osteoarthritis (degenerative arthritis) but can also be performed for other types of hip arthritis, including the following:

- Inflammatory arthritis
  Rheumatoid arthritis (adult or juvenile)
  Lupus
  Psoriatic arthritis
  Ankylosing spondylitis
- Avascular necrosis (osteonecrosis)
- Fractured hips with pre-existing arthritis

- Osteoarthritis secondary to forms of developmental dysplasia ranging from congenital dislocation of the hip to hip subluxation to more mild hip dysplasia
- Post-traumatic arthritis (i.e., osteoarthritis after proximal femur or acetabular fractures)
- Postinfectious arthritis
- Benign and malignant bone tumors
- Osteoarthritis secondary to Paget's disease

Many of these categories overlap. Their common feature is pain and stiffness due to the loss of hip cartilage, the hallmarks of hip arthritis. For the subsequent replacement to be effective, the surgeon must be certain that hip arthritis rather than another condition is responsible for the bulk of the preoperative hip pain. Other conditions that can mimic the pain from hip arthritis include sequelae of spine arthritis (e.g., spinal stenosis, degenerative disk disease), trochanteric and iliopectineal bursitis, and occult fractures or tumors.

Alternatives to hip replacement include the following:

- Observation
- Altered activity
- Ambulation supports
- Wheelchair
- Physical therapy
- Analgesics
- Injections
- Arthroscopic debridement
- Femoral osteotomy
- Pelvic osteotomy

Some of these alternatives can be useful to delay or even avert hip replacement. Choosing them over hip replacement is a complex decision based on the age of the patient, the expected effectiveness of these alternatives, and the risk involved with hip replacement.

The timing of surgery varies greatly and is ultimately a cost-benefit decision made by the patient: Is the pain and lack of function experienced severe enough to warrant major surgery and its risks? There is no specific amount of cartilage loss that causes the surgeon to decide to operate.

There are no discrete age limits. In the young, considerations center mainly on whether the hip replacement will last a lifetime and the subsequent consequences of requiring revisions throughout the patient's life. In the elderly, considerations center on whether the patient's medical condition allows him or her to withstand the surgery and whether the patient's expected remaining years of life warrant such surgery.

Once the patient chooses hip replacement surgery, the surgeon's preoperative goal is to optimize the patient's condition such that he or she can likely tolerate the surgery. Medical clearance is obtained, infections are cleared, and blood can be autologously donated. The surgery is performed under spinal, epidural, or general anesthesia.

## Approaches for Total Hip Replacement

Each surgeon is faced with a number of compromises when choosing an approach for THR. Factors in the decision making include the following:

- Adequacy of the exposure
- Consequences for the patient in obtaining such exposure
- Ease of the hip replacement
- Ease of the repair of the interval through which the surgery is performed
- The training and customs of the surgeon

This chapter divides approaches into two major groups—anterior and posterior—depending only on how the femur is positioned when the stem is inserted. Approaches are further divided as to how the abductors and trochanter are handled. This is done because most postoperative problems depend on whether it is the anterior or posterior intervals that are dissected and how the abductors are mobilized and repaired. Such a division simplifies the nomenclature and makes the titles of the approaches more precise.

The traditional nomenclature can be quite confusing. Approaches that are termed *anterior* in this chapter are frequently called *lateral* or *anterolateral* to distinguish them from the traditional anterior approach that is rarely used in North America. Similarly, this chapter uses *posterior* to refer to approaches that are frequently termed *posterolateral*. Furthermore, the names of the original descriptors of these approaches are frequently used to denote them. Surgeons have modified the subdivisions of these approaches as well and frequently refer to their modifications with various titles. Table 5-1 compares the division of approaches used in this chapter to other terms frequently used.

## Anatomic Considerations in Total Hip Replacement

The anatomy of the hip has been presented in Chapter 1. With regard to surgically exposing the acetabulum and proximal femur, the main anatomic considerations include the following:

- Retracting the gluteus maximus

**Table 5-1**    Anterior and Posterior Surgical Approaches

| Traditional terms | Described in this chapter as |
| --- | --- |
| Traditional anterior (Smith-Peterson 1917) | Anterior approach (not covered) |
| Anterolateral (Watson-Jones approach) | Anterior approach: no osteotomy |
| Standard trochanteric osteotomy | Anterior approach: standard trochanteric osteotomy |
| Direct lateral (Hardinge 1982) | Anterior approach: no osteotomy |
| Modified trochanteric osteotomy (Dall approach) | Anterior approach: modified trochanteric osteotomy |
| Posterior | Posterior approach |
| Posterolateral (Austin-Moore approach) | Posterior approach |

- Mobilizing the gluteus medius and minimus
- Excising or mobilizing the capsule
- Avoiding substantial bleeding
- Avoiding stretch or direct trauma to the sciatic or femoral nerves

With regards to optimizing the end result, anatomic issues relate to the following:

- Repair of the abductors (and trochanter or both) and capsule
- Ensuring proper tissue tension
- Reproducing or enhancing offset of the abductor musculature (Figure 5-1)

The main obstacle to proper exposure of the hip joint is the abductor mechanism: the gluteus medius and minimus. The gluteus maximus overlies the hip joint as well but is easily bypassed by either splitting its fibers proximally or releasing its tendon distally. The medius and minimus, however, cover the anterior capsule and femoral neck and must be either avoided with a posterior approach or repaired after an anterior approach. The cost of failure of repair is a greater tendency toward limp or dislocation. The posterior approach averts this risk by dividing the short external rotators instead of the abductors but increases the risk of dislocation.

Thus, both anterior and posterior approaches can provide excellent exposure of the hip in standard arthroplasty, but each introduces a different risk. Surgeons base their choice of approach on the following:

- Which risk, dislocation or limp, they think is more important

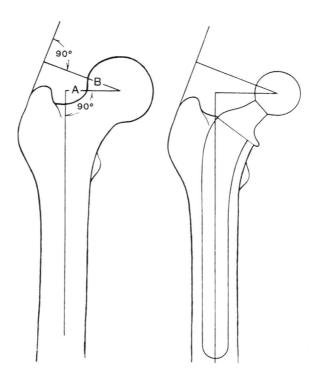

**Figure 5-1** Diagram of measurement of the offset of the abductor mechanism before and after hip replacement. *Offset* refers to the perpendicular distance (A) between the center line of the femoral component and the center of rotation of the femoral head. *Abductor lever arm* refers to the perpendicular distance (B) between the center of the femoral head and the line through which the abductor muscles work. (Reprinted with permission from B Steinberg, WH Harris. [1992] The "offset" problem in total hip arthroplasty. *Contemporary Orthopaedics* 24, 557.)

- How well they think they can control the other risks
- How expeditiously the procedure can be performed
- How familiar the surgeon and the operating room staff is with the approach

These factors are interrelated: A surgeon and staff accustomed to an approach perform the surgery with more alacrity and are more adept at minimizing the limitations of the approach (i.e., the risk of dislocation with a posterior approach or of limp with an anterior approach).

### Posterior Approach

As mentioned in the previous section, the great advantage of the posterior approach is its avoidance of the abductor mechanism. The price it pays is a higher dislocation rate, triple that of the anterior approaches (Morrey 1992).

The patient is placed in a lateral decubitus position. The standard posterior approach uses a curved incision extending from the buttock, over the greater trochanter, and along the lateral aspect of the proximal femur. After the skin incision and division of the subcutaneous tissue, the iliotibial tract is incised distally in line with the incision. The gluteus maximus then overlies the hip. It can then be either incised in line with its fibers or retracted posteriorly after developing the interval between it and the tensor fascia lata. When the greater trochanter is reached, its bursa is incised.

The anterior and posterior borders of the gluteus medius then become evident. With the superior aspect of the right greater trochanter viewed as 12 o'clock, the posterior border of the medius is in the 10 o'clock position, and the anterior border is at about 4 o'clock. The abductors rest far more anteriorly than posteriorly (Figure 5-2). The interval between the short external rotators and the posterior border of the medius is then developed. The most superior short external rotator, the piriformis, is identified by its stout tendon inserting near the posterior greater trochanter and is incised at its insertion. With the piriformis retracted, an interval between the posterior capsule and the more inferior muscles (i.e., the superior and inferior gemelli and the obturator internus) is developed. These three muscles are similarly incised at their attachments to the femur and are retracted posteriorly. While the piriformis usually lies superficial (posterior) to the sciatic nerve, the gemelli and obturator internus lie deep (interior) to it (Beaton and Anson 1937). Thus, gentle posterior retraction of these three muscles forms a layer of protection over the nerve, which in standard primary cases lies about halfway between the greater trochanter and the ischial tuberosity. Two more short external rotators then require incision: the muscular quadratus femoris and the tendinous obturator externus. The quadratus contains the largest blood supply to the femoral head, the medial circumflex artery; thus, the surgeon encounters this vessel or its branches when incising the quadratus. After the obturator externus is incised, a sponge can be used to bluntly separate the inferior capsule from more inferior structures.

With a retractor placed beneath the gluteus minimus and medius superiorly and the sponge inferiorly, the surgeon now has access to over half of the hip capsule. If capsular excision is chosen, the capsule is removed from the femoral neck and excised down to the rim of the acetabulum both infe-

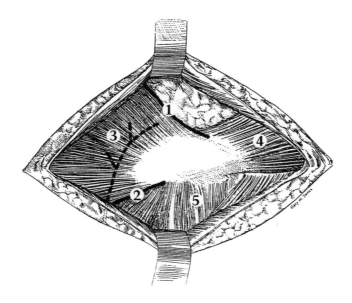

**Figure 5-2** Drawing of the abductors inserting on the greater trochanter of the right hip. 1. The anterior border of the abductors. 2. The posterior border of the abductors. 3. The course of the superior gluteal nerve and its branches within the abductors. 4. The vastus lateralis muscle distally. 5. The short external rotators. (Adapted from ID Learmonth, PE Allen. [1996] The omega approach to the hip. *Journal of Bone and Joint Surgery* 78, 559.)

riorly and superiorly. If capsular retention is chosen, it must be similarly removed from the femoral neck, then incised in line with the femoral neck, and retracted with sutures placed in its corners. Its presence makes the placement of reamers in the acetabulum more difficult.

Before the next step, dislocating the hip, many surgeons create reference points on the pelvis and the femur, so that the amount of change in leg length, offset, or both can be gauged when trial components are placed. These are usually created by placing pins in the pelvis, marking the femur with electrocautery, and making a measure between these two points.

The hip is dislocated with internal rotation, flexion, and lateral pull on the femoral neck. An estimation of the proper femoral neck length to preserve when the head is removed is then made. The surgeon can then either place a metal template on the back of the femur and measure from the top of the femoral head or greater trochanter or can mark the femoral neck at a predetermined distance superior to the lesser trochanter. The femoral neck is then cut with a saw, and the head is removed.

The anterior capsule must be released or excised to retract the femur anteriorly away from the acetabulum when reaming it. The acetabulum is then prepared by reaming with the femur retracted anteriorly. If an uncemented cup is chosen, its metal shell is fixed with screws or by precise fit (i.e., press fit), and a plastic liner is fitted. If the surgeon chooses to cement, the acetabulum is filled with bone cement. Usually, an all-plastic cup is then placed.

The femoral canal is then prepared with the leg held in internal rotation. If the surgeon chooses to place a femoral component without cement, the canal is first reamed, and the proximal metaphyseal bone is sculpted to allow good fit of the trial components. (If the surgeon chooses to cement, reaming of the canal is usually not necessary.) The proximal bone is then sculpted, and trial components are placed. A judgment is made as to the stability of the reconstruction and the length of the leg. If adequate, the final components are then placed by tamping an uncemented stem into the canal or by filling the canal with cement and then placing a stem. Fracture of the femur can occur with either type of reconstruction, but it is more common with uncemented stems due to the necessity of fitting the stem tightly in the canal. If fracture occurs and is recognized, the split femur is exposed by stripping the vastus musculature from it and is usually fixed with circular cables or wires.

When the reconstruction is complete, the split in the posterior capsule is sutured if it has been preserved. It can then be attached to the greater trochanter through drill holes. The piriformis, gemelli, obturator internus, or any combination of these can be reattached to the gluteus medius or to the trochanter through drill holes. The obturator externus and quadratus are generally not repaired to the femur and are left unattached. The fascia overlying the gluteus maximus, its tendon (if cut), and the iliotibial tract are repaired anatomically.

### Posterior Approach Strengths

The great strength of the posterior approach is its preservation of the abductor attachment, which thus requires no repair and also aids rehabilitation.

### Posterior Approach Weaknesses

The greatest weakness of the posterior approach is its propensity for dislocation. Surgeons attempt to prevent dislocation while still using the posterior approach by preserving the capsule, repairing of the short external rotators, or completely excising the capsule. The choice between these options depends on what the surgeon views as the main cause of dislocation. If the surgeon thinks that posterior laxity from the absence of capsule is the cause, he or she preserves and repairs the capsule. On the other hand, if he or she believes that excessive soft tissue present around the hip joint causes impingement and dislocation, he or she excises the capsule. If the surgeon thinks that weakness of external rotation plays a role, he or she repairs the short external rotators. These measures may not be as important as proper component positioning, which is facilitated by wide exposure, which is itself aided by capsular excision. Each surgeon weighs these factors and his or her estimation of their practicality.

The proximity of the sciatic nerve, which can be stretched by excessive lengthening of the leg or excessive retraction of the short external rotators, is also a weakness of the posterior approach. Direct injury with this approach is rare with standard primary surgery. The sciatic nerve's position, however, is much less predictable in revision surgery; thus, the risk of direct injury in revisions is much greater.

Additional weaknesses of the posterior approach include the following: (1) The position of the incision, as compared to that used in anterior approaches, is closer to the rectum. This is especially a concern in patients likely to have fecal incontinence postoperatively. (2) The leg must be held in internal rotation during femoral preparation, which is much more difficult and can compromise sterility. (3) Substantial bleeding from the medial circumflex vessels lying within the quadratus femoris is possible.

## Anterior Approaches

The traditional "anterior" approach, which involved positioning the patient supine and removing the abductors from their origin on the iliac crest (Smith-Petersen 1917), is rarely used in North America for hip replacement; therefore, it is not discussed in this chapter. The common feature of the anterior approaches discussed in this chapter is the mobilization of the abductor mechanism, which allows the surgeon to place the femoral stem with the hip held in external rotation. This positioning is of great advantage during the surgery, as the foot and calf point downward and not near the assistant's face as with the posterior approach. The assistant can keep the leg reliably still and sterile in a bag attached to the front of the table.

The great postoperative advantage of the anterior approaches is the reduced rate of dislocation, which probably results from the preservation of the posterior capsular and muscular structures. The solid repair of the anterior structures is more feasible with some of these anterior approaches than with others; however, even when the repair is not solid, the dislocation rate is lower than with posterior approaches. This probably relates to the different mechanism by which the hip is dislocated postoperatively with anterior and posterior approaches. Though anterior and posterior dislocations occur with either approach, the greater danger is posterior dislocation with posterior approaches and anterior dislocation with anterior approaches. Internal rotation is generally the culprit with posterior approaches, while external rotation is the culprit with anterior approaches. With either position, adduction plays a key role in actually dislocating the hip. It is much easier to adduct the hip in internal rotation than in external rotation; thus, the posterior approach provides a greater risk of the patient accidentally malpositioning his or her hip.

The main anatomic issue with the anterior approaches is how the abductors are mobilized. The abductors can be incised at their insertion on the greater trochanter; the greater trochanter can be separated from the femur (osteotomy) with the muscular insertion intact; or a portion of the abductors can be left on the greater trochanter with the remainder attached to the greater trochanter osteotomy fragment. If the surgeon chooses to osteotomize the trochanter, he or she can leave the inferior musculature attachment (vastus lateralis origin) intact or incise it. The posterior structures are generally left intact.

The patient is placed in a lateral decubitus position with the operative hip facing upward. The incision generally resembles that of the posterior approaches: It is directed along the lateral border of the femur distally and then is curved proximally according to the preference of the surgeon. (As the hip is usually flexed while the femoral stem is placed, curving the incision posteriorly with either an anterior or posterior approach allows for better access to the femur. Most surgeons, though, tend not to curve the incision posteriorly while using an anterior approach.) The iliotibial tract is incised in line with the incision, the trochanteric bursa is incised, and the interval between the tensor fascia lata and gluteus medius is developed.

### Standard Trochanteric Osteotomy

If the surgeon chooses standard trochanteric osteotomy, the periosteum overlying the vastus tubercle of the greater trochanter is cut with electrocautery. The distal end of the anterior insertion of the gluteus medius is identified, and the osteotomy proceeds with all of the medius and the underlying minimus attached to the osteotomy fragment. Portions of the anterior and posterior capsule are adherent either to the osteotomy fragment or the femoral neck, depending on the depth of the osteotomy. This capsule can be excised or retracted superiorly. Similarly, the posterior musculature, the short external rotators, is variably adherent to the trochanteric fragment and can be incised at its insertions if necessary.

Repair of the osteotomy at the end of the procedure is performed with either metal wire or cables. The wires can be placed longitudinally through the femoral canal before cementing. The surgeon can then drill holes in the trochanteric fragment. Wires or cables can also be placed horizontally around the femur and around or through the osteotomy fragment, especially when the stem is not cemented. The grip of the wires or cables on the osteotomy fragment can be enhanced by a clamp device or mesh placed on the superolateral border of the fragment.

### Modified Trochanteric Osteotomy

The most common modified trochanteric osteotomy used keeps only the anterior half of the abductors (about 40% of the medius and 80% of the minimus) attached to the osteotomy fragment (Dall 1986). It leaves the remainder attached to the femur and thus involves a split in the abductors. The split is carried out at the anterosuperior corner of the trochanter and must not exceed 5 cm. If the split exceeds 5 cm, the dissection damages the superior gluteal nerve (see Figure 5-2), which innervates the abductors and the tensor fascia lata and produces a limp. To aid in the repair of the osteotomy, the vastus lateralis origin is left intact with the osteotomy fragment. To retract the fragment anteriorly and not exceed the above mentioned 5-cm split, the vastus lateralis is elevated from the femur distal to its origin. This produces a band of tissue and bone anteriorly: portions of the medius and minimus attached proximally to the osteotomy fragment, which is in turn attached to the vastus lateralis distally. This distal attachment should help prevent superior migration of the fragment when repaired and preserve its distal blood supply. Greater amounts of the abductors can be left with the fragment; however, anterior retraction of the fragment is then more difficult, as more of the posterior portion of the abductors are left attached to the fragment (Figure 5-3). The anterior capsule can be left intact with the osteotomy fragment or excised. The posterior capsule and muscles are left intact.

The osteotomy is repaired as with the standard trochanteric osteotomy, except that the wires generally do not need to be placed longitudinally. Horizontal wires suffice, as the vastus lateralis helps to prevent superior migration of the fragment.

### No Osteotomy

If no osteotomy is chosen, the anterior aspect of the gluteus medius and minimus is incised at its insertions on the anterior greater trochanter. Superiorly, they can be split as with a modified trochanteric osteotomy, or they can be removed along their entire insertions on the superior aspect of the trochanter. The underlying capsule is incised or excised. Repair of the musculature is affected with sutures through the tendon rem-

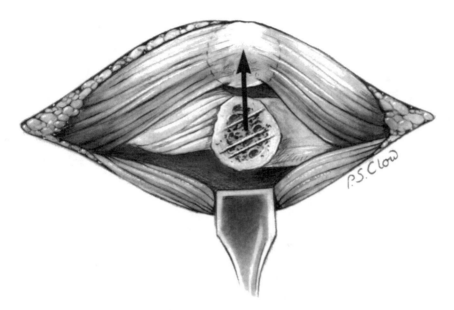

**Figure 5-3** Drawing of a modified trochanteric osteotomy of the right hip, in which all of the abductors (left of the arrow) have been left attached to the trochanteric fragment, which is attached distally to the vastus lateralis (right of the arrow). In the modified osteotomy described in the text, only about half of the abductors are left attached. (Reprinted with permission from HU Cameron. [1992] *The Technique of Total Hip Arthroplasty* [p. 153]. St. Louis: Mosby–Year Book.)

nant still attached to the trochanter or through drill holes in the bone. This approach is often referred to as the *anterolateral* or *Watson-Jones approach* (Hoppenfeld and deBoer 1994).

The origin of the vastus lateralis can be stripped from the trochanter in continuity with the split or detached abductors. Doing so constitutes the *direct lateral approach of Hardinge* (Hardinge 1982), which differs from the modified trochanteric osteotomy approach mainly in cutting the abductor tendons rather than taking a trochanteric fragment.

### All Anterior Approaches

Regardless of the means used to mobilize the abductors, once done, the hip is dislocated with external rotation, flexion, and lateral pull. Gauging of the leg length and preparation of the acetabulum proceeds as with posterior approaches, though the femur is retracted posteriorly while reaming the acetabulum. The femoral stem is prepared and inserted as with the posterior approaches, except that the hip is held in external rotation, with the leg directed downward in a sterile bag. Repair of the trochanter or abductors is as discussed earlier in this section. The interval between the gluteus maximus and tensor fascia lata is then repaired as with posterior approaches.

### Weaknesses of Anterior Approaches

The mobilization and reattachment of the abductors is the main disadvantage of the anterior approaches. During mobilization, the superior gluteal nerve can be injured, which denervates the portion of the abductors distal to the site of injury and produces a limp. Even if not denervated, a similar functional result can occur if the repair is inadequate. The scar that forms when the abductors are sutured can be weak or elongated, or the repair of the osteotomy fragment can fail and produce a trochanteric mal- or nonunion. Thus, if the abductor attachment does not adequately repair, soft tissue tension and muscular control will be reduced, and the odds of dislocation or limp or both will be greater.

### Strengths of Anterior Approaches

The following are the strengths of anterior approaches:

- Even with the risk of repair failure, the overall risk of dislocation with anterior approaches is half that of posterior approaches. Unlike posterior approaches, the area of weakness is anterior; thus, excessive external rotation in extension should be avoided postoperatively.
- The sciatic nerve is at less risk with these approaches, though it can be snared with wires or cables used to fix the trochanter. The femoral nerve is at similar risk as with the posterior approaches.
- The leg is held in external rotation during femoral preparation, which keeps it away from the assistant's face and makes positioning much easier than with internal rotation.

## Choice of Fixation and Implants

It is beyond the scope of this chapter to fully cover the choice of component fixation (cement versus uncemented) and how the age of the patient influences it. Indeed, much of the vast literature on THA deals with these topics. Most surgeons use an uncemented acetabular component; however, surgeons choose cemented and uncemented femoral components in about equal numbers. There is no uniform consensus; thus, surgeons differ in how they acquire and analyze the vast information present and how they weigh advantages and disadvantages of each technique and implant.

The issues that concern surgeons are as follows:

- The short-term result. Will this component fully relieve the patient of pain and improve his or her function? Will it dislocate? Will it loosen prematurely? Will an uncemented component cause the patient to have thigh pain? Will it become infected? If any of these events necessitate revision of the hip, how difficult and successful will the revision operation be?
- The long-term result. How long will it be before the component requires revision? How quickly will the plastic wear, and what will be the consequences of the wear? Will the plastic wear debris cause the pelvis or the femur to develop osteolysis (a reactive cyst in the bone), which can then cause fractures or loosening?
- After the long-term result. How difficult will it be to revise this component? Will the cement present make it such that the component will never need to be revised, or will the presence of cement make the inevitable revision more difficult and less successful?
- Reproducibility. Will the surgeon be able to duplicate excellent results on a daily basis using this technique and implant? How much intraoperative flexibility is offered by this technique? Is the surgeon able to adjust a component after placing it?

To understand such concerns, one must have a rudimentary understanding of the basic issues. Modern metal components (acetabular cups and femoral stems and heads) are made of either titanium or cobalt chrome. Generally, uncemented cups and stems take advantage of the greater flexibility of titanium, which then allows the surrounding bone to take more of the stress. Most cemented stems are cobalt chrome, a stiffer metal that causes the surrounding cement to face less stress. Femoral heads are also usually made of cobalt chrome, which has more resistance to scratching than titanium. The head is fit to the stem by a press-fit mechanism, and liners are usually fixed to cups by a snap fit. Liners of the cup are made of the plastic polyethylene, as generally are cemented acetabular components. Femoral and acetabular components are fixed to bone in three ways:

1. Cement. The component is "glued" to the bone with acrylic cement.
2. Press fit. A larger component is tamped into a smaller space in the bone. The difference in size causes the bone to grip the component. In the acetabulum, surgeons can insert screws through holes in the metal shell to augment, or take the place of, the press fit. Surgeons in North America uncommonly use stems or cups that are purely press fit (without porous coating for bony ingrowth).

3. Bony ingrowth. A porous coating on the stem allows bone to grow into it over time, if the motion between the stem and bone (micromotion) is sufficiently minimized. The motion can be shear or "out of plane" (Burke et al. 1991). A shear motion occurs when the stem moves up and down relative to the bone, as when weight is placed directly over the top of the stem. Alternatively, an out-of-plane motion occurs when a patient flexes the hip, as in arising from a chair or ascending stairs, and the prosthesis twists relative to the bone. These motions are minimized by using press fit to achieve fixation until the bone grows in. Various stems have various shapes to achieve a lock with bone and minimize this micromotion.

The three means of fixation bear great similarities but have important differences. Cement can be viewed as the ultimate press fit or the ultimate bony ingrowth method. The cement fills the interstices of the bone, such that the fit is even better than that of press fit, and the construct resembles a fully ingrown stem when the cement hardens. Of course, the technique is vastly different in that the surgeon relies on the cement rather than the metal achieving a lock with the bone. It also introduces an interface between the prosthesis and the cement, as well as one between the cement and bone.

Before the components loosen from the bone, wear occurs between any parts that move. The parts that move most relative to each other are the femoral head and the plastic liner. Minute particles are created every time the hip moves. Over millions of cycles in a patient's life, the load of debris can be quite great. The liner wears about 1–2 mm over 10 years (Isaac et al. 1992), which is worse with more activity. The plastic liner can also wear over its back surface. Furthermore, different particles are created from between the component and bone, between the cement and component, between the cement and bone, and among different parts of the components if present. More particles are created with more motion between any of these interfaces. Thus, the number of particles created increases when the components loosen and move more against the bone or cement. These metal or cement particles can enter the articulation between the femoral head and plastic and accelerate the wear of the plastic.

All the particles can then enter the interfaces between the cement and bone, or the prosthesis and bone, and cause a reaction in the bone. The distance the particles travel (the effective joint space [Schmalzried et al. 1992a]) is greater with more pressure created in the joint by excessive exercise. The reaction in bone to the particles (mainly of the plastic) can be loosening of whatever portion of the prosthesis was well fixed or osteolysis, cysts that form within the bone. These cysts can be small and grow slowly or can be massive and quickly progress (Schmalzried et al. 1992a). This reaction to the particles routinely loosens cemented acetabular components after many years, especially if the seal between the pelvis and the cement is poor. The linear lysis travels slowly around the rim of the cup up to the dome as years go by (Schmalzried et al. 1992b). When it occurs around uncemented femoral and acetabular components, the course it takes is more variable. It can grow into large cysts in the bone, which can fracture, or make relatively smaller cysts that remain the same size for many years without causing symptoms.

Cemented femoral components are relatively protected from this process by the seal of the cement, which is generally better than that achieved with cemented cups. Lysis does occur, but usually is of much lesser nature with a well-fixed cemented stem than with an uncemented one (Goetz et al. 1994). Cemented stems loosen by debonding from the cement many years after implantation (Jasty et al. 1991). The cement can then fragment and cause lysis as discussed previously in this section.

Uncemented stems loosen by bone not growing into the stem or by the aggressive lysis mentioned previously in this section (Goetz et al. 1994). The lysis occurs near the top of the stem with stems that are fully porous coated and down the shaft with those that are porous coated only proximally. Limiting the porous coating to the top of the stem allows the femoral bone to bear more weight and thus not experience stress shielding. When a large metal stem is fit tightly into a canal, the stem carries the weight of the body, and the bone is unstressed, causing the body to resorb this bone (Engh and Bobyn 1988). The bone then present for future revision is very poor and weak.

Surgeons do not agree on the optimal components and fixation techniques to use. Many surgeons choose one technique of fixation or implant in the young and another in the more elderly. Many use one technique for the acetabular component and another for the femoral component. Furthermore, not all techniques are equal. Cementing a femoral stem has been categorized as "first, second, or third generation" (Harris 1993), depending on how well the canal is cleaned, how much cement is used, and how greatly cement is pressurized when inserted. Improvements in these techniques have yielded improved results.

When the surgeon cements the stem and not the cup, the technique is known as *hybrid* (Harris and Maloney 1989). As more surgeons have come to view this method as optimal, it has grown in popularity. Choices continue to evolve as more long-term information becomes available and as cost pressures take their toll. Tables 5-2 and 5-3 summarize the issues related to cementing and noncementing the acetabular component and femoral component respectively.

**Table 5-2** Acetabular Component

| Variable | Cemented | Uncemented |
|---|---|---|
| Track record | Much longer | Promising but shorter |
| Short-term loosening | Rare | Rare |
| Long-term loosening | Frequently loosened by 15 years, but uncommonly requires revision by this time | Hope that bone ingrown into the component prevents long-term loosening (not proven) |
| Wear | Less wear of the plastic by the head of the femoral component | Greater wear of the plastic by the head of the femoral component |
| Bony ingrowth | None needed | Required |
| Fracture risk during insertion | *Very* unlikely | Rare |
| Screw holes | None | Possible conduit for debris to travel if present |
| Speed of insertion | Must wait for cement to dry and ensure that all excess is removed | Much quicker |
| Ease of insertion | Bone must be dried of blood, which is exceedingly difficult in this cancellous bone | Much easier |
| Ability to readjust component | None | Easily done by reinserting it or by placing a tilted or offset liner |
| Use in revision situations | Fairly poor track record due to the smooth bone present after a failed cup is removed, but useful when bone graft is used | Reliably good fit and fixation even in revisions |
| Use with bone grafts | Useful | Bone grafts do not grow into it |
| Cost | Much less expensive | More expensive but takes less operating room time |

**Table 5-3**    Femoral Component

| Variable | Cemented | Uncemented |
|---|---|---|
| Track record | Longer; excellent results at 20–25 years using certain implants and techniques even in young, active people | Excellent with some designs, though information is absent beyond 15 years and rare beyond 10 years |
| Thigh pain | None | Frequent with many designs |
| Stress shielding | Less than with very large or extensively coated uncemented stems | Less than with a cemented stem if the uncemented stem is not coated at its distal portions |
| Micromotion | Basically none between the stem and bone; one-piece stem avoids new interfaces among parts of the stem that can wear and produce debris | Variable; between the stem and bone or between parts of the stem, producing metal debris that can enter the interface between the head and liner and cause increased wear |
| Canal sealing | Cement retards travel of the plastic wear debris that occurs between the liner and head of the femoral component; this results in less osteolysis | Less sealing, since the bone does not grow into the prosthesis completely, allowing travel of debris and subsequent osteolysis where the debris settles |
| Femoral preparation | Less sculpting of the proximal bone, usually no reaming of the distal cortical bone | Extensive canal preparation with most designs |
| Reliance on the shape of the femur | Little; as room is left for cement, the stem can be rotated to a proper position more easily even in a deformed femur | Important; stem must be custom or modular when the femur is deformed |
| Fracture | Much less likely | Can occur during preparation or implantation |
| Operative time | More; cement must dry, and excess cement must be removed | Less |
| Bone stock for revision | Cement fragments when the stem loosens and creates a cystic reaction of the bone to the cement (i.e., "cement disease"); removing adherent cement also destroys bone | Uncemented stems can leave more, but when osteolysis (i.e., cementless disease) occurs, little bone may be left for reconstruction |
| Ease of revision | If loose, one must still remove the cement after removing the stem; if well fixed, it is extremely | If loose, it is much easier to remove If well or somewhat fixed |

| Variable | Cemented | Uncemented |
|---|---|---|
| | difficult to remove | to the bone, it can be extremely difficult to remove |
| Cost | Slightly less expensive | More expensive, but takes less operating room time |

## Postoperative Care

Medical care after THR includes the following:

- Controlling pain with narcotics
- Following hematocrit or hemoglobin and replenishing (if needed)
- Anticoagulating to help prevent clots
- Antibiotics to help prevent infection
- Managing pre-existing medical problems (often with the assistance of medical doctors)

Nonorthopedic potential complications include the following:

- Urinary retention
- Excessive bleeding, hematoma formation, or both
- Ileus
- Gout
- Healing problems

The stay in the hospital varies nationally but is usually about 5 days. Often, a social worker discusses the home situation with the patient and helps provide services. Occasionally, patients require transfer to a rehabilitation facility. Before discharge, x-rays are often taken, and some surgeons screen for deep vein thrombosis using ultrasound or a venogram. Before withholding physical therapy, it should be ascertained whether the screening study is routine. Most surgeons do not want therapy withheld while results are pending.

## Revision Total Hip Arthroplasty

Replacing a previously placed prosthesis is much more difficult and less uniform in nature. Each case substantially differs from all others and has unique problems and risks. In all cases, the risks are much greater than with primary surgery. The recovery is usually longer, and the results are less certain. Revision surgery, however, has greatly improved over the years. Even if the outcome is not always as good as with first-time surgery, great improvements in pain and function often result.

Many surgeons who use one approach for primary surgery use a different one for revision surgery. The tissue planes are compromised in previously dissected areas, and surgeons usually begin the exposure in normal tissue planes and proceed to dissect the scarred region.

More exposure is generally needed; thus, standard trochanteric osteotomy is more frequently used. The exposure of the acetabulum is thereby greatly facilitated, and room for large reamers or bone graft is made available. Of course, repair of the trochanter is necessary after osteotomy, which can be exceedingly difficult when lateral femoral bone stock is deficient. If so, the trochanter is advanced distally to allow it to reach an area of bone for repair. This is performed by placing the hip in wide abduction intraoperatively. Postoperatively, an abduction contracture is present, which produces an apparent lengthening of the operative leg. A lift in the other shoe may be necessary until the abductors stretch, which generally commences rapidly.

Acetabular reconstruction in revisions is complex and varies greatly. Most often, it is performed in an uncemented fashion, using screws for initial fixation. The fixation of these reconstructions is usually good but not as secure as that of primary cemented or uncemented acetabula. Defects are usually filled with small pieces of bone graft, but rarely is it necessary to use large bone grafts to actually support the cup. Large grafts, usually femoral heads of cadavers (allografts), are generally fixed to the pelvis with plates or screws. The cups then are usually cemented into the pelvis and graft, as there is no potential for bone from the graft to grow into the cup. Bulk allografts in acetabular revision are avoided, however, if possible (Shinar and Harris 1997).

If extensive exposure of the femoral shaft is required, the vastus lateralis, vastus intermedius, or both can be elevated off the femur. This exposure allows for repair of defects in the cortex of the femur by placing allograft cortical strut grafts over the defects and securing the struts with cables or wires. The fascia of the vastus is repaired at the conclusion of surgery.

Access to the interior of the femoral canal to remove cement or an ingrown stem can be achieved by a number of methods. Most often, the surgeon removes as much of the proximal cement or ingrown bone from the stem as possible and then removes the stem by pounding it out. This method is not always successful, and a femoral fracture can result. If so, the fracture is treated with wires or cables. Increasingly, surgeons are using a method called *extended trochanteric osteotomy* (Younger et al. 1995). Some of the vastus musculature is elevated, and the femoral shaft is split longitudinally both anteriorly and posteriorly. Distally, a horizontal bone cut is made, which connects these two splits, and the lateral fragment is lifted off the stem or cement. The fragment is continuous with the trochanter proximally and is retracted anteriorly or superiorly to give access to the acetabulum, as well as the interior of the femoral shaft. After removing the stem and cement (if needed) and replacing the acetabulum, the canal is ready for reconstruction. If an uncemented stem is chosen, it is fixed into the canal distal to the horizontal cut, and the split of the femoral shaft is wired or cabled over the stem. If the surgeon opts to cement a stem, the split is reassembled first with wires or cables, and the stem is then cemented down the new canal.

Revision surgeries are a much more heterogeneous group than primary surgeries. Thus, they have a much more variable postoperative course. In general, however, the complication rates are much greater in all areas: limp, nerve injury, dislocation, leg length discrepancy, infection, and trochanteric nonunion. The patient and the therapist must be even more vigilant in dislocation precautions.

## Hemiarthroplasty

This discussion of one treatment for femoral neck fractures, hemiarthroplasty, is included in the section "Total Hip Replacement" because the operative procedure and aftercare resemble that of THR. Indications are discussed in "Hip (Proximal Femur) Fracture Repair." The procedure involves replacing the femoral head with a metal ball attached to a stem inserted down the shaft. The ball is either in one piece (*unipolar* or *endohead*) or two that articulate with each other (*bipolar*). The larger head of the unipolar or bipolar construct is inherently less likely to dislocate than the smaller head of a THR, but patients receiving hemiarthroplasty are generally less able to follow dislocation precautions. When the acetabulum displays arthritis that existed before the fracture, the surgeon can opt to replace the acetabulum as well, yielding a THR. If this situation exists, and the patient has an intertrochanteric fracture, a THR can be performed; however, a stem that replaces the region around the lesser trochanter (i.e., the calcar) is needed. These prostheses are termed *calcar replacement stems*.

Surgeons use both anterior and posterior approaches for treating femoral neck fractures with hemiarthroplasty. The decision is based on the same considerations as in "Total Hip Replacement." Some surgeons consider the risk of dislocation among this group of generally more debilitated patients to be higher and thus choose an anterior approach. Such a choice has the further advantage of keeping the incision more anterior in this group of patients who more often suffer fecal and urinary incontinence. Many surgeons, however, think the recovery is quicker with a posterior approach and believe that they can perform the procedure more expediently with a posterior approach in this medically frail group. These approaches are as described in "Total Hip Replacement," except that less acetabular exposure is necessary. Thus, the capsule is usually saved and repaired.

## Physical Therapy Issues in Hip Replacement

Details of postoperative physical therapy are covered in Chapter 6. This chapter discusses considerations with regard to the variations in hip replacement surgery. Ideally, the physical therapist has a clear understanding of the issues with each surgery from the surgeon's postoperative orders or from personal communication. When not available, the operative note should be scanned for these details. An idea of the stability of the reconstruction can be gleaned from the intraoperative range of motion of the hip. Strength of fracture or graft fixation usually is stated but also can be implied by mentions of bone quality (Figure 5-4). When the surgeon uses the term *osteoporotic bone*, it usually means that the fixation is less strong. Leg length changes, obvious nerve injuries, and other complications should also be sought in the operative report.

### Instability

Precautions to prevent both anterior and posterior dislocations are necessary with any hip replacement, but it is worthwhile to understand which should be stressed. Adduction should be avoided with any approach, but particularly in association with flexion when a posterior approach has been used.

Excessive extension and external rotation should be carefully avoided after anterior approaches. Excessive extension is particularly likely to occur when the patient attempts to arise from a supine position by raising his or her buttocks to move distally in bed. A trapeze is instrumental in assisting the patient to avoid this position. Excessive external rotation in extension is likely to occur when turning while ambulating, particularly if the patient's foot catches on the ground. Taking turns slowly and carefully with many steps is helpful. External rotation in flexion is generally safe, particularly with a posterior approach.

OPERATIVE REPORT A
PREOPERATIVE DIAGNOSIS: Left hip intertrochanteric
                                    fracture
POSTOPERATIVE DIAGNOSIS: Same

OPERATION: Closed reduction, insertion of left sliding hip screw
(90 mm) and placement of a 140-degree four-hole plate ... The plate
was fixed to the femoral shaft with a clamp and then four screws
were put in standard fashion. The first two screws were 36 mm in
length, the second two 34 mm in length. The plate and screw were
checked both in the anteroposterior and lateral directions, and
these demonstrated that the plate and hip screws were all in proper
position. The fracture remained slightly distracted, and therefore
a compression screw was placed through the plate and into the sliding hip screw. This was compressed until a bite was extremely
strong. X-rays were checked, and this demonstrated that the fracture was reduced nearly anatomically. The compression screw was
then removed. The wound was copiously irrigated with antibiotic
solution. The vastus ...

OPERATIVE REPORT B
PREOPERATIVE DIAGNOSIS: Left hip intertrochanteric
                                    fracture
POSTOPERATIVE DIAGNOSIS: Same

OPERATION: ... under direct x-ray vision, an 85-mm screw was
placed. The plate was then placed over the screw and held to the
bone with a clamp. The screws were then placed in standard technique and their position checked on the x-ray, and it was found
that the screws were in good position. At least three of the
screws were completely below the fracture site. The wire was then
placed through the lesser trochanteric fragment and tightened
around the plate superiorly, and this was checked with x-rays and
found to bring the lesser trochanter into good opposition with the
medial femur. Two cables were then placed in standard fashion,
being careful not to tighten too much due to the weak bone, but
they were found not to be loose either. They were crimped
directly over the plate and cut at their junction with a crimping
device. The wound was thoroughly irrigated and the whole device
was checked with x-ray, and it was found that the screw did not
penetrate the femoral head cortex. The fracture site appeared ...

**Figure 5-4** *Excerpts* from two operative reports for intertrochanteric hip fracture repair. Underlined are terms that suggest stable fixation (A) versus less
solid repair (B).

Any internal rotation should be avoided after a posterior approach. It is particularly dangerous, because it is easiest to rotate one's hip internally in a position of flexion and adduction, the exact position used to dislocate the hip intraoperatively. This position is likely to occur when the patient is seated and reaches for an object improperly. The patient should be instructed to turn his or her pelvis to face the object directly ahead and to move toward the object, rather than excessively flexing his or her hip to reach forward. Alternatively, the patient can cautiously use grabbers. The patient can also replicate the dangerous position by reaching to pick up an object on the outside of his or her legs and should be instructed to avoid picking up objects altogether (or only between his or her legs). Excessive flexion is likely to occur when a patient sits on too low a chair, a soft chair or sofa, or a low toilet seat. It can also occur with sitting or rising too rapidly without the use of handrails.

The risk of dislocation decreases with time as scar tissue forms around the located hip replacement, but the risk is always present. Patients should be instructed to always be cautious and to understand that it is much more difficult to be cautious when performing quick motions, as in sports or falls. All risks of falling should be minimized (see Table 6-5). Common culprits are throw rugs, uneven carpet edges, single steps in bilevel houses, and pets on leashes.

### Weightbearing Status

Weightbearing restrictions relate to the reconstruction and to the repair of the surgical approach. When all components are cemented, no weightbearing restrictions are necessitated by the reconstruction. Exceptions occur when fractures occur or when bone graft is used. Bone graft heals slowly by growth of bone across the gap between the living bone and the dead bone. Regardless of whether auto- or allograft is used, the graft is basically dead bone. The surgeon bases the duration of restricted weightbearing on his or her estimation of the duration of the healing period. The amount of stability present between the graft and host is variable and is dependent on the size and shape of the graft and the fixation used. The surgeon bases the degree of allowed weightbearing on his or her estimation of the strength of the construct's fixation. Similar considerations relating to the degree and duration of weightbearing restrictions apply to fixation of intraoperative acetabular and femur fractures and repair of an extended trochanteric osteotomy.

Uncemented acetabular and femoral components depend on screws or press fit for initial stability. If micromotion is appropriately limited, the bone grows into the porous metal coating on the component. Surgeons generally limit weightbearing for 6 weeks or longer for this to occur.

## Position and Strengthening of Repaired Structures

When trochanteric osteotomy is performed (standard or modified), surgeons prohibit abductor exercises or stretching until the osteotomy heals at 6–12 weeks. Stretching is limited by the use of a cane or crutches and by avoiding stretching exercises. With some anterior approaches, portions of the abductors have been repaired with sutures into their stumps or into the trochanter. Surgeons often limit abductor strengthening and stretching while the repair heals (i.e., for about 6 weeks) to prevent failure of the repair. The abductor muscles are also stretched by external rotation, and stretching in this direction should also be avoided while healing occurs.

Surgeons generally do not limit quadriceps strengthening after takedown of the vastus lateralis, as the muscle usually heals in an adequate position even with exercise.

The abductors are not incised with a posterior approach, and surgeons generally allow strengthening of these muscles immediately postoperatively. Of course, an adducted position of the hip for stretching or strengthening is not permitted, as dislocation can occur. The abductors are usually stretched with the surgery, as the reconstruction often has a greater offset (see Figure 5-1) than is present preoperatively. The leg is frequently lengthened by the surgery, and the abductors are also stretched by this means. The repair of the iliotibial tract tends to abduct the hip, and gentle stretching is necessary to overcome this effect. The rhumba and hula are helpful exercises (Chandler 1987) (see Chapter 6).

## Alternatives to Hip Replacement

### Osteotomy

Before the advent of THR, the hip surgeon could offer the patient only relatively crude methods of hemiarthroplasty: a loose uncemented femoral stem (Austin-Moore prosthesis) replacing the proximal femur or a loose metal cup (cup arthroplasty) interposed between the reamed femoral head and socket. These methods were later supplanted by modern THR or hemiarthroplasty. Even before the development of hip replacement methods in the 1960s, surgeons were able to offer patients promising alternatives (i.e., acetabular [pelvic] and femoral osteotomies).

Femoral osteotomies rotate the cartilage of the femoral head to allow new and better cartilage to bear weight. Furthermore, the cartilage of the hip joint experiences a surprisingly beneficial response to the cutting of the proximal femur. The results of these procedures were good in properly selected patients (Miegel and Harris 1984) but were not as reliable as those of THR. When it was found that early hip replacements did not fare as well in young people, femoral osteotomies ideally served to temporize in the young until they reached a proper age for THR. It is becoming clear that the results of hip replacements using cemented femoral stems are not affected by young age (Barrack et al. 1992; Ballard et al. 1994; Neumann et al. 1996), and the indications for femoral osteotomy are dwindling. In the very young, hip replacement cannot optimistically be seen as likely to last the patient's entire life. In this group, osteotomy remains a viable option. Furthermore, no long-term restrictions on activity are imposed after the osteotomy heals, which suits the young particularly well.

Early pelvic osteotomies, designed to place new bone over the dislocated or dysplastic femoral head, have achieved moderate success. More modern variants (i.e., periacetabular osteotomy and dial osteotomy) differ by rotating the acetabular cartilage and the underlying bone to face the femoral head more normally. They have achieved excellent results in well-selected cases and hold promise for eliminating the need for THR altogether in young people with minimal arthritis who have an acetabulum that can be made normal with rotation. The procedure is difficult and complicated, though, and can hold grave complications for these relatively asymptomatic patients. Hence, they are commonly performed by only a few surgeons in North America.

All osteotomies involve intentional fracture of the femur or acetabulum and are approached in a similar manner to unintentional fractures (Figure 5-5G). Approaches and therapy are thus covered in the following sections, "Hip (Proximal Femur) Fracture Repair" and "Acetabular Fracture Reconstruction." Postoperative care and physical therapy are identical to that of unintentional fracture repair with one exception—osteotomies usually involve young people with good bone stock. Repair of these intentional fractures is solid, and more weightbearing is sometimes allowed.

## *Hip (Proximal Femur) Fracture Repair*

Fractures of the proximal femur occur in three main groups: in the elderly after falls, in younger patients experiencing high-speed trauma, and in femoral osteotomies when the surgeon intentionally fractures (osteotomizes) the femur. Attempts are usually made to repair rather than replace all fractures in the young. In the elderly, surgeons more often opt for replacement, either hemiarthroplasty or THR. Fractures can also occur through bone tumors, which frequently necessitate hemiarthroplasty.

Fractures are classified as to the location and the displacement of the fracture (Figure 5-5D). The location can be within the femoral head, at the junction of the head and neck (subcapital), within the femoral neck, at the base of the femoral neck (basicervical), between the trochanters (inter-

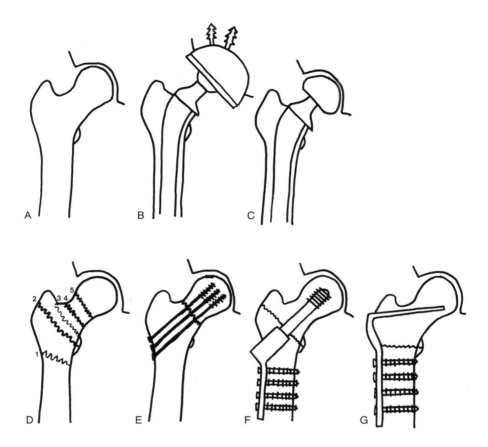

**Figure 5-5** Drawings of various hip reconstructions. A. Normal hip joint. B. Total hip arthroplasty. C. Hemiarthroplasty. D. Levels of proximal femur fractures: 1. subtrochanteric, 2. intertrochanteric, 3. basicervical, 4. transcervical (femoral neck), and 5. subcapital. E. Multiple screw fixation of a femoral neck fracture. F. Screw-and-plate fixation of an intertrochanteric hip fracture. G. Blade-plate fixation of a proximal femoral osteotomy—no rotation of the proximal fragment was performed.

trochanteric, where femoral osteotomies are made), or below the trochanters (subtrochanteric). Displacement is variable, from nondisplaced to completely detached.

For displaced fractures, surgeons weigh the risk of dislocation and bleeding with hemiarthroplasty against the risks of nonunion, malunion, and avascular necrosis with fracture repair. For nondisplaced fractures, surgeons weigh the risk of future displacement with nonoperative treatment against the risks of surgery. Furthermore, surgeons weigh the consequences of the delayed weightbearing that is necessary with nonoperative treatment or with fracture repair against the lesser weightbearing restrictions that follow hemiarthroplasty. Generally, surgeons choose as in the following outline:

1. Hemiarthroplasty (Figure 5-5C). Displaced femoral head, displaced subcapital, and some displaced femoral neck fractures
2. Screw fixation (Figure 5-5E). More mildly displaced femoral neck fractures
3. Compression screw and plate (or sliding hip screw) (Figure 5-5F). Basi-cervical, intertrochanteric, and some subtrochanteric fractures (sometimes augmented with bone graft). (Other subtrochanteric fractures are treated with intramedullary devices, as with femoral shaft fractures, or with special compression or blade plates [see Figure 5-5G].)
4. Nonoperative approach. Nondisplaced fractures

Approaches and physical therapy considerations for hemiarthroplasties are covered in "Total Hip Replacement," and those for fracture fixation are covered in the following section.

### Approaches for Hip Fracture Internal Fixation and Femoral Osteotomies

The approaches for femoral osteotomies and hip fractures are similar, though their indications are vastly different. Intertrochanteric fractures are repaired with a screw and plate device that allows controlled impaction of the fracture to allow early healing, motion, and ambulation while the fracture heals. The device is usually composed of two main parts, a large screw that is inserted up the femoral neck into the femoral head, and a special plate that has a barrel at its most superior portion that articulates with the shaft of the screw (see Figure 5-5F). Minimally displaced femoral neck fractures are similarly treated, except that multiple smaller screws are placed across the fracture site without using a plate. The screws are usually hollow (cannulated) to allow them to be placed over smaller wires that can be removed and adjusted before placing the screws (see Figure 5-5E). Using multiple, smaller screws rather than a screw-plate device allows for a smaller exposure and better rotational control of the fracture. However, the procedures and devices are often mentioned in operative reports and hospital charts by the brand name or type of device, which can be confusing. Physical therapists can check the preoperative diagnosis and description of the procedure in the operative note to find which type of procedure was performed.

Proximal femoral osteotomy is performed to rotate the cartilage of the femoral head, such that different cartilage is bearing weight, or to achieve the positive effect that an osteotomy has on the hip arthritis. It usually involves removing a wedge of bone at the intertrochanteric level and fixation of the "fracture" site with a blade-plate device (see Figure 5-5G). This device is composed of a blade inserted into the femoral neck that is attached to a plate that is screwed to the lateral femur. As the wedge of bone removed is triangular in shape, closing the site where it is removed tilts the femoral head to allow different cartilage to bear weight.

The patient is positioned on the fracture frame in a supine position with the contralateral hip flexed in a well-leg holder. (Some surgeons prefer a lateral decubitus position on a radiolucent table.) If fractured, the hip is reduced under fluoroscopic guidance before surgery.

A straight incision is made laterally starting from the tip of the greater trochanter. The fascia lata is incised in line with the skin incision. The vastus lateralis and its fascia are then encountered. If single screws are to be placed across a femoral neck fracture, little exposure of the femoral shaft is required, the origin of the vastus lateralis on the vastus tubercle of the greater trochanter is detached, and a small amount of the vastus is elevated distally. After placing the screws, minimal closure of the vastus is needed, and the iliotibial tract is closed.

If a plate and screw for an intertrochanteric fracture is needed, or if an intertrochanteric osteotomy is to be performed, more extensive exposure of the lateral shaft of the femur is necessary. After incising the iliotibial tract, the vastus is either split or retracted anteriorly and then split closer to its insertion on the linea aspera. Multiple perforating vessels must be cauterized. The vastus is then closed over the plate after the fracture or osteotomy is fixed.

As these procedures do not involve the hip joint per se, dislocation is not a risk postoperatively, as in THR and hemiarthroplasty. The amount of weightbearing allowed is at the discretion of the surgeon; however, in general, partial weightbearing is allowed for intertrochanteric fractures and osteotomies, while toe-touch weightbearing is usually required for fixed femoral neck fractures. These restrictions contrast with the weightbearing for THR and hemiarthroplasties, which are generally full weightbearing for cemented reconstructions and partial weightbearing for uncemented components.

### Core Decompression

Core decompression is a procedure that aims to relieve the increased pressure within the femoral head that is present in the condition of avascular necrosis, which is also called *osteonecrosis*. Generally, it is performed before the death of the femoral head has caused significant arthritis of the hip. The procedure opens a tract from the lateral proximal femoral cortex less than a centimeter wide into but not through the femoral head. Making this tract reduces the pressure within the head of the femur, which helps relieve pain, relieves pressure (and thus retards further bone death), and allows a tract for new bone and blood vessels to grow.

The procedure resembles that of pin fixation in that only a small area near the origin of the vastus lateralis needs to be opened to perform the procedure. It resembles that of compression-screw placement in that a single tract up the femoral neck is drilled. After drilling, the layers are closed.

Physical therapy postoperatively involves 6 weeks of toe-touch weightbearing.

## Hip Fusion

The scope of this chapter does not allow extensive detail about the rarer procedures of hip fusion, resection arthroplasty, and acetabular fracture reconstruction; however, they are discussed here briefly.

Hip fusions are performed to eliminate hip pain by eliminating the joint (Figure 5-6). They are usually performed in younger men who are involved in heavy labor or in patients with previous sepsis in whom the surgeon chooses not to place a joint replacement. Its main disadvantages are the chance for nonunion, an awkward gait, and increased chance of eventual arthritis in the low back and instability in the ipsilateral knee. The advantages of fusion over arthroplasty are less restrictions of activity after healing of the fusion, reduced risk of infection, and lesser consequences of infection.

Hip fusion is performed by exposing and dislocating the hip joint, clearing the remaining cartilage, and fixing the femur to the pelvis. The approach is usually anterior or by trochanteric osteotomy. Fusion is performed by either transfixing the two bones with hardware placed through the femoral neck and head into the pelvis or by placing a plate on the lateral surface of the pelvis and femur and compressing the two bones longitudinally. The forces across this fusion are immense, and most surgeons thus require spica cast or brace immobilization postoperatively until healing commences (in about 2–4 months). Weightbearing across the fusion is usually restricted for a similar period. If a removable brace is placed, the surgeon generally allows passive motion of the ipsilateral knee with the hip held steady.

## Resection Arthroplasty

Resection arthroplasty (Girdlestone) procedures are most often indicated after failed or infected hip replacements. They involve removing

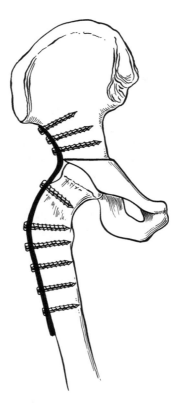

**Figure 5-6** Drawing of a technique for hip fusion in which a plate is placed over the lateral border of the proximal femur and the pelvis. (Reprinted with permission from HU Cameron. [1992] *The Technique of Total Hip Arthroplasty*. St. Louis: Mosby–Year Book.)

the prosthesis and infected tissues through the approach used for previous surgery. If infected, the wound is often left open to allow drainage and formation of granulation tissue. Usually, no repair has taken place, and partial weightbearing is allowed postoperatively. Sometimes, the surgeon places the patient in traction for a number of weeks while scar tissue forms in the "dead space." When infection has cleared, the surgeon may opt to reimplant a prosthesis. The approach in so doing resembles that of revision surgery, which is detailed in the section "Revision Total Hip Arthroplasty."

Occasionally, a resection arthroplasty is performed in place of a hip replacement for infection or arthritis not amenable to arthroplasty. The approach used can be any of those mentioned in "Total Hip Replacement," and weightbearing restrictions are usually partial weightbearing.

### Acetabular Fracture Reconstruction

Acetabular fracture reconstruction is directed to the area of the acetabulum involved. (See Table 2-8 for acetabular fracture classification.) If the main portion of the fracture is posterior, an approach similar to the one described in "Posterior Approach" is used. It differs in that the blood supply to the femoral head is preserved by not dissecting the quadratus femoris or the capsule. A trochanteric osteotomy can be necessary for exposure. Weightbearing is usually restricted (i.e., touchdown weightbearing [TDWB] or nonweightbearing if patient cannot maintain TDWB) until fracture healing at 6–8 weeks.

Anterior acetabular fractures are usually fixed through an ilioinguinal approach. It involves peeling the iliopsoas from the interior of the pelvis; retracting the abdominal musculature and contents in the groin medially; dissecting on both sides of the femoral artery, vein, and nerve; and mobilizing the spermatic cord or round ligament medially. Access is thus obtained to the inner wall of the hip joint; the joint itself is not violated. Plates are placed along the pelvic brim and pubic ramus. Weightbearing restrictions apply as with posterior repairs.

As with the comparison of femoral osteotomies and simple intertrochanteric fractures, acetabular osteotomies are equivalent to simple acetabular fractures with regards to fixation and physical therapy. The approach usually used is the traditional anterior, in which the abductors are stripped off the lateral wall of the iliac wing, and the iliacus is stripped off the inner (medial) wall. Bony cuts are then made around the acetabulum, and the socket is redirected to better cover the femoral head. The fragment containing the acetabulum is then fixed to the remainder of the pelvis with plates, pins, or screws. The abductors are then repaired either to the abdominal musculature, the iliacus on the other side of the iliac crest, or to the iliac bone itself. Minimal weightbearing (toe-touch or light-partial) is generally allowed postoperatively. Abductor strengthening is delayed until healing commences at 6 weeks. Very gentle range of motion exercises are allowed.

Fractures of both the anterior and posterior acetabulum can be approached through either of the anterior or posterior fracture approaches described in this section or through the extended iliofemoral approach. The extended iliofemoral approach peels the abductors from the entire outer surface of the pelvis, where plates are placed. Problems with healing of the abductors and heterotopic ossification are common. Abductor strengthening is delayed until the repair of the abductors is felt to be secure. It is usually delayed in other approaches, as well, to protect the trochanteric osteotomy if performed and to lessen the compressive forces across the hip joint while the fractured joint surface heals. Gentle active and passive range of motion of the hip joint is usually allowed.

Severe fractures or fractures in those not medically clear for surgery can be treated with traction.

## Summary for the Physical Therapist

When planning an individualized program or generalized protocol of physical therapy, the following questions ought to be considered:

- What is the weightbearing status? It is generally dictated by the surgeon's perception of the stability of the operative construct, but can also be chosen to allow bony ingrowth into a prosthesis. Check with the surgeon if the choice of status seems out of order or if the patient cannot maintain it. It sometimes needs to be altered.
- In which direction is the hip more likely to dislocate? The physical therapist can glean this answer from the operative report by finding what surgical approach the surgeon used. He or she can also find how stable the surgeon thought the components were through the mentioned range of motion of the implants before soft tissue closure. Stricter dislocation precautions are required with some patients.
- What was done with the abductors? Were they avoided by a posterior approach, incised through muscle or tendon, or mobilized by a trochanteric osteotomy? The answers to these questions dictate whether the physical therapist should avoid resistive contractions and stretch. Unless they were avoided, the abductors were repaired. If repaired, it is important to avoid resistive contraction until healed (at least 6 weeks), and it is worthwhile to teach the patient to rest the hip in 10–20 degrees of abduction. This position prevents stretch and deters dislocation.
- Was an uncemented femoral component used? Surgeons generally do not make restrictions with regards to whether the acetabular component was cemented but do so with the femur. Most surgeons want the amount of micromotion between the stem and femur minimized during the early period of bony ingrowth (at least 6 weeks and even for the first 6 months).
- How secure was the fixation? Is the bone osteoporotic? Slow progression of weightbearing is indicated when the fixation is not secure, especially if its hold in osteoporotic bone is poor.

- Were there operative or postoperative complications or complexities? Leg length discrepancy, intraoperative femur or acetabular fracture, femoral perforation, nerve injury, dislocation in the recovery room, use of bone graft, and other complexities alter the postoperative management.
- What individual considerations are at play? The patient's compliance and attitude toward physical therapy, insurance restrictions (e.g., length of stay, equipment allowed, discharge facility, postdischarge therapy allocations), nursing staffing, and therapist staffing individualize every patient's postoperative course.

## Conclusion

This chapter is intended to expose the physical therapist to the vast array of information involved with surgeries about the hip. It should do the following:

- Highlight the rationale for postoperative rehabilitation protocols
- Assist the therapist in developing an effective yet safe rehabilitation program for uncommon cases
- Demonstrate the essential information the therapist should acquire from the surgeon or operative report before implementing or progressing a rehabilitation program

Though this chapter covers multiple other issues, it focuses on the surgical approaches and details the manner in which the soft tissues are incised, excised, dissected, and repaired. These tissues are responsible for movement and function, the basis of the physical therapist's work. Thus, the therapist should be aware of which alterations of soft tissues were performed during surgery and of the possible consequences of such alterations. The expert therapist appropriately applies surgical information to postoperative activity and thereby acts as a vital agent in reducing postoperative complications and improving functional outcomes.

# 6

# Postoperative Physical Therapy

Timothy L. Fagerson

Hip surgery patients are the largest orthopedic inpatient population. In a study on health care use by all fracture types, 52% of hospital bed days and 56% of physical therapy sessions were for hip fracture patients (Garraway et al. 1979). Of joint replacement cases, total hip replacement (THR) accounts for 50.2% of patients, with the next most common, knee replacement, accounting for 32.1% (Cauley 1994). Physical therapy after hip surgery occurs in many different settings (e.g., hospitals, rehabilitation facilities, nursing homes, home care, and outpatient clinics). Knowledge and skill in evaluation and treatment of the hip is, therefore, essential for physical therapists working in these settings.

Some surgeons are cautious about referring their patients to physical therapy because of an added risk and added cost. Admittedly, some patients do well without skilled physical therapy after hospital discharge. However, *appropriate* physical therapy should decrease risks, decrease overall costs, and improve the short- and long-term outcome. More research is obviously necessary to test these views and to determine the optimal role for physical therapy in the management of hip disorders. Nevertheless, the wise surgeon refers patients to physical therapists who know about the hip, know what they are doing with hip patients, and who will communicate with the surgeon.

An important component of clinical judgment is cost-benefit analysis (also called risk-benefit analysis). As illustrated in Figure 6-1, decision making after hip surgery involves balancing the risk of *failure* with the benefit of regaining best possible *function*. It also involves controlling *forces* (loads) through the hip with the regaining of best possible *form* (e.g., range of motion [ROM], strength, gait, transfers, endurance, balance). Long-term consequences should be a factor in addition to short-term outcomes. This may involve avoiding some activities because of a long-term concern about prosthetic loosening, and adding certain interventions to prevent contractures or weakness or both that may not become apparent until the patient is ambulating without an assistive device. In

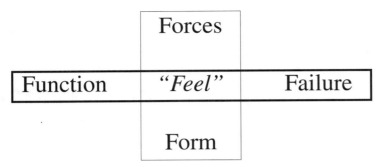

**Figure 6-1** The "F" balance—a model for clinical decision making.

the midst of this thinking-process is the patient, who should be central to decision making (i.e., how does the patient "feel"?) (see Figure 6-1). Making the right decision will depend on the circumstances, but it also heavily depends on the clinician's depth of knowledge and clinical reasoning skills.

This chapter presents the foundations for postoperative physical therapy management regardless of hip surgery type or clinical setting. Although it is written with an early postoperative bias, additional information for later stage rehabilitation (e.g., full weightbearing, no precautions) can be gleaned from Chapters 3 and 4.

## Generic Inpatient Goals

### Short-Term Goals

The patient should be able to demonstrate the following before physical therapy discharge:

- Independent and safe bed mobility and transfers
- Independent and safe ambulation on level surfaces with appropriate assistive device and weightbearing status
- Independent and safe ascent and descent of stairs while maintaining prescribed weightbearing status
- Independent with home exercise program
- An understanding of precautions (e.g., dislocation precautions, weightbearing precautions, activity-level precautions)
- Independence and safety performing activities of daily living (ADL) (if not, may be an indicator for occupational therapy evaluation and intervention)

The physical therapist should also perform the following:

- Evaluate the need for adaptive devices, such as a raised toilet seat and transfer tub bench, and ensure that these are provided or obtained for the patient.
- Evaluate the need for inpatient rehabilitation (e.g., acute, subacute, nursing facility), home physical therapy, or outpatient physical therapy. Necessary discharge paperwork should be completed.

### Long-Term Goals

The primary long-term goal is to restore the patient to his or her predisability level of functional mobility. For most hip patients, this means return to pain-free and stiffness-free ambulation, work, and ADL. In some cases, it may take as long as 6 months to 1 year for this goal to be fully realized. A higher-level goal of return to recreational activity is desirable for many patients and can be the reason they chose surgery. The physical therapist should be able to explain the options (e.g., which sports or recreational activities are realistic) and risks and be able to effectively rehabilitate and prepare patients for return to sport. Communication with the orthopedist is important when making decisions regarding return to sport.

## Physical Therapy Management: Overview

When staffing and timing of admission allows, preoperative assessment is recommended. From the preoperative assessment, the therapist is able to formulate a baseline of the patient's medical and functional status. Breathing exercises, coughing techniques, isometric exercise, and restricted weightbearing with an assistive device (e.g., walker or crutches) are taught. The initial evaluation (either pre- or postoperatively) should include a patient profile, description of current condition and surgery, past medical history review, physical examination findings, and social history. Postoperative evaluation and intervention should commence on postoperative day (POD) 1, unless contraindicated by medical condition.

A doctor's order is required at most institutions for initiation of postoperative physical therapy. Following initial evaluation, bed exercises, including ankle pumps, quadriceps sets, gluteal sets, and incentive spirometry, are taught. Mobilizing from bed to a chair should be attempted on POD 1. However, low hematocrit, low blood pressure, or both can result in lightheadedness and dizziness that limits the time tolerated out of bed. The old adage "first of all, do no harm" should always take precedence over the need to meet length-of-stay quotas. Postoperative complications that occur most commonly are deep vein thrombosis, atelectasis, pneumonia, pressure sores, and postanesthetic confusion. Complications are relatively rare, since preventative measures, such as early mobilization, calf-compression sleeves, anticoagulation, incentive spirometry, and epidural anesthesia, are employed at most centers.

Short-term goals listed in the earlier section should ideally be achieved by POD 5. However, for many hip replacement and hip fracture patients the achievement of all these functional goals in 5 days is unrealistic. My recommendation is that, if within a few days of surgery it seems that discharge home cannot be achieved by POD 5, then triage to a rehabilitation facility should be planned as soon as the patient is medically stable. With managed-care pressures, length of acute hospital stay for hip patients may be reduced to 2 or 3 days! Caution needs to be exercised to ensure that the burden of care is not merely shifted from one facility to another, and that quality of care does not suffer (Fitzgerald et al. 1988; Strömberg et al. 1997). Predictive criteria and critical pathways can be used to enable effective and efficient patient care and discharge planning (Figure 6-2).

## Subjective and Objective Assessment

### Preoperative Assessment

Because the length of hospital stay has been dramatically reduced to save health care dollars, preoperative assessment and teaching should be improved as a means of maintaining quality. Currently, arenas for preoperative physical therapy assessment are the doctor's office, outpatient department (individual or group class), and the home setting. Educational pamphlets and videos are used in many institutions.

The preoperative assessment and intervention should include the following:

- A brief evaluation of the patient's general health and physical condition
- A social history
- Description of the procedure and likely postoperative progression with physical therapy
- Fitting of the patient with crutches and teaching in their use on level surfaces and stairs
- Education as to the postsurgery precautions (e.g., dislocation risk and weightbearing status)
- Instruction in postoperative exercises, in particular breathing exercises and simple bed exercises (e.g., ankle pumps, quadriceps sets, gluteal sets)
- Home environment assessment and removal or adaptation of architectural barriers

## Physician's Orders for Physical Therapy

To improve the continuity of care and enable safe and effective physical therapy intervention, the surgeon should include the following in his or her orders:

- Diagnosis and surgery (with date of surgery)
- Reason for referral (e.g., gait training, ROM, strengthening)
- Weightbearing status
- Precautions (e.g., dislocation risk, no active hip abduction)
- Clarification of orders (e.g., hip abduction brace can be off in bed but must be donned for transfers and ambulation)

Although many states allow physical therapists to practice without referral, a doctor's order is often necessary for insurance reimbursement.

## Medical Record (Chart) Screen

Before meeting the patient, the following information should be noted from the medical record:

- Presenting complaint
    Reason for admission
    Surgery: type, date, and complications
- History of presenting complaint
    Onset: approximate date and mechanism
    Previous treatment: surgery (including dates), physical therapy, and so on
- Medical history: past and present (systems screen)
    Cardiovascular
    Pulmonary
    Nervous system
    Musculoskeletal
    Gastrointestinal
    Visual
    Hearing
    Behavioral
    Communication
- Social history
    Persons at home
    Occupation
    Stairs to climb
    Types of chairs

| | Preoperative Evaluation and Education | Operation Day | POD 1 | POD 2 | POD 3 | POD 4 | POD 5 |
|---|---|---|---|---|---|---|---|
| **Consults** | | | | | | | |
| **Surgeon** | | Anticoagulation needs | If there are long-term anticoagulation needs, make anticoagulation appointment for POD 3 | | | | |
| **Case Management** | D/C needs | | | | | | |
| **Nursing** | SF-36 | | | | | | |
| **Anesthesia** | | Pain Service if the patient has an epidural | | | | | |
| PT | | | Perform the postoperative evaluation See "Activity and exercise" section for treatment progression | | | | |
| OT | | | | | OT consult if | | |

| Tests | Chest x-ray EKG Blood work | Prothrombin time → | → | → the patient has comorbidities, is going home, or has functional limitations | → | D/C if lower extremity ultrasound for DVT is negative |
|---|---|---|---|---|---|---|
| | | HCT | → | → | → | |
| **Medication** | Nursing assessment | Pain medication (epidural or PCA) | → or PO pain medication | PO pain medication | → | |
| | | Cefazolin for 36 hrs | D/C | | | |
| | | | Premedicate before activity PRN | | → | |

**Figure 6-2** Total hip replacement clinical pathway. This clinical pathway is designed to be useful for medical purposes only. It is not intended to be used as a diagnostic decision-making tool and must not be used to replace or overrule a physician's judgment or diagnosis in each case. The responsibility for decisions regarding individual patient care rests solely with the physician treating the patient. (POD = postoperative day; D/C = discontinue; SF-36 = short form 36 questions (health survey); PT = physical therapy; OT = occupational therapy; EKG = electrocardiogram; HCT = hematocrit; DVT = deep vein thrombosis; PCA = patient controlled analgesia; IV = intravenous; PRN = as required; PO = by mouth; NPO = nothing by mouth; DSD = dry sterile dressing; BID = twice a day; PWB = partial weightbearing; ADL = activities of daily living; SNF = skilled nursing facility; ROM = range of motion; OOB = out of bed; AAROM = active-assistive range of motion; AROM = active range of motion; THR = total hip replacement.) (Adapted from J Siliski, J Empoletti, J Pedro. *Orthopedic Service*. Boston: Massachusetts General Hospital.)

| | Preoperative Evaluation and Education | Operation Day | POD 1 | POD 2 | POD 3 | POD 4 | POD 5 |
|---|---|---|---|---|---|---|---|
| | | Coumadin | ↑ | ↑ | ↑ | ↑ | D/C if ultrasound is negative |
| | | IV therapy | → or PRN lock | PRN lock | D/C | | |
| **Nutrition** | Nursing assessment | NPO → clear liquids | → diet as tolerated | | | ↑ | ↑ |
| **Wound and skin** | Nursing assessment | Assess need for pressure relieving overlay | Assess skin every shift→ | | ↑ | | |
| | | Assess alignment and position in traction | Assess skin of extremity in balance and pillow suspension | | D/C balance and pillow suspension | The patient should wear an abduction wedge at night | |
| | | Hemovac | D/C | | | | |
| | | Primary dressing | ↑ | Change to DSD | DSD PRN | ↑ | ↑ |
| **Elimination** | Nursing assessment | | Encourage fluids→ | | ↑ | ↑ | ↑ |
| | | | Bulk laxative BID, PRN | | ↑ | ↑ | ↑ |

| | | | | | |
|---|---|---|---|---|---|
| **Discharge planning** | Assessments are performed by physician, nursing, PT, and OT. If rehabilitation placement criteria are met, make rehabilitation referrals | D/C plan is initiated. If criteria are met, refer to SNF. Evaluation performed by an acute rehabilitation facility | Finalize D/C disposition | Initiate D/C referrals. If the patient is going home, identify nursing, PT, and OT needs. Identify and alert home health care agency of tentative D/C date. Determine which agency will be used. Determine the date PT will be available | D/C to acute rehabilitation. Order bathroom and ADL equipment. Order ambulatory equipment. If outpatient services are needed, arrange the location and the initial PT visit |
| | | | | | D/C home or to SNF |
| **Activity and exercise** | **PT** Assess and initiate treatment plan: Dislocation precautions | ↑ | ↑ | ↑ | ↑ |
| | | | | | ↑ |

**Figure 6-2** *Continued*

| | Preoperative Evaluation and Education | Operation Day | POD 1 | POD 2 | POD 3 | POD 4 | POD 5 |
|---|---|---|---|---|---|---|---|
| | | | Circulatory exercise | ↑ | ↑ | ↑ | ↑ |
| | | | Breathing exercise | ↑ | ↑ | ↑ | ↑ |
| | | | ROM exercise | AAROM, progress to AROM | ↑ | ↑ | ↑ |
| | | | Motor-control exercise | Submaximal isometrics and isotonics | ↑ | ↑ | ↑ |
| | | | OOB to chair | Transfer training | Encouraging independent transfers | ↑ | |
| | | | PWB with walker | Gait training | Progress to crutches; Begin stairs training; Determine walking-device needs for D/C | | |
| | | | ADL training and equipment | | OT consult for ADL | Assess raised toilet seat and tub seat needs for home | |
| | | | Communicate and post exercise and activity plan | ↑ | ↑ | ↑ | ↑ |
| **Nursing** | | | Reinforce activity plan, hip precautions, and exercises | ↑ | ↑ | ↑ | ↑ |
| **Physician** | | | Reinforce daily activities and goals with patient and family; Use clinical pathway | ↑ | ↑ | ↑ | Determine if D/C today is appropri- |
| **Patient education** | Physician's office; Video | | | | | | |

| | | |
|---|---|---|
| Education pamphlets Patient clinical pathway | | ate and complete D/C teaching |
| **Nursing** Pain management | → **Nursing** Pain management → | Instruct and provide with medications, prescriptions, and dressing needs Provide patient and family teaching |
| | Incentive spirometry → | |
| **PT** THR precautions Mobility | → **PT** THR precautions → Bed exercise → | Instruct regarding safety issues Instruct in a PT program for the home |
| **OT** Safety at | → **OT** Encourage use → | Review self-care tech- |

**Figure 6-2** *Continued*

| | Preoperative Evaluation and Education | Operation Day | POD 1 | POD 2 | POD 3 | POD 4 | POD 5 |
|---|---|---|---|---|---|---|---|
| | home ADL | | of ADL devices in the bed or chair as needed | | | niques and safety techniques with equipment | |
| | | | Patient's pain should not exceed 4 of 10 on pain scale | | | | |
| **Goals** | Assessments Patient education | — | Initiate rehabilitation plan | Finalize D/C location | Complete referrals to acute rehabilitation | — | Assess the home medication needs |
| | | | Patient demonstrates awareness of correct lower extremity | Patient demonstrate precautions | | | Patient should be independent with transfers and ambulation on level surfaces and stairs |
| | | | | | Patient should ambulate with crutches short distances with | Patient should ambulate increasing distances with crutches | Patient should perform ADL independently or with home sup- |

| positioning and hip precautions | | assistance | | port |
|---|---|---|---|---|
| | Patient should be OOB for meals | Patient should ambulate increasing distances with a walker | Stair training should be initiated | Provide a written home exercise program |
| | Patient should perform bed exercises at frequency prescribed by PT | | Patient demonstrates ADL skill with OT equipment | Discharge the patient if safety and home-support criteria are met |

**Figure 6-2** *Continued*

Bed height from floor
Whether there is a raised toilet seat
Whether there is a transfer tub bench
Whether there are assistive ambulatory devices
Recreational pursuits

## Laboratory Test Results of Importance

It is important for the inpatient physical therapist to review the operative report and radiographic reports. Heart rate, blood pressure, and respiratory rate should be monitored before and after out-of-bed activity. When necessary, percent oxygen saturation should also be monitored. Temperature, hematocrit, and prothrombin times should be reviewed. Knowledge of white blood cell count, erythrocyte sedimentation rate, rheumatoid factor, and blood sugar is important in certain cases. Medications that the patient is on and their effects and side effects should be known. Analysis of such information aids treatment planning and helps explain clinical responses. Refer to appropriate texts for further information on this subject.

## Subjective Assessment

The physical therapist should use the patient interview as a means of confirming and enhancing the chart review. A confident and clear introduction of yourself as the physical therapist and your role is essential.

## Objective Assessment and Physical Therapy Intervention

Efficiency is the key to surviving in today's health care environment. Thus, incorporating treatment and education in the same session as the initial evaluation may be necessary. A sequence for performing the objective assessment and providing intervention strategies is listed in Table 6-1.

Red flags to consider before attempting to mobilize a patient out of bed are as follows:

- Does the patient have any medical issues that limit or prevent the physical therapist from getting him or her out of bed (e.g., Is he or she on bed rest for evaluation of suspected myocardial infarction or deep venous thrombosis? Does the patient require oxygen for ambulation

**Table 6-1** Initial Evaluation Sequence

| Objective assessment (physical examination) | Treatment and intervention |
| --- | --- |
| Posture and position of whole body and limbs | Clearly introduce yourself. Explain to the patient the nature of surgery and what physical therapy involves. Take a patient history. |
| ROM | |
| Ankles | Teach ankle pumps. |
| Knees | Teach AROM of uninvolved LE joints. |
| Hips | Teach AA flexion ROM of involved hip. |
| Upper extremities | Teach AROM and resistive exercise for UEs or have the physical therapy assistant or aide teach later. |
| Strength (MMT) | |
| EHL | — |
| Tibialis anterior | — |
| Quadriceps | Teach quadriceps sets. |
| Gluteus maximus | Teach gluteal sets. |
| Gluteus medius | — |
| (Test resisted hip abduction only on noninvolved hip in first few postoperative days.) | |
| Hamstrings | Teach hamstring sets (optional). |
| Upper extremities (quick tests for ROM and strength) | Teach UE strengthening and ROM if necessary. |
| Sensation (gross assessment of light touch) | — |
| Proprioception | — |
| (Test if there are balance problems with standing and gait.) | |
| Circulation | Ankle pumps (as above). |
| (Check for capillary refill to toes and color and temperature. Ask the patient if he or she has calf pain. Perform Homans test.) (Documentation abbreviation: CSM = circulation, sensation, and movement; NVI = neurovascular intact.) | Calf compression pumps may be in use. Patient is also likely to be on prophylactic anticoagulation (e.g., warfarin sodium [Coumadin]). |

**Table 6-1** *Continued*

| Objective assessment (physical examination) | Treatment and intervention |
|---|---|
| Mental status<br>(If patient's answers to questions seem inappropriate, perform the short mental status exam to assess alertness and orientation to person, place, and time.) | — |
| Transfers<br>Supine-sit, sit-stand, and sit-supine (document assistance required) | Teach most appropriate method in terms of safety, precautions, and ease of function. |
| Balance<br>Sitting (static and dynamic) and standing (static and dynamic) (In the early postoperative period, tests such as the one-leg stance time [OLST] are not usually performed due to limited weightbearing.) | Often in the early postoperative phase, balance is impaired for reasons associated with the surgery (e.g., dizziness from low hematocrit, low blood pressure, pain, or postoperative confusion).<br>In the majority of cases, balance improves as other rehabilitation parameters improve. |
| Posture<br>Sitting and standing | Encourage upright sitting and standing.<br>Common faults are slouched sitting; flexed knees, hips, and lumbar spine; and forward head. |
| Gait<br>(Determine what walking aid is required and whether the patient already owns one. Base decision on physician's orders, patient's physical condition, and the strength of the patient's other limbs.) | A walker is useful as a means to initiate standing and gait due to its inherent stability.<br>Use of crutches is preferable if the patient can safely maintain weightbearing status and balance. |
| Stairs<br>(Determine whether the patient has stairs to negotiate at home, and whether there are sturdy rails. With few exceptions, patients should be taught how to ascend and descend steps while maintaining the prescribed weightbearing status.) | Use of crutch or handrail is more supportive than crutches only and is preferable for safety; however, both methods should be taught in case rail-less steps or curbs are encountered.<br>Initiate stair training after patient is safely ambulating on level surfaces.<br>Patients who are safe with a walker on level surfaces may be able to safely do stairs with a crutch and banister, if someone is with them to carry the walker. |

LE = lower extremity; AA = active assistive (range of motion); ROM = range of motion; AROM = active range of motion; UE = upper extremity; MMT = manual muscle test; EHL = extensor hallucis longus.

due to a pulmonary condition? Does the patient's mental status indicate that he or she should not be left unattended?)

- What are the doctor's orders? Are they appropriate given the chart information extracted?
- What are the orthopedic precautions (e.g., weightbearing status, dislocation precautions, presence of a trochanteric osteotomy, whether any muscles were "taken down" that should not be stressed, need to wear a brace)?
- Are there any other fractures, surgeries, or conditions at other sites that should be considered?

Discussion with the nurse, physician, or both about the patient before physical therapy evaluation and treatment can be valuable in helping plan an efficient, effective, and safe physical therapy intervention.

## Postoperative Positioning Devices

Postioning devices after hip surgery include:

- Pillow suspension: for comfort, elevation, and to ease movement of the patient in bed.
- Balanced suspension: allows movement of the patient in the bed without affecting the position of the involved lower extremity. It consists of a half-ring Thomas knee splint and a Pearson attachment to allow knee flexion.
- Buck traction: a temporary means of traction for hip fracture or after hip replacement as dislocation prophylaxis and for comfort.
- Skeletal traction: uses a pin through bone to deliver traction. For hip and acetabular fractures, a Steinmann pin can be placed through the distal femur or the proximal tibia.
- Russell traction: used for temporary traction of a fractured hip in the elderly. It consists of skin traction attached to weights.
- Abduction wedge or pillow: for dislocation prophylaxis after hip replacement. (For more information, see "Dislocation Precautions.")
- External rotation strap: used in cases in which the hip rolls into internal rotation after surgery. This strap keeps the hip in neutral rotation or slight outward rotation.

Note that, except for the abduction wedge, all of these devices require a bed frame for attachment.

## Functional Mobility Scale

Independent and safe performance of the following tasks (key functional milestones) should ideally be achieved before discharge home (Guccione et al. 1996):

- Supine-to-sit transfer
- Sit-to-supine transfer (Getting into bed is generally more difficult than getting out of bed.)
- Sit-to-stand transfer (Sitting down is always easier than standing up; therefore stand-to-sit is not included in this key functional milestone list.)
- Ambulation on level surfaces with walker
- Ambulation on level surfaces with crutches
- Stairs with crutch and banister
- Stairs with crutches only

Patients do not need to achieve independence in all of the above functions, if they have maximal help at home and no stairs. Other patients need to be independent at an even higher level, involving many more tasks than the basic seven listed above. In such cases, the following factors should be considered:

- Person available at home to help
- Walking distances necessary inside and outside house to enable function
- Types of surface to walk over (e.g., Is the path up to the house flat and paved or is it cobbled and on an incline?)
- Number and type of stairs to negotiate

## Weightbearing Status

Teaching weightbearing status is a very important component of the physical therapist's role. The definitions and the rationale for why a particular weightbearing status is used are given below.

- Nonweightbearing (NWB). The affected limb does not bear any weight. This is usually prescribed for hip patients who would be unable to maintain touchdown weightbearing.
- Touchdown weightbearing (TDWB). The foot touches down for balance only. Some studies have operationally defined this as not more than 10-lb weight through the affected limb. Other terms to describe this concept are *weight-of-limb weightbearing*, *feather weightbearing*, and *toe-touch weightbearing*. Although literal toe touching is occasionally warranted, hip patients should be encouraged to use as normal a gait pattern as pos-

sible while maintaining this weightbearing status. Acetabular fractures, tenuous hip fracture repairs, allograft reconstruction, and hip fusions are prescribed TDWB. *If performed correctly*, it creates the lowest hip loads by keeping ground reaction forces and muscular forces to a minimum (Fagerson et al. 1995; Givens-Heiss et al. 1992).

- Partial weightbearing (PWB). PWB is sometimes described as one-third of body weight and sometimes described as one-half of body weight. Some doctors prescribe a particular poundage (e.g., 20-lb PWB). How accurately restricted weightbearing can be taught and how consistently it can be maintained is debatable. The majority of patients probably partial weightbear as tolerated (PWBAT), and recent research suggests that PWBAT is a sensible weightbearing restriction for most THR, hemiarthroplasty, and hip fracture repairs (Fagerson et al. 1995). PWBAT implies that the surgeon would prefer PWB, but regaining of function should not be limited if the patient cannot maintain PWB.
- Weightbearing as tolerated (WBAT). With WBAT, loading the limb as pain tolerates is allowed, but assistive devices are used for protection. THR and hemiarthroplasty patients may be permitted to weightbear as tolerated, especially older patients who otherwise would be unable to mobilize.
- Full weightbearing (FWB). With FWB, 100% weightbearing is permitted. The physical therapist should clarify with the surgeon if an assistive device should be used for "protected" weightbearing. Crutches tend to slow a patient down and protect against accidental stumbles that may be detrimental to the prosthesis (Bergmann et al. 1993). Some surgeons allow THR patients to full weightbear. Indeed the father of hip replacement surgery, the late Sir John Charnley, allowed his cemented THR patients to full weightbear based on the rationale that "newly cemented implants are stronger than they will ever be at any later stage, so that the load of body weight is not important" (Charnley 1979, p. 304). Charnley was concerned, however, with avoiding powerful contraction of the hip abductors due to the trochanteric osteotomy he routinely performed as part of his surgical technique. He advocated a four-point gait pattern as a means to minimize abductor muscle contraction (Charnley 1979). However, recent research indicates that less in vivo acetabular contact pressures are generated with a three-point crutch gait pattern than with a four-point crutch gait pattern (Fagerson et al. 1995).

These descriptions of weightbearing status are not universally accepted, so adherence to your institution's definitions is recommended.

## Monitoring Limb Load

Most frequently, assessment of weightbearing is done by patient report (e.g., "I am putting about 25% weight through the operated leg"); visual analysis, which involves looking for correct use of assistive device and technique (reliable for NWB but not for grading of weightbearing); and tactile assessment, in which the therapist places a hand under the patient's foot and asks him or her to replicate the required amount of weightbearing.

A more accurate method of providing limb-load feedback is to have the patient stand on a bathroom scale with the operated leg, with the unaffected leg on a level surface. A pair of bathroom scales is used in some centers. This method provides accurate information as to the weight that is loaded through the involved extremity. However, the bathroom-scale method measures a static situation and has no direct carryover to gait, where it is most needed.

A limb load monitor can be used to provide feedback during gait of limb load (Betts and Watson 1992; Gapsis et al. 1982). The device is most widely used for research purposes. It consists of a sensor insole placed in the shoe with a wire connecting to a monitor. The device beeps when a predetermined load is exceeded or in some cases, such as with neurologic patients, when a required amount of weight is not maintained. The monitor is set at the desired weight, while the patient stands on bathroom scales. During gait, if this maximum or minimum weight is exceeded or not achieved, the device beeps.

A technique called *summary knowledge of results* applies motor-learning principles to the task of learning PWB and helps with carryover of what is learned outside of the clinic. One method involves the patient ambulating PWB and stepping on a scale set in the floor. After a few attempts, feedback is given to the patient as to whether he or she is maintaining the prescribed level of PWB. Progressively, over more and more trials, the feedback becomes less frequent to prevent patient dependence on the summary knowledge of results (Winstein et al. 1993). The accuracy can be improved when pain is included as a factor.

## Assistive Devices

The hierarchy of orthopedic assistive devices from most to least supportive is as follows:

- Parallel bars
- Walker with platform attachments
- Walker (standard, folding, or rolling)
- Crutches with platform attachment
- Crutches (axillary or forearm [elbow or Canadian])

- Quad cane (large base or small base)
- Cane

Most hip patients are discharged from the hospital with crutches. A walker is often employed for its stability in the first few postoperative days. The patient is then progressed to crutches, unless, for safety reasons, he or she should continue to use a walker. Axillary crutches are the most widely used, probably because they are least expensive and they also encourage the patient to stand up straight. Forearm crutches are useful for patients with hip orthoses and patients with conditions such as status postmastectomy. Sir John Charnley (1979) encouraged the use of forearm crutches, as they enable easier progression to canes. Most centers do not progress THR patients as rapidly to canes. Devices less supportive than crutches are unlikely to provide consistent weightbearing relief. Involvement of upper extremities (e.g., wrist fracture) can necessitate the use of a platform walker or platform crutches.

## Levels of Assistance (Guarding)

During transfers, gait, and other forms of functional training, the amount of assistance provided to the patient should be documented. From most to least protection, these are as follows (Kauffman et al. 1987):

- Maximum assist: assistance of one or more persons. More than one-half of the patient's body weight (BW) requires support.
- Moderate assist: assistance of one or two persons. One-fourth to one-half of the patient's BW needs support.
- Minimum assist: assistance of one person. Up to one-fourth of the patient's BW requires support.
- Contact guard: hands in contact with patient ready to supply more assistance if needed. Some centers consider this *minimum assist*.
- Hand-hold assist: therapist holds patient's hand for reassurance and slight balance assist. This is only possible if the patient can fully weightbear. Some centers consider this *minimum assist*.
- Stand-by guard: therapist is in very close proximity with patient but not touching. Therapist is ready to provide assistance at a moment's warning. Some centers call this *close supervision*.
- Supervision: therapist feels obliged to observe patient for safety reasons and possibly for verbal cues, but no human assistance is required.
- Verbal cues: Therapist needs to give patient verbal feedback and instruction for safety. This can be required during any of the above levels of assistance.

**Table 6-2** University of Iowa Level of Assistance Scale with Associated Ordinal Grades

| Grade | Definition |
|---|---|
| 0: Independent | No assistance or supervision is necessary to safely perform the activity with or without assistive devices, aids, or modifications. |
| 1: Standby | Nearby supervision is required for the safe performance of the activity. No contact is necessary. |
| 2: Minimal | One point of contact is necessary for the safe performance of the activity, including helping with the application of the assistive device (part of ambulation), getting leg(s) on or off the leg rest, and stabilizing an assistive device. |
| 3: Moderate | Two points of contact are necessary (by one or two persons) for the safe performance of the activity. |
| 4: Maximal | Significant support is necessary at a total of three or more points of contact (by one or more people) for the safe performance of the activity. |
| 5: Failed | Patient attempted the activity but failed with maximal assistance. |
| 6: Not tested | Due to medical reasons or reasons of safety, the test was not attempted. The test was attempted and was not completed at less than maximal assistance. |
| Contact | Any physical contact between the therapist and the patient or the assistive device (e.g., walker, crutches, gait belt). |

Source: Reprinted with permission from RK Shields, KC Leo, WF Dostal, R Barr. (1994) An acute care physical therapy clinical practice database for outcomes research. *Physical Therapy* 74, 463–470.

- Independent: therapist is comfortable with patient performing function without any assistance.

The number of people required for assistance, guarding, or both should be documented. Use of a gait belt is encouraged in many centers.

A modification of this widely used level of assistance scale has been developed at the University of Iowa (Table 6-2) and has been "shown to be highly reliable, valid, and responsive" (Shields et al. 1995, p. 169).

## Transfer Training

*Transfer* refers to the act of moving from one position to another (e.g., supine-to-sit or sit-to-stand). Precautions need to be heeded with some surgical procedures, usually relating to dislocation precaution, weightbearing status, or trochanteric osteotomy. Some practitioners advocate a specific way to perform transfers and are dogmatic about it. It was once taught that THR patients should get out of bed on the same side as the operation, as they are less likely to hip adduct and therefore less likely to dislocate. This advice is often impractical, as it requires the patient to get into bed on the other side! It is better for the patient to have a full understanding of his or her precautions and then apply that understanding to different situations. Orthopedic patients should be given the minimum amount of assistance required for safe performance of a task. The goal, after all, is functional independence. A useful reminder are the words of Abraham Lincoln, "do for no person what he can do for himself."

Some useful transfer tips are as follows:

- With heavy patients (i.e., greater than 200 lb), frail patients, or neurologically impaired patients, always consider obtaining assistance for the transfer, so as not to put yourself or the patient at risk.
- Provide assistance for the operated leg in supine-to-sit transfers during the first few postoperative days, as this gives much needed confidence and pain relief.
- If the patient is having difficulty with supine-to-sit transfers, consider help at home, supply with a leg-lifter device, or both.
- With sit-to-stand transfers, advise the patient to keep the operated foot in front. This has been shown to reduce acetabular contact pressures (Fagerson et al. 1995).
- Hip chairs are highly recommended for minimizing acetabular contact pressures during standing up and sitting down.
- A patient in a hip spica cast or brace does best with an overhead bar or trapeze attached to the bed (at home as well as in hospital). This sometimes necessitates renting a hospital bed for the home.

## Gait Training

Gait training of orthopedic hip patients involves teaching protective weightbearing with the use of an appropriate assistive device and ensuring that the prescribed weightbearing status is maintained efficiently and safely. In the inpatient setting, the goal of gait training is primarily to ensure safe and independent function, whereas, in the outpatient setting, greater emphasis is placed on the quality of the locomotion. There are different types of gait pattern that can be taught:

- Three-point gait. This is usually the first gait pattern taught to post-surgery hip patients. It can be used to teach TDWB to FWB gait. Often a walker is used first, with progression to crutches as able. Three-point gait involves forwarding the assistive device just before the operated extremity. The body weight is then shared between the involved leg and the upper extremities, while the noninvolved leg steps to or steps past the involved leg.
- Four-point gait. The sequence for this gait pattern is crutch (or cane) and then contralateral lower extremity (e.g., right crutch, left leg, left crutch, right leg). Since only one assistive device or leg is off the ground at one time, it leaves three supports in contact with the ground. This makes it a good gait for patients with bilateral lower extremity involvement (e.g., after bilateral THR).
- Two-point gait. The patient advances one assistive device (crutch or cane) and the opposite foot at the same time. One leg and one assistive device always provide two points of support on the ground at one time. A minimum weightbearing status of more than 50% BW is required for two-point gait. Two-point gait is a progression of four-point gait and is closer to the natural rhythm of walking.
- Step-to gait. Step-to gait is a three-point gait in which the noninvolved foot steps to the same level as the involved limb.
- Step-through gait. In the step-through gait, the noninvolved foot steps past the position of the involved foot. This sequence approximates a normal gait sequence and attention should be focused on step length, timing, and normal gait features. The prescribed weightbearing status should always be maintained.

The terms *step-to* and *step-through* should not be confused with *swing-to* and *swing-through*. A swing-to and swing-through gait (most commonly used by paraplegics) involves momentarily bearing weight on both lower extremities, while the assistive device (crutches or walker) is forwarded. The legs then swing together either to or through the position of the assistive device. This type of gait pattern should only be shown to a hip patient who has poor use of both lower extremities, who is in such excruciating pain that the opposite leg acts as a splint, or who is unable to step because he or she is wearing a hip spica cast.

When weightbearing is permitted through both lower extremities (with or without assistive devices) the quality of the gait pattern should be assessed. The clinician should observe the swing and stance phase of both extremities:

- Swing phase. This is the open kinetic chain phase of gait. It is usually broken down into three stages: initial swing, midswing, and terminal swing. Sufficient hip, as well as knee, flexion should be ensured. Compensation by hip hiking is common to allow foot clearance, but normal hip and knee flexion should be encouraged instead.

- Stance phase. This is the closed kinetic chain phase of gait. It involves five instants: initial contact, load response, midstance, terminal stance, and preswing. Normal heel strike, foot flat, and toe off should be encouraged.

The physical therapist should compare the operated side with the contralateral side and encourage symmetry. Loss of hip motion often results in the compensatory mechanisms of increased knee movement on the same side and increased hip movement on the opposite side.

## Common Post–Hip Surgery Gait Faults

The most common gait faults after hip surgery are either caused by or contribute to hip flexion contractures. A Trendelenburg or compensated Trendelenburg gait is usually masked by use of an assistive device postsurgery. The physical therapist should observe the postoperative patient for the following gait faults (Chandler 1987):

- Uneven step length. The patient takes a large step with the operated leg and a short step with the noninvolved leg to avoid discomfort in the groin caused by stretching the leg into hip extension.
- Knee flexion at late stance phase. The patient breaks the knee out of extension at late stance phase to avoid hip extension. Encourage the patient to keep the knee extended throughout stance phase. Over time and as the patient walks faster, the subtle changes that occur in knee flexion during stance phase are usually regained.
- Flexing forward at the waist. This is done at mid and late stance to avoid hip extension. Encourage thrusting the pelvis forward and the shoulders back with the knee in extension during mid and late stance to counteract this. Trunk flexion is more common with patients using forearm crutches.
- Overstriding the crutches. Encourage the patient to place the forefoot of the operated leg level on an imaginary line between the two crutches when using a three-point pattern.

## Stairs

Once independent with gait on level surfaces and before discharge, the patient receives instruction in ascending and descending stairs. In general, all patients who are to be discharged home should be independent on stairs even if they do not have stairs at home. Curbs are a form of step, and patients have to negotiate them in the community. Patients who are house bound and never face stairs can be excused from stair training, as should patients who are not medically or physically ready for stairs. These patients can be transported home by ambulance and receive further rehabilitation in the home. Stair training can then be done when the patient is ready.

Stair climbing is taught using the following sequence:

1. Ascent: unoperated leg first, then operated leg, and then crutches
2. Descent: crutches first, then operated leg, and then unoperated leg.

The prescribed weightbearing status should be maintained. A sturdy banister, if available, should be used for support instead of one of the crutches. The crutches should be doubled up in one arm or one given to a companion to carry while using the railing. Use of a banister and a crutch is a good precursor in training before teaching use of both crutches.

Some patients are safer on stairs with railing and crutch combination than they are with crutch gait on level surfaces. Therefore, patients who can ambulate safely with a walker should not be excluded from doing stairs with railing and crutch, even if they are not safe with crutches on level surfaces. There are techniques for negotiating stairs with a walker, but they are not recommended, and the patient needs to be permitted weightbearing as tolerated.

## Dislocation Precautions

Following hip replacement (hemi- or total) there is an increased risk of dislocation. Hemiarthroplasties (especially bipolar) tend to be more stable than total hip arthroplasties because of a larger femoral head. THRs are essentially performed via a posterior or an anterior approach (see Chapter 5). The terms *direct lateral, anterolateral*, and *posterolateral approach* are also used clinically (Barber et al. 1996; Hardinge 1982; Hoppenfeld and deBoer 1994). However, even with direct lateral approach, the hip must be dislocated either anterior or posterior to insert the total hip components; therefore, it should be thought of as either an anterior or posterior approach. The lateral approach is considered to have a lower dislocation rate than the posterior approach due to preservation of the posterior capsule (Barber et al. 1996). Dislocation risk is usually in the direction of the surgical approach (e.g., posterior approach carries with it a posterior dislocation risk). Dislocation precautions are listed below for the various surgical approaches.

- Posterior. Avoid hip flexion greater than 90 degrees, adduction, and internal rotation.

- Anterior. Avoid combined hip extension and external rotation and avoid adduction.
- Lateral. Avoid hip adduction. Also avoid the combined movements comprising posterior precaution or anterior precaution, depending on the direction of femoral head dislocation at surgery.

Dislocation is a relatively rare complication: The average incidence of dislocation after THR is 2–3% (Morrey 1992). If dislocation occurs, however, it is serious and can become a recurrent problem. Prevention is therefore key. The physical therapist should explain and demonstrate the risks clearly to the patient, but, unless the risk is high, the patient should not be made to feel paranoid about dislocating. Satisfaction for the patient usually entails enabling a high level of pain-free function while maintaining safety and not compromising the artificial joint's stability in the socket.

In the early postoperative phase, a knee immobilizer can be used when in bed on the operated leg (especially with noncompliant or confused patients) to minimize the risk of hip flexion combined with internal rotation or adduction. The patient's operated hip is usually too weak and too painful for it to be flexed by straight leg raising. An abduction wedge with straps is a more secure method of holding the operated hip in abduction than a pillow between the legs. The abduction wedge can be used in conjunction with a knee immobilizer to provide strict posterior dislocation prophylaxis. This can be cumbersome, however, and a pillow between the legs can suffice as a reminder not to cross the legs in fully alert patients. Balanced suspension is often used for the first 2–3 PODs. Balanced suspension keeps the operated hip in abduction, keeps the leg elevated, and allows some early hip movement through a small range.

To improve patient compliance with dislocation precautions, the precautions should be explained in a meaningful and relevant way to each patient (Roush 1985). Simply ensuring that the patient can recite the precautions may not be consistently effective. Dislocation precautions should be explained and applied in terms of getting dressed, getting in and out of a car, gardening, sexual intercourse, and so on. Explaining the mechanism of dislocation by movement of the trunk over the hip (closed chain) is as important as the mechanism of dislocation by movement of the leg on the hip (open chain), as in the following examples:

- A posterior dislocation can occur by flexing the knee toward the chest (usually beyond 90 degrees). It can also occur, and this is the more common mechanism, when getting out of a chair when the hip flexes past 90 degrees by movement of the trunk flexing over the leg. The risk is greatly increased and can occur at less than 90-degrees flexion when there is a component of adduction, internal rotation, or both (i.e., combined movement). In bed, posterior dislocation can occur by flexing, adducting, and internally rotating the hip by moving the leg. It can also occur by twisting the trunk toward the at-risk side. Rolling onto the nonoperated side places the operated hip at risk of both adduction and internal rotation; therefore, an abduction wedge or a couple of pillows between the legs is essential when rolling on to the side (for all hip replacement approaches).

- An anterior dislocation can occur by extending and outwardly rotating the hip by moving the leg. It also occurs in standing (hip is already in extension) by rotating the trunk away from the operated side. Likewise in bed, anterior dislocation occurs by the leg rolling outwards at the hip (the hip is already in almost full extension when the patient is lying supine). This risk is further increased when a patient uses a bedpan or when twisting the trunk away from the operated side. Keeping the leg in abduction with a pillow and neutral rotation with a rolled towel tucked under the length of the outside of the leg decreases the risk of anterior dislocation in bed.

Patients often ask, "When can I stop worrying about dislocation?" Orthopedic texts generally state that after 3–6 months the risk is much less due to healing of soft tissues and formation of a pseudocapsule. However, there will always be a greater risk of dislocation in THR patients compared to the normal population. It may be wise, therefore, to tactfully instruct a THR patient to heed the precautions for the rest of his or her life. I often explain the true story of one fully functional woman (who even played tennis) who, 6 years following hip replacement, was at a barbecue when she felt a mosquito on the outside of her ankle. She moved to swat it and subsequently dislocated her hip due to the movement of flexion, adduction, and internal rotation performed quickly. It is comforting to let the patient know that after 3–6 months it usually takes a combination of movements (e.g., flexion, adduction, and internal rotation) performed suddenly to dislocate, and also that, over time with conscious effort, the precautions become subconscious.

Physical therapists have an important role to play in the education of patients following hip replacement. Most of the details described in this chapter are not included in postoperative physical therapy orders. The astute physical therapist gathers from the surgeon information that is important for effective and safe rehabilitation. Developing a mutual respect with the surgeon enables the appropriate sharing of information and enhances patient care.

## Orthotic Devices

Sometimes after hip surgery, it is necessary to have the patient wear an orthotic device to protect the hip during function. A removable orthosis is most often prescribed after hip dislocations, some hip revision surgeries, hip reconstructions, and fusions. An orthosis may be preferable to a spica cast if healing of incisions and pressure care are a primary concern. For the noncompliant patient, or when immobilization of the hip is the primary concern, or both, a spica cast is preferred.

Types of hip orthoses are as follows:

- Hip spica brace or cast: is commonly used after a hip fusion or after a delicate hip reconstruction, when it is critical to keep the hip immobilized. If complete immobilization is required, both thighs should be incorporated in the hip spica. A higher level of functioning can be achieved when only one thigh is included; however, movement of the pelvis results in some stress to the protected hip. The hip spica usually immobilizes the hip in 10–25 degrees of flexion and 5–15 degrees of abduction. By extending the brace to the foot on the operated side, hip rotation can be effectively controlled.
- Mini hip spica (one-half hip spica): incorporates the trunk and one thigh. It does not provide as secure a stability as the full spica.
- Hip abduction orthoses: to control hip motion in the coronal and sagittal planes, a hip abduction orthoses can be prescribed. Most frequently, these are used after reduction of a dislocation or after revision arthroplasty. They usually come prefabricated and consist of a thigh cuff attached to a waist belt. Adjustments can be made to provide a comfortable and correct fit. A shoulder strap can be added in cases in which the brace slips out of position. The hip is usually positioned in 15–30 degrees of abduction, and a flexion stop is used for posterior dislocation protection and an extension stop for anterior dislocation risk. The surgeon should prescribe the limits he or she thinks are necessary. Patients and caregivers should be shown how to don and doff these braces safely. In general, the hip abduction orthosis should be used at all times except when standing to shower, and in some cases when the physician allows substitution with an abduction pillow while in bed.
- Hip-knee-ankle-foot orthoses (HKAFO): extends to the foot so that it provides good rotational control of the lower extremity. This amount of control is usually not required after hip surgery, except in some cases of femoral allograft, internal hemipelvectomy, or tenuous hip reconstructions. Obviously, the larger and heavier the brace, the more difficult it is for the patient to maneuver. Some HKAFOs provide weightbearing through the ischial tuberosity to theoretically decrease loads through the hip and femur. Hodge and colleagues (1989) found that an ischial-bearing long-leg brace is as effective as PWB with

crutches in reducing in vivo maximum acetabular contact pressures. Bergmann and colleagues (1990b), using a force instrumented THR, found that an ischial weightbearing orthosis provided the same reduction in in vivo forces as use of a contralateral crutch, but that two crutches reduced the load on the femoral head much more. They concluded that good clinical results with an ischial-bearing brace are more likely due to the reduced physical activity in such patients and not the load-reducing effect of the brace.

The hip is a difficult joint to brace due to its size and available ROM. A certain amount of mobility and stability needs to be available to permit donning and doffing of a removal orthotic, such as the abduction brace. Considerations, such as patient compliance and help at home, need to be taken into account.

Patients in hip spica casts and orthoses need to learn unconventional functional techniques. They also need to be trained and supplied in the use of appropriate assistive devices. These methods include long-handled ADL devices, overhead bed frames, whole-body diagonal transfers in bed followed by direct supine-to-stand transfer or prone-to-stand transfer, and swing-through gait patterns.

## Activities of Daily Living Devices for Hip Patients

In environments in which there are occupational therapists, it is worth delineating whose role it is to order and instruct in the use of the various types of adaptive equipment. In general, the physical therapist provides equipment related to functional training (e.g., raised toilet seat and transfer tub bench) and the occupational therapist provides equipment related to ADL (e.g., dressing and washing aids).

It is important to ask specific questions as to the bathroom set up and consider size of the patient before ordering bathroom equipment. For example, a large patient may not fit comfortably in a raised toilet seat with arms, therefore a raised toilet seat without arms and a separate side rail should be ordered. A raised toilet seat should be provided before discharge home, as it may be needed right away. A shower and tub seat may be best ordered by the community therapist, if the patient has home care.

The following are types of ADL equipment to consider:

- Raised toilet seat
- Transfer tub bench
- Hip chair
- Long-handled reacher

- Dressing stick
- Flexible sock and stocking aid
- Long shoehorn
- Elastic shoelaces (or slip-on shoes)
- Long scrub sponge
- Shower hose

There are also techniques for tying shoes and picking objects from the floor without assistive devices.

## Therapeutic Exercise for Hip Surgery Patients

The goals of exercise are to increase ROM, reduce stiffness and prevent joint contracture, increase muscle strength, increase circulation, lubricate joint cartilage when it is present, prepare for functional activity, and provide psychological benefits.

Common postoperative exercises taught to hip patients are listed below. (The most appropriate exercises to be commenced during the inpatient stay for hip replacement are italicized.)

- *Ankle pumps*
- *Quadriceps sets*
- *Hamstring sets*
- *Gluteal sets*
- *Short arc quadriceps and terminal knee extension*
- *Hip flexion, supine with knee flexing* (heel slide)
    Supine with knee straight (straight leg raise)
    Sitting (make sure legs apart)
    Standing
- *Hip extension, standing (open chain and closed chain)*
    Prone (with knee flexed and with knee straight [straight leg raise]) (To roll to prone position, the patient should have hips abducted with pillow between legs and should roll via operated side.)
    Sitting on edge of bed, leaning back on arms
- *Lying flat (prone or supine) for 30 minutes per day to stretch hip flexors*
- *Thomas test stretch*
- *Hip abduction, supine* (Red flag: active hip abduction exercise should be avoided after trochanteric osteotomy)
    Standing
- *Hip rotation (internal and external), supine* (Red flag: For internal rotation with posterolateral approach, make sure the patient is lying

flat with legs apart. Avoid hip rotation with hip fracture open reduction internal fixation patients unless physician permits.)
  Prone
- *Hip hiking (the hula), supine* (Red flag: active hip abductor exercise should be avoided after trochanteric osteotomy unless surgeon permits)
  Standing
- The "rhumba" (Chandler 1987), standing (closed-chain hip abduction and adduction by side gliding the pelvis)
- *Knee flexion and extension, supine and sitting*
  Prone (for rectus femoris stretch)
- All fours, buttocks to heels (Red flag: this involves flexing hips well over 90 degrees flexion and should not be done with posterior approach cases. It should only be done if the surgeon permits.)
- Stationary bicycle (Full revolutions performed only when comfortable, with no resistance during first 2 weeks. It has been shown to generate low acetabular contact pressures [Hodge et al. 1989]. With lateral approach, the patient can do "jockey" riding to increase flexion.)
- Pool therapy (see Chapter 4)

The initiation of postoperative exercises should be staged. Ankle pumps and isometric contractions should be started on POD 1 to maintain circulatory status and deep-breathing exercise should be started to prevent chest complications. Active-assisted ROM can be started on POD 2, with ROM increasing and assistance decreasing as tolerated each postoperative day.

On discharge, the home program should be performed two to three times per day, with 10 repetitions of each exercise at first. Intensity, frequency, and duration of exercise should be modified appropriately. Not until bone and soft tissues have healed sufficiently should resistive exercise or passive stretching be considered by an outpatient physical therapist and not without clearance of the surgeon.

## Discharge Planning

In the 1990s, when length of stay following hip surgery has been reduced to 3–5 days, it is imperative that discharge planning be initiated immediately after the operation. Most THR patients go directly home. Figure 6-3 provides a useful algorithm for physical therapy discharge planning.

Hip fracture patients tend to be elderly and in poor general health and may need rehabilitation or nursing-home placement before discharge home. A small proportion may have already been nursing-home residents, and, in such cases, prompt return (within approximately 10 days) is necessary to prevent loss of their bed. Multiple factors should be considered in planning discharge, and some of the most important are listed below. These are most applicable to the hip fracture population.

The following are factors with the potential for affecting hip surgery outcome:

- Age. The likelihood for discharge directly home after hip surgery decreases with increasing age, particularly after 65 years of age (Barnes and Dunovan 1987; Guccione et al. 1996; Mossey et al. 1990; Thorngren et al. 1993).
- Prefracture ambulatory status. Independent ambulators are more likely to go directly home than those who depended on assistive devices, human assistance, or both before surgery (Guccione et al. 1996; Koval et al. 1995).
- Prefracture living situation and social supports. Living with someone who is healthy, having supportive relatives and friends, being involved in church or social clubs, and not having to climb stairs are factors that increase the likelihood of discharge directly home (Ceder et al. 1980; Zuckerman 1996).
- Comorbid conditions (e.g., stroke, depression, dementia, recent myocardial infarction). The presence of one of these conditions decreases the likelihood of discharge directly home (Ensberg et al. 1993; Greenfield et al. 1993; Guccione et al. 1996). Other factors to consider are arthritis, additional fractures, poor eyesight, frailty, poor balance, and side effects of medication (e.g., dizziness and weakness) (Michelson et al. 1995).
- Type of surgery. In elderly patients, surgical fixation that permits immediate FWB (or WBAT) is more likely to enable return to independent ambulation with assistive device than surgery that requires NWB, TDWB, or PWB. For example, a cemented hemiarthroplasty or THR is more stable than a pin or screw system, allowing for early FWB. A lateral approach for joint replacement is less likely to dislocate than a posterior approach. (Incidentally, the more stable approaches are also more costly, and the surgeon usually weighs the costs and benefits in his or her choice of surgery decision. Surgeons tend to use the most stable approach possible with more debilitated patients to enable early return to function [Lhowe 1990].)
- Lower extremity joint contractures of greater than 10 degrees. Particularly hip and knee flexion deformities and ankle plantar flexion contractures can impair return to function (Barnes and Dunovan 1987).
- Hip abductor weakness. This has been correlated with slower regaining of function (Barnes and Dunovan 1987). Hip abductor strengthen-

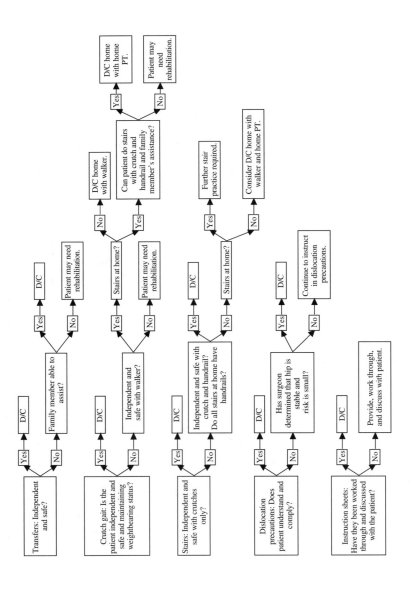

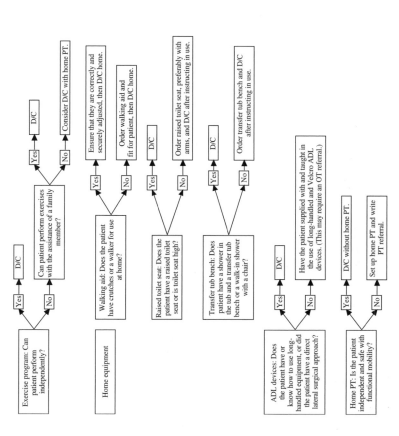

**Figure 6-3** Hip surgery discharge planning algorithm. This figure illustrates the thought process that a physical therapist should use when planning to discharge a patient home. All of the questions on the left of the figure should be asked. If the algorithmic end-point for each question is not "D/C home" then other discharge arrangements should be considered. (ADL = activities of daily living; D/C = discharge; PT = physical therapy; OT = occupational therapy.)

ing should be performed (provided the surgery did not involve a trochanteric osteotomy) to help improve function, as well as to decrease the likelihood of a Trendelenburg lurch when the patient is ready to be weaned from a cane.

- Postoperative complications (e.g., upper respiratory tract infection, deep venous thrombosis, urinary tract infection, wound infection). Such complications can increase the length of acute hospital stay and decrease the odds of being discharged directly home (Guccione et al. 1996).
- Intensity of postoperative physical therapy. Physical therapy should start the day after surgery and ideally occur more than one time per day (Guccione et al. 1996). Efforts to shorten acute-care hospitalization for hip fracture patients since the implementation of prospective payment resulted in decreased quality of care and increased cost, as more patients were triaged to nursing homes, albeit never to return home (Fitzgerald et al. 1987, 1988). Intensive and skilled early mobilization can therefore prevent long-term institutionalization. It should be noted that the findings of Fitzgerald and colleagues (1988) were challenged by another study of similar design (Palmer et al. 1989).

Bonar and colleagues (1990) identified the following as factors that contribute to a patient's ability to return home within 6 months of placement in a skilled nursing facility (SNF) following hip fracture: orientation, younger age, ability to bathe independently, family involvement, ability to ambulate or transfer independently, and greater number of available physical therapy hours. Likelihood of returning home increased from 7% in those with less than two of the factors to 82% for those with four or more factors.

## Minimizing Hip-Joint Loads

Patients who have acetabular fractures or tenuous hip-joint reconstructions should be instructed in methods to minimize hip-joint loads (see Chapter 1, Table 1-5). In vivo acetabular contact pressure studies using pressure instrumented prostheses have led to the following conclusions regarding means to *minimize* hip pressures (Fagerson et al. 1995; Givens-Heiss et al. 1992; Hodge et al. 1989; Krebs et al. 1991; Strickland et al. 1992):

- Chairs. The patient should sit in high (hip) chairs with arms and keep operated foot in front during sit-stand transfers.
- Gait. The patient should use NWB or TDWB gait with walker or crutches.
- ROM. The patient should use passive, active-assisted, or powder-board ROM.

- Isometrics. The patient should perform submaximal contractions and hold for only a few seconds.
- Strengthening. The patient should keep to slow, gravity-eliminated exercise and avoid maximal contractions.
- Stairs. The patient should ensure that TDWB or NWB is maintained.

It has been demonstrated that TDWB, if performed correctly, produces less acetabular contact pressure than NWB (Givens-Heiss et al. 1992). However, there may be a tendency with elderly, weak, or noncompliant patients for TDWB to become WBAT (Fagerson et al. 1995). In such cases, if minimal hip loads are desired, NWB is advocated.

With patients who have tenuous surgical fixation or acetabular fractures, the physical therapist should ask himself or herself questions such as, Is exercise necessary at this stage? He or she should always weigh the benefit of an intervention against the risk (see Figure 6-1).

Although muscle-strengthening exercises produce acetabular contact pressures of similar magnitude to FWB gait (Krebs et al. 1991), this should not discourage use of strengthening exercises after *routine* hip arthroplasty, especially if increased strength improves the patient's function.

Stair climbing and rising from a low chair create higher pressures than bed exercises (Fagerson et al. 1995; Hodge et al. 1989; Krebs et al. 1991) (see Table 1.5). Accidental loss of balance and stumbling have resulted in high hip pressures and forces (Bergmann et al. 1993; Fagerson et al. 1995), suggesting that balance and safety measures should be important components in a rehabilitation program.

Recent research indicates that high pressures do not damage a natural joint when the opposing cartilage surfaces are congruent, because the load in a well-fitted joint is not supported by the cartilage at all but rather by the hydrostatic pressure of the fluid in the cartilage tissue (Macirowski et al. 1994). This has implications for surgeons who implant total and hemi-hip arthroplasties—they must ensure as congruent a fit as possible. However, as amazing as arthroplasty of the hip is, it will probably never be as perfect as a natural healthy hip joint. Failure of hip prostheses mostly results from wear. Wear results in the breaking away of polyethylene, cement, or bone particles resulting in (1) direct loosening of a prosthesis from micromotion at the cement-bone interface or cement-prosthesis interface (which is the most common mechanism of *femoral* component loosening [Jasty et al. 1991]) or (2) indirect loosening by initiating the process of osteolysis (the most common mechanism of *acetabular* component loosening [Schmalzried et al. 1992a]). Wear also leads to degeneration of the acetabular cartilage in hemiarthroplasties (Dalldorf et al. 1995). Physical therapists cannot expect a patient not to function, after all the reason a patient has a THR is to relieve pain and restore function. The effects of wear can be reduced by optimizing the internal mechanics (the surgeon's role) and by rehabilitating the patient to optimal function using and teaching methods that minimize wear (the physical therapist's role). Moderation in activity is practical advice for most patients. In time, with improvements in prosthetic design, the level of activity for THR patients should be able to safely increase.

## Leg Length Discrepancy

Detecting, measuring, and treating a leg length discrepancy (LLD) is an important component of the physical therapist's role. Occasionally after hip surgery, a patient presents with a significant LLD. The discrepancy could be new or it could be long standing, and it may be intentional by the surgeon to optimize hip mechanics (Johnston et al. 1979). If the LLD is a result of the surgery, tact must be used in presenting potentially disturbing news to the patient. It may be best to allow the surgeon to inform the patient about a LLD, because in certain states this is the primary reason for litigation after THR (McGann and Hungerford 1996). Some patients perceive a difference in leg length postoperatively even when clinically there is no difference. Most often this occurs in patients who had an apparent LLD preoperatively, such as from an abduction contracture. Emphasizing rehabilitation and downplaying the LLD is advised initially as the perceived difference usually fades with time (Abraham and Dimon 1992). Measurements of leg length should be made in standing using blocks to even the iliac crest height, in addition to supine measurement of apparent and true leg length. The surgeon should be informed of findings and of the proposed intervention. An LLD of 0.25 in. is considered within normal limits. A discrepancy of less than 1 in. in the immediately postoperative patient probably does not need compensation. A 0.25 in. heel insert is preferable cosmetically, but, when LLD is greater than 1 in., an external shoe lift is necessary for mechanical symmetry. A supportive shoe with a rubber or leather sole is required when adding a lift.

## Postoperative Instructions for Hip Replacement Patients

The advice listed in Tables 6-3 and 6-4 applies to THR and hemiarthroplasty patients who had a posterior surgical approach. The advice is, however, useful for most patients after hip surgery with minor modifications.

**Table 6-3** Instructions for Patients After Hip Replacement

Walking

Use two crutches and partial weight on the operated leg.

Step first with crutches, then operated leg, then nonoperated (good) leg.

Dislocation precautions

Avoid bending more than 90 degrees at the hip.

Do not cross your legs.

Do not turn your operated leg inwards.

Above all, avoid a combination of bend, cross, and twist of the operated leg.

Avoid bending over in sitting to tie shoe laces.

Avoid leaning forward too far when getting up from sitting.

Be careful to observe dislocation precautions at all times, especially when getting in and out of a car, when turning in bed, and in the bathroom.

Stairs

Going up: Step with the good leg first, then operated leg, and then crutches.

Going down: Step with crutches first, then operated leg, and then good leg.

"The good go up, the bad go down" may help you remember.

Crutches always go on the lower step.

Use a banister in one hand, if available, and crutches in the other.

Exercises

Perform the exercise program you have been given at least two or three times per day.

Do not perform an exercise if it is painful.

Sitting

Sit in a chair that is high and has arms (consider purchasing a hip chair).

Slide the operated leg out in front before you sit or stand.

Sit down slowly and with control.

Avoid bending forward as you sit or stand.

Avoid sitting too long, not more than 1 hour at a time.

Lying in bed

Sleep on your back the first 6 weeks.

If you must rest on your side, place a couple of pillows between your legs to prevent the operated leg from crossing and twisting in.

To get onto your stomach, turn onto the operated side; keep a pillow between your legs.

Bathroom

A raised toilet seat with arms is recommended.

**Table 6-3** *Continued*

A shower chair or tub bench can be useful.

A nonslip mat in the shower and sturdy handrails are recommended for safety.

Dressing

Dress the operated leg first.

Use long-handled equipment to prevent the hip flexing more than 90 degrees.

Elastic laces may be helpful.

Rest

Rest in bed for at least 3 hours per day.

Spend at least 20 minutes, two times per day, lying flat on your back or on
your stomach.

## Preventing Falls

A large proportion of postoperative hip patients have undergone surgery to repair a hip fracture. Most of these hip fractures are the result of a fall. Fall-prevention education and training need to become a routine component of the physical therapist's role to curb the rate of hip fractures. This applies not only to education in the community and through the media but also to those patients being treated for a current hip fracture. A cognizant patient will be receptive to methods of preventing further falls. Table 6-5 illustrates the type of information that should be given to patients and reinforced by the home therapist.

A series of studies conducted at Yale University, called the *FICSIT\* trials*, have tested a wide range of treatment strategies and found that the risk of falls are reduced by the following (Kiel 1994; Tinetti et al. 1988):

- Improving physical capacities
- Optimizing healthy behaviors (use of nutritional strategies and pharmacologics)
- Improving the safety and living environments of community dwellers and long-term care residents

---

*FICSIT = Frailty and Injuries: Cooperative Studies on Intervention Techniques.

**Table 6-4** Common Questions After Hip Replacement

How do I get into the car?

It is best to sit in the front passenger seat of a large family car. Sports cars and trucks should be avoided. The following technique is recommended:

Push the front passenger seat all the way back and recline it somewhat.

A pillow or two helps raise the height of the seat.

Slide the operated leg out in front before you start to sit.

Slowly lower yourself onto the car seat (get your head in first so you do not bend too far forward).

Once seated, move your buttocks back toward the driver's seat and then lift your feet into the car, being careful not to cross or inwardly twist your operated leg.

Can I drive?

When your surgeon says so. If you had your left hip replaced and you drive an automatic, then you could probably be driving again within 2–4 weeks. Otherwise, do not plan to be driving until you are off crutches (approximately 6–8 weeks). You definitely should not drive at any time if your judgment is impaired by medication.

Can I sit in a tub?

Definitely not, unless you are sitting on a raised tub seat. Sitting in a bathtub would involve flexing more than 90 degrees and getting out could be very difficult.

When can I shower?

After the wound is clean and dry. If you do not have a walk-in shower, a raised transfer tub bench may be necessary.

What about sex?

Hold off for 6–8 weeks if you can, and not too vigorous at first. The safest position for your hip is on your back with your legs apart. Ask your physical therapist or doctor for a "safe positions" pamphlet. Check the World Wide Web site "Totally Hip" at http://www.telapex.com/saman1/hip.html.

How long will I be on crutches?

It can vary from person to person, but on average crutches are used for 6–8 weeks, then a cane is used in the opposite hand until you can walk without pain or limp. Your surgeon will advise you when to progress from crutches to a cane.

How long do I have to be careful about dislocating?

Be particularly cautious the first 3–6 months. Avoid a combination of bend, cross, and twist for the rest of your life!

What about sports?

Low-impact activities, such as walking, swimming, cycling, bowling, golf, social tennis, intermediate skiing (if you are advanced and never fall), are fine.

Higher-impact sports, such as running, competitive tennis, mogul skiing, basketball,

**Table 6-4** *Continued*

squash, racquetball, horseback riding, and lifting heavy weights, are not recommended. Obviously, there are different levels of intensity for every sport, so ask your surgeon if you have a particular concern. McGrory et al. (1995b) presented recommendations for return to specific sports after total hip or total knee replacement based on a review of the literature and a survey of 28 orthopedic surgeons at the Mayo Clinic. Participation in golf, swimming, cycling, bowling, sailing, and scuba diving were recommended. Twelve intermediate- to moderate-intensity activities were recommended with modification of technique. Ten sports not recommended were handball, racquetball, running, hockey, baseball, water skiing, karate, basketball, soccer, and football.

How can I prolong the life of my artificial hip?

Avoid high-impact sports and activities that involve twisting and turning. Minimize your use of stairs. Sit in armchairs that are high (consider buying a hip chair). Moderation in all things is key.

## Summary

The postoperative physical therapist plays a key role in the ultimate success of hip surgery. Communication with the surgeon is essential. Effective teaching of precautions and techniques for safe functioning, and prescribing the appropriate exercise program requires knowledge, skill, and clinical experience. Innovative means to deliver quality care in a cost-efficient manner—for example, critical pathways (see Table 6-1)—must continue to be developed. Ensuring the patient has a good understanding of and can demonstrate home instructions and exercises is paramount. If the patient does not demonstrate independent and safe functioning, follow-up therapy is justifiable. Although this chapter is geared toward acute inpatient physical therapy, it is applicable to the rehabilitation facility, nursing home, and home care.

The words of a great orthopedic surgeon make a fitting close to this chapter:

> With proper instruction and diligent performance of the prescribed exercise program, the patient can transform a merely good result into an excellent one (Chandler 1987, p. 401).

## Patient Educational Resources

American Academy of Orthopaedic Surgeons. (1995) *Total Hip Replacement, Patient Education Booklet.* Rosemont, IL: American Academy of Orthopaedic Surgeons.

**Table 6-5** Tips for Preventing Falls

General

  Ensure good lighting at all times.

  Use easily accessible light switches, especially from the bed.

  Remove scatter rugs and tack down carpets.

  Eliminate or avoid slippery surfaces (e.g., highly polished, wet, or icy surfaces).

  Remove obstacles from corridors and paths (e.g., electric or phone cords, low furniture, toys, pet dishes).

  Clearly mark threshold moldings.

  Make sure chairs, sofas, toilet seats, and beds are of a height that aids sitting down and standing up.

  Minimize risky behaviors such as standing on chairs.

  Keep frequently used items within easy reach.

Bathroom

  Use securely fastened grab bars by toilet, bathtub, and shower.

  Use nonslip mat or strips in tub and shower.

Kitchen

  Use a sturdy step stool for reaching high shelves.

Stairs

  Ensure that a securely fixed handrail goes the whole length of the stairs.

  Remove thick carpet and under padding.

Outdoors

  Give yourself plenty of time to cross the street.

  Use pedestrian crossings.

  Have ice and snow promptly cleared from walkways.

Personal

  Wear supportive and well-fitting shoes.

  Wear cleats in potentially icy conditions.

  Use a cane if you have bouts of unsteadiness and stay close to supportive structures.

  Position telephones in accessible locations.

  Stay alert.

  Keep physically fit.

Source: Modified from SR Flanagan, KT Ragnarsson, MK Ross, DK Wong. (1995) Rehabilitation of the geriatric orthopaedic patient. *Clinical Orthopaedics and Related Research* 316, 84.

Krames Communications. (1996) *After a Hip Fracture: Getting on Your Feet Again*. San Bruno, CA: Krames Communications.

Krames Communications. (1996) *Total Hip Replacement: Returning to Movement*. San Bruno, CA: Krames Communications.

Krames Communications. (1996) *After Total Hip Replacement: Living with Your New Hip*. San Bruno, CA: Krames Communications.

McCullen G, Miller R. (1996) *Hip and Knee Replacement: A Patient's Guide* (illustrated). New York: Norton.

Public Broadcasting Video. (1989) *The Implant: Hip Replacement Surgery* [video]. Tempe, AZ: KAET.

Total Hip Replacement Online Support Group. "Totally Hip." http://www.telapex.com/saman1/hip.html.

# 7

# Diagnostic Imaging of the Hip

Timothy L. Fagerson and
Scott L. Jones

Accurate diagnosis of hip disorders requires data from a thorough history, detailed physical examination, and appropriate imaging studies. Diagnostic imaging should be performed to confirm a suspected diagnosis, rule out serious pathology, and discover the presence of anatomic anomalies before the initiation of treatment. The physical therapist (PT)'s role regarding diagnostic imaging is to (1) recognize when referral to a physician is necessary for imaging and inspection; (2) provide the physician and radiologist with clinical information to assist in the choice of study and in the interpretation of findings; and (3) interpret radiologic studies to assist in physical therapy evaluation and treatment. Even if it appears to the therapist that viewing radiologic studies will not change the type of treatment, the images provide useful information to the therapist regarding "things under the skin." Given the reported poor reliability of many palpation and physical examination techniques for determining the integrity of anatomic structures, PTs should use radiologic information that is available to enhance the effectiveness of management for any given patient.

The following are common diagnostic imaging techniques for the hip-joint complex:

- Plain film radiography (x-rays)
- Conventional tomography (tomograms)
- Computed tomography (CT)
- Nuclear imaging (bone scan)
- Magnetic resonance imaging (MRI)
- Fluoroscopy (real-time x-ray; procedure with x-ray guidance)
- Sonography (ultrasound)
- Arteriography and venography (arteriogram and venogram)
- Arthrography (arthrogram)

PTs are not expected to have a radiologist's or orthopedist's level of skill at interpreting imaging tests; however, knowledge at both the conceptual and practical level assists the clinician's clinical decision making, education of patients, treatment effectiveness, and communication with physicians. When viewing hip films—even those that are "negative"—the clinician should look for changes in alignment of the pelvis and lumbar spine (as well as at the hip), which can confirm physical exam findings or provide evidence that leads the clinician down another path of investigation. Physicians and radiologists are primarily concerned with "major" problems (e.g., fracture, degenerative joint changes, pathology) when reading plain films. PTs should, in addition, look for more subtle features that can influence treatment planning and aid in establishing treatment goals. To make reasonable interpretations, however, the PT must have an understanding of the radiologic techniques and procedures used. Knowing the positions that images are taken from is essential to making comments about normal versus abnormal alignment (e.g., weightbearing versus nonweightbearing, flexion versus extension films of the spine).

## Plain Films

The plain x-ray is the most valuable imaging study for the patient with hip disease and dysfunction (Petty 1991). Routine radiography has been described as the "gold standard" for hip and pelvis imaging, because it is relatively inexpensive, readily available, most clinicians are familiar with it, and it provides a good foundation of information for clinical decisions (Pitt et al. 1990).

Plain film radiography refers to the general process of creating images by exposing body parts to x-rays. These images are called *radiographs*, *radiograms*, or *roentgenograms* but are commonly known as *x-rays* or *plain films*. Tissue types absorb differing amounts of x-rays based on their attenuation properties and radiographic densities. Bony tissue has the highest absorption of x-rays, and air has the lowest. Radiographic density, or radiodensity, depends on the composition of a structure and its thickness. The more radiodense a substance, the whiter it appears on x-ray.

An understanding of the correlation between anatomy and the radiographic image of that anatomy is crucial to interpretation of each type of radiologic study. The hip complex is a geometrically complex structure. The pelvis has many curves, irregular surfaces, and varying densities and thicknesses of cortical and trabecular bone. Routine x-rays superimpose and summate these intricate features. The following hip x-ray features represent summations: the tear-drop or U figure, the acetabular roof (*sourcil*), and the ilioischial line (Pitt et al. 1990). Bones have a three-dimensional shape and standard radiographs only provide a two-dimensional image; therefore, at least two different x-ray views are required for adequate interpretation of the image. Routine hip x-rays should include an anteroposterior (AP) view of the pelvis, an AP view of the hip, and a lateral view of the hip. Specialized views or other modalities may be necessary to accurately diagnose a specific lesion.

## General Observations for Interpretation of Radiographs

The following information should be gleaned from a plain film:

- Patient's name
- Date of film
- Body part
- Radiographic view (e.g., AP, lateral)
- Side of body (right or left)
- Comparison with other side
- General bony architecture (e.g., normal versus abnormal anatomy and number of bones)
- Density of each image

  Black     air

                fat

                soft tissue (tendon)

                $H_2O$

                bone

                calcific deposition

                radiopaque dye

  White     prosthetic implant
- General and local bone density (e.g., trabecular patterns)
- General contour, shape, and size of images
- Cortical outline and medullary of bones
- Articulating relationships between bones
- Articular cartilage and potential space
- Joint capsules
- Soft tissues

## Routine Hip Views

Routine x-ray views for the hip are:

- Routine AP pelvis: A symmetric view of the pelvic girdle from low lumbar segments to the proximal third of the femurs should be seen

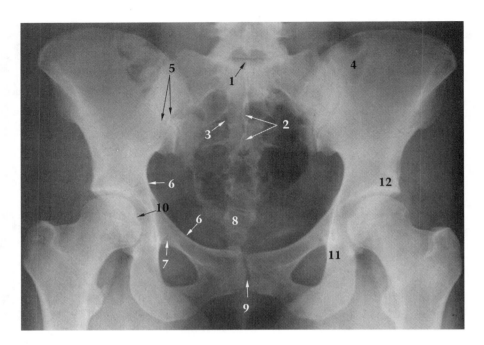

**Figure 7-1** Anteroposterior radiograph of the adult female pelvis. 1. Sacral promontory. 2. Sacral spinous crest. 3. Margin of anterior sacral foramen. 4. Gas in pelvic colon. 5. Sacroiliac joint. 6. Pelvic brim. 7. Obturator groove. 8. Coccyx. 9. Symphysis pubis. 10. Fovea of the femoral head. 11. Tear figure. 12. Acetabular roof. (Reprinted with permission from PL Williams, R Warwick, M Dyson, LH Bannister. [1989] *Gray's Anatomy* [37th ed] [p. 520]. Edinburgh, UK: Churchill Livingstone.)

(Figure 7-1). This view provides information about the lumbosacral spine, both sacroiliac joints, and both hip joints.

- Routine AP hip: This view gives better visualization of the affected hip than an AP pelvis view (Figure 7-2 A, B, and C). The radiographic information that should be assessed on the AP view is listed in Table 7-1.
- Routine lateral (shoot-through lateral): This true lateral view is taken approximately 90 degrees to the AP (Figure 7-2 G, H, and I). It is the preferred lateral view after trauma and surgery. The x-ray beam is directed at the medial femoral neck with the unaffected leg flexed.

Some practitioners advocate that standard AP pelvis and AP hip views be taken with the hip(s) in 15 degrees internal rotation to enable a good view of the femoral neck(s) without foreshortening (Long and Rafert 1995). Others do not advocate internal rotation positioning for standard views but recommend the

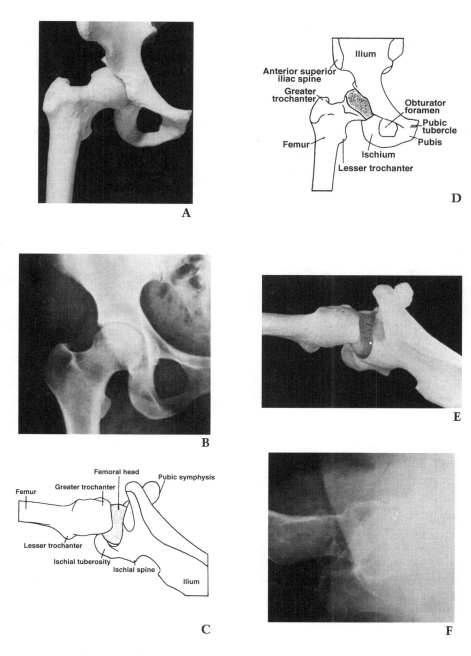

**Figure 7-2** The normal hip: photographic, diagrammatic, and radiographic anatomy of the hip in the AP (A, B, C), frog lateral (D, E, F) projections. (Reprinted with permission from BNW Weissman, CB Sledge. [1986] *Orthopedic Radiology* [pp. 386–387]. Philadelphia: Saunders.)

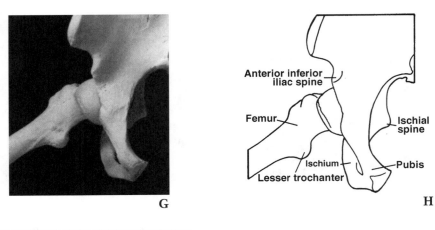

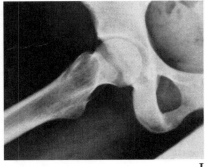

**Figure 7-2** *Continued* The normal hip: photographic, diagramatic, and radiographic anatomy of the hip in the true lateral (G, H, I) projection. Reprinted with permission from BNW Weissman, CB Sledge. [1986] *Orthopedic Radiology* [pp. 386–387]. Philadelphia: Saunders.)

"internal rotation view," especially when osteotomy is considered, as this allows accurate measurement of the neck-shaft angle (Zukor and Lander 1995). Maximal abduction and maximal internal rotation of the hip is described by Pitt and colleagues (1990) to be the best position to radiographically estimate the angle of inclination, because the femoral neck is perpendicular to the AP beam.

### Specialized Views

#### Hip

Specialized x-ray views for the hip include:

- Frog-leg lateral: This view is taken with the involved hip flexed, abducted, and externally rotated (see Figure 7-2 G, H, and I). Some

**Table 7-1** Radiographic Evaluation of the Hip: Anteroposterior View

Skeletal anatomy

    Iliopubic line

    Ilioischial line

    Radiographic U (teardrop)

    Acetabulum

        Dome

        Posterior rim

        Anterior rim

Angles

    Center edge angle of Wiberg (normal 20–40 degrees, average 36 degrees)

    Neck-shaft angle (normal 120–135 degrees; >135 degrees: coxa valga; <120 degrees: coxa vara)

Fat planes

    Obturator line

    Iliopsoas line

    Capsular line

    Gluteal line

Source: Adapted from TH Berquist, MB Coventry. (1986) The Pelvis and Hips. In TH Berquist (ed), *Imaging of Orthopedic Trauma and Surgery* (p. 197). Philadelphia: Saunders.

surgeons use this as a routine hip view. It gives a better view of the anterolateral femoral head and is useful in suspected Legg-Calvé-Perthes or avascular necrosis. Due to the flexed position of the hip, a lateral view of the acetabulum is not obtained (an AP projection of the acetabulum is achieved).

- Modified frog-leg lateral (table-down lateral): This method is more reproducible and more comfortable than the standard frog-leg lateral (Gold et al. 1991). This position is also described as the modified Lauenstein lateral (Long and Rafert 1995). It involves having the lateral border of the involved thigh resting on the table while the pelvis and trunk are rotated away.
- 40-degrees cephalad AP: This position is useful for subtle femoral neck fractures and pubic fractures (Eisenberg et al. 1981).
- Functional views: These views are AP views taken with the hip in (1) maximal abduction and (2) maximal adduction. They are used when planning osteotomy to determine the position of best coverage and containment of the femoral head within the acetabulum. Use of tracings and

fluoroscopy are also recommended when planning an osteotomy to determine the most congruent position for the hip-joint surfaces (Poss 1984).

- Contour views of Schneider: These views are useful in detecting abnormalities of the posterior and anterior aspects of the femoral head. CT gives the best image of the femoral heads, but, when it is not available, the contour views are a nice substitute. The anterior contour view is taken with the patient supine with hips flexed 45 degrees and the central ray positioned vertically over the femoral head. The posterior contour view is taken with the patient supine and the central ray directed caudally at the hip 30 degrees to the vertical (Zukor and Lander 1995).
- False-profile view: This is a lateral view of the hip taken with the patient standing. It is useful when planning an osteotomy, as it provides an estimate of anterior and posterior coverage of the femoral head in weightbearing (Zukor and Lander 1995).

### Pelvis

If a problem of the acetabulum or pelvis is suspected, pelvis views are necessary. Because these are not standard hip views, they are considered here as specialized views.

- AP frog-leg (modified Cleaves) pelvis: This view gives additional information to the AP pelvis, especially of both femoral necks. It is taken with both legs in frog-leg position and was first described by Cleaves in 1941.
- Inlet pelvis: This view is ordered in cases of pelvic trauma to detect pelvis fractures. It is an AP view of the pelvis with the beam directed caudally.
- Outlet (tangential) pelvis: This view is also ordered in cases of pelvic trauma. It is an AP view of the pelvis with the beam directed cranially.
- Judet oblique views: These are obtained when an acetabular fracture is suspected.
  - Iliac (posterior) oblique: Using a wedge, the patient is positioned 45 degrees from supine with the involved side up. The x-ray beam is centered directly above the hip. This view provides a good visualization of the posterior column and anterior rim of acetabulum, as well as the iliac wing.
  - Obturator (anterior) oblique: Using a wedge, the patient is positioned 45 degrees from supine with the involved side down. Again, the x-ray beam is centered directly over the hip. This view provides a good visualization of anterior column and posterior rim of acetabulum, as well as the obturator foramen.

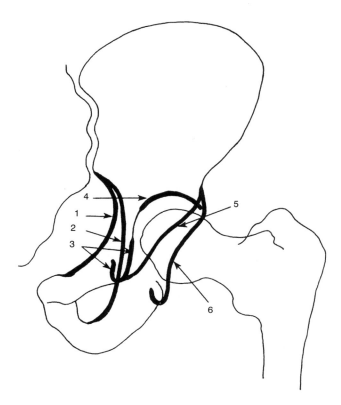

**Figure 7-3** Line drawing of anteroposterior radiograph of the hip. 1. Arcuate or iliopectineal line. 2. Ilioischial line. 3. Pelvic teardrop. 4. Superior acetabular margin. 5. Anterior margin of acetabulum. 6. Posterior margin of acetabulum. (Reprinted with permission from MK Dalinka, LM Neustadter. [1991] Radiology of the Hip. In ME Steinberg [ed], *The Hip and its Disorders* [p. 57]. Philadelphia: Saunders.)

When viewing x-rays, a working knowledge of anatomy (clinical and radiographic) is of utmost importance. On a normal AP radiograph six landmarks (Figure 7-3) should be noted on the acetabular side of the hip (Dalinka and Neustadter 1991). They are as follows:

1. Iliopectineal or arcuate line: represents the anterior column of the acetabulum.
2. Ilioischial line: represents the posterior column of the acetabulum.
3. Pelvic teardrop: a U-shaped structure that forms the anteroinferior portion of the acetabular fossa at the acetabular notch.

4. Superior acetabular margin
5. Anterior margin of acetabulum
6. Posterior margin of acetabulum

Disruption of any of these acetabular lines is suggestive of a fracture or other problem.

## The ABCS of Plain Film Interpretation

The ABCS approach described by Forrester and Brown (1987) provides a simple but useful framework for systematic interpretation of radiographs:

*A*lignment
*B*ony mineralization
*C*artilage space
*S*oft tissues

### Soft Tissues

The reason that soft tissues are described first is that Forrester and Brown (1987) stated that soft tissue evaluation is an important first step in examining radiographs because, in some cases, the definitive diagnostic clue is in the soft tissues. These clues are with tissue mass (too much or too little) or tissue density (radiolucency or calcification).

Joint effusions at the hip are difficult to diagnose due to the deeply situated nature of the hip capsule and its relative nondistensibility. Three different radiographic signs indicate fluid in the hip joint (Forrester and Brown 1987):

1. Lateral dislocation of the femoral head. This most commonly occurs in children, and the most frequent cause is juvenile rheumatoid arthritis. It takes a large effusion to subluxate or dislocate the femoral head from the acetabulum.
2. Absence of a vacuum effect. This technique can be used to detect small effusions of the hip. It is done by providing manual traction to the hip, while the x-ray is being taken. In a normal hip, traction creates a negative pressure in the joint, and the gas that is released is observed as a radiolucent crescent between the joint surfaces. The frog-leg view sometimes exhibits the vacuum effect. This phenomenon does not occur when there is extra fluid in the joint.
3. Demineralization of subchondral bone. Fading of the sharp subchondral white line of the femoral head is indicative of a synovitis of the hip—an inflammatory process. It is caused by demineraliza-

tion, which results in a fuzzy, ill-defined outline and apparent joint-space widening.

The presence of calcification should be noted about the hip joint. It may be seen in muscle, about the joint capsule, and in bursa and tendons (calcific bursitis or tendinitis). The finding of calcification is fairly nonspecific, but it can suggest an underlying process like rheumatoid arthritis, systemic lupus erythematosus, heterotopic ossification, or a response to trauma in the past.

Four fat lines are described about the hip: (1) obturator line, (2) iliopsoas line, (3) pericapsular line, and (4) gluteal line. They often provide the clue that leads to detection of subtle fractures or diagnosis of a rheumatic disorder. Considerable skill and experience are required for detection and accurate interpretation of fat lines. Reference should be made to texts such as Weissman and Sledge (1986) and Berquist (1986) for further information with illustrations.

### Alignment

An abnormal shaft-neck angle is the most common *congenital* abnormality of alignment at the hip (see Table 7-1 and Figure 1-3). However, *traumatic* disturbance of alignment from fracture or dislocation is more common (Forrester and Brown 1987). Hip fractures and dislocation are described in Chapter 2.

When viewing x-rays about the hip, the PT should pay special attention to alignment of the lumbar spine and sacroiliac joints. Of all the factors in the ABCS, soft tissues and alignment are the x-ray features that a PT can potentially impact. Therefore, when analyzing films, ask the following questions:

- Is the alignment an effect of the patient's posture or positioning when the film was taken?
- Is the alignment fixed, like a fixed-flexion deformity, or is it deformable (i.e., is the deformity partially or fully reversible with stretching and mobilization techniques)?
- How long has the malalignment been present? (Ask the patient and compare with previous films.)
- Is the observed alignment compensating for malalignment elsewhere in the lumbo-pelvic-hip chain or is it, for example, because of muscle spasm, hip hiking, or leg length discrepancy?

Radiographic assessment of alignment is generally more reliable than physical exam assessment of alignment (e.g., the scanogram is the gold standard for measuring leg length discrepancy). However, it is recommended that physical exam findings and radiographic findings be compared to yield the most valid interpretation.

The following alignment issues should be considered when viewing plain films of the hip:

- Fracture. Suspected fracture requires immediate orthopedic referral. See Chapter 2.
- Dislocation. Suspected dislocation requires immediate orthopedic referral. See Chapter 2.
- Angle of inclination. Angle of inclination is measured from an AP pelvis or hip view with the hip internally rotated approximately 15 degrees. Table 7-1 lists normal values.
- Center edge (CE) angle of Wiberg. The CE angle is a measure of inferior tilt of the acetabulum. It is the angle to vertical of a line connecting the lateral edge of the acetabulum with the center of the femoral head. Mean values are 38 degrees for men and 35 degrees for women with a range of 22–42 degrees (Anda et al. 1986).
- Acetabular index. The acetabular index is considered a more reliable measure of acetabular inclination than the angle of Wiberg. It is the angle to horizontal of a line connecting the medial and lateral inferior margins of the acetabulum (Figure 7-4). It is also known as Hilgenreiner's angle. The greater the angle, the less stable the femoral head within the acetabulum. Normal range is 20–30 degrees.
- Femoral offset and abductor lever arm. Femoral offset and abductor lever arm is an important concept related to hip replacement surgery and is illustrated in Chapter 5 (see Figure 5-1). Greater femoral offset after total hip replacement has been shown to allow greater hip abductor strength and abduction range of motion (Gore et al. 1977; McGrory et al. 1995a). Conversely, a less than optimal femoral offset distance could potentially result in irreversible abductor muscle weakness due to a mechanical disadvantage not corrected or unable to be corrected at surgery. Such information is useful to the PT in understanding why some patients take so long to regain abductor strength or never regain sufficient strength to overcome a positive Trendelenburg sign. Such patients may benefit from long-term use of a cane (Blount 1956).
- The interteardrop line. This is the preferred horizontal reference line for adult radiographs (see Figure 7-4).
- "Teardrop" sign. This is observed by drawing a line between the tips of each teardrop and extending this line into the femoral heads. If the extended line first meets the femoral neck and not the inferior point of the femoral head, it is suggestive of migration of the femoral head upwards into the pelvis (see Figure 7-4). If one proximal femur is greater than 10 mm superior compared to the other, it is a definite positive finding on that side (Magee 1992).

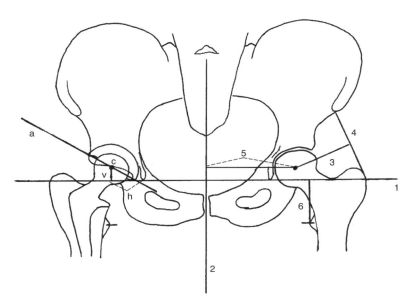

**Figure 7-4** Line drawing of an anteroposterior radiograph of the pelvis illustrating selected alignment measurements. For illustration purposes, each measurement is shown on one side only, but in practice both sides of the body should be compared. The line drawn between the lateral and medial margins of the base of the acetabulum is indicated by a. The angle of acetabular inclination is formed where this bisects the interteardrop line (1). This is a line joining the most inferior margins of the right and left teardrops. The center of the hip is indicated by c and the horizontal position of hip center by h. This is the horizontal distance from distal tip of the teardrop to a perpendicular line dropped from the hip center. The vertical position of the hip center is indicated by v. This is the vertical distance from the interteardrop line to the hip center. 2. Midline. 3. Abductor lever arm. See Figure 5-1 for an illustration of femoral offset. 4. Approximate length of abductor muscles. 5. Body weight lever arm. Note that in normal one-leg stance (i.e., no trunk lean), the line of body weight falls even further away from the hip center than the midline (2) (see Figure 1-13). 6. Proximal femur length (leg length measurement). This is the perpendicular distance from the lesser trochanter to the interteardrop line.

- "Absent teardrop." Absent teardrop, or "absent sourcil," is suspicious for metastatic disease (Pitt et al. 1990), as with an absent (nonvisualized) pedicle on lumbar radiographs.
- Bryant's triangle and Nélaton line. Bryant's triangle and Nélaton line are both described and illustrated in Chapter 3 (see Figures 3-8 and 3-9). These measurements can be applied to a true lateral x-ray of the hip in the same way that they are applied to surface anatomy in physical exam. A positive finding in each case is suggestive of a dislocated hip.

- Hilgenreiner and Perkins lines. Hilgenreiner and Perkins lines are bisecting lines that are drawn on an AP pelvis x-ray when developmental dysplasia of the hip (DDH) is suspected. Under normal circumstances, the ossification center of the femoral head is located in the inferomedial quadrant formed by the two lines. In DDH, the ossification center is in the superolateral quadrant (see Figure 2-5).
- Hilgenreiner line. This is a horizontal line drawn at the inferior border of the ilium (see Figure 2-5).
- Perkins line. This is a vertical line drawn from the most lateral point of acetabulum (see Figure 2-5).
- Shenton line. This is a curved line that can be drawn on an AP pelvis radiograph from the medial edge of the femur arcing smoothly upwards and then down to meet the inferior edge of the pubis. It is usually applied to pediatric assessment (see Figure 2-5).
- "Sagging rope" sign. This is one of the "head-at-risk" signs observed in Legg-Calvé-Perthes, where the normal upwardly convex curve of the capital femoral epiphysis curves downward (now upwardly concave) like a sagging rope.

Figure 7-4 illustrates additional features and measurements that can be made on an AP pelvis view.

### Bony Mineralization

Conditions that manifest themselves with changes in bony mineralization about the hip include inflammatory synovitis, osteoporosis, and avascular necrosis.

- Inflammatory synovitis. A loss of the sharp cortical line of the epiphysis is indicative of inflammatory synovitis. Inflammatory synovitis is associated with rheumatic diseases and with acute transient synovitis that occurs in children.
- Osteoporosis. Thinning of the cortex and loss of trabeculae is indicative of osteoporosis. The term *osteopenia* is used to describe local x-ray findings in the absence of widespread bone density changes. The Singh index is a method of grading the degree of osteopenia (see Figure 2-1). Note that osteopenia is not recognizable on plain films until there has been approximately a 40% loss in bone mineral density (Chew 1989).
- Avascular necrosis. Plain film indicators of avascular necrosis are scattered lucencies and areas of sclerosis. On the frog-leg view there can be breaks in the cortex and the characteristic rim sign (a subcortical black lucent line). At a later stage, collapse of the femoral head is observed. Legg-Calvé-Perthes, which is essentially avascular necrosis occurring in

childhood, has similar radiographic findings. X-ray findings of avascular necrosis may not be present until the process is far advanced. MRI is the most sensitive detector of avascular necrosis (see Table 2-6).

### Cartilage

The roentgenogram features indicative of cartilage abnormality are as follows:

- Joint space narrowing
- Osteophytes
- Subchondral cysts
- Subchondral sclerosis
- Subluxations

Diagnosis of hip diseases based on radiographic appearance alone is sometimes difficult, because most hip diseases progress to demonstrate osteoarthritis x-ray changes that obscure the original cause. To solve this dilemma, a radiologist or orthopedist can view all films taken since the start of a hip complaint, which should help greatly to determine the cause of the problem based on the pattern of progression of the x-ray changes. The radiographic appearance of osteoarthritis can be the end stage of the following disorders: rheumatoid arthritis, ankylosing spondylitis, psoriatic arthritis, infection, tuberculosis, and avascular necrosis. Uniform narrowing of the joint space and protrusio acetabuli at the end stage is indicative of rheumatoid arthritis. Osteoarthritis tends to cause narrowing in areas of major lines of force with presence of osteophytes. A new radiographic classification of primary osteoarthritis separates x-ray findings into three groups (Bissacotti et al. 1994):

1. Medial osteoarthritis: loss of medial joint space. Eventually progression can result in protrusio acetabuli.
2. Superior-lateral: loss of superior joint space. Lateral subluxation can be present in conjunction with medial osteophytes. This is the most common form of osteoarthritis.
3. Global osteoarthritis: uniform loss of joint space is seen, and there can be cystic changes but very few osteophytes. There is no clinical or pathologic sign of rheumatoid arthritis.

## General Overview of Imaging Studies Used in Hip Diagnosis

Many imaging studies are used to evaluate the hip joint. This chapter provides a fairly detailed review of plain films, which are the most fre-

**Table 7-2** Suggested Imaging Techniques for Various Adult Pathologies of the Hip Complex

| | Ultra-sound | X-ray | Bone scan | Tomog-raphy | Computed tomog-raphy | Magnetic reso-nance imaging | Arteri-ography and ve-nography |
|---|---|---|---|---|---|---|---|
| Fracture | — | + | + (stress) | + (stress) | + (pelvic) | + (stress) | — |
| Healing fracture | — | + | — | — | + (com-plex fx) | + (com-plex fx) | — |
| Prosthetic joint | — | + | + (if painful) | — | + | + (with arthrogram) | — |
| Trauma | — | + | — | — | + | + | — |
| Avascular necrosis | — | + | + | — | + | + (best) | + |
| Degenera-tive joint disease | — | + | — | — | — | — | — |
| Tumors (cancer) | — | + | + | — | + | + (best) | + |
| Osteomye-litis | — | + (late changes) | + (early changes) | — | — | — | — |
| Soft tissue injury | + | + | — | — | — | + | — |
| Osteoporo-sis | — | + | + | — | + | — | — |
| Joint laxity | + (infants) | + (fluor-oscopy) | — | — | — | — | — |

+ = frequently used for this problem; — = not often used for this problem; fx = fracture.

quently used and least expensive orthopedic imaging studies. However, it is beyond the scope of this book to comprehensively describe every method. This section is a general overview of imaging studies used in hip diagnosis. Table 7-2 summarizes the multimodality approach to diagnosis of adult hip disorders.

## Plain Film Radiography

*Plain film radiography* is the general process of creating images by exposing body parts to x-rays. Characteristics of plain film radiography are as follows (Merritt and Bluth 1985):

- Very sharp detail of bony structures
- Poor detail of soft tissues
- Two-dimensional summation image
- Difficulty detecting subtle changes in bone structure
- Easily obtained
- Can be portable
- Rapid
- Inexpensive

The plain film radiograph is a first-line study in diagnostic workup of hip disorders.

## Tomography

*Tomography* is a technique for obtaining a series of radiographs at consecutive planes through a body part. It is used to focus in on a particular area of interest. The following are characteristics of conventional tomography:

- Good contrast resolution
- High radiation
- Not portable
- Fairly expensive

Tomography is rarely used in hip workup because it has been superseded by CT and MRI.

## Computed Tomography

*CT* is computerized enhancement of a series of radiographs at consecutive planes through a body part. The following are characteristics of CT scans (Merritt and Bluth 1985):

- Three-dimensional, sectional images
- Good spatial resolution
- Good contrast resolution
- Best for identifying foreign bodies
- Usually requires contrast agents
- Not portable
- Moderately expensive

CT is the preferred method for assessment of osseous-based abnormalities of the hip, such as after trauma (especially useful for acetabular fractures) and in congenital disorders, like hip dysplasia (Conway et al. 1996). A new method called *helical (spiral) CT* enables the CT examination to be performed much more quickly (in 30–40 seconds of scanning) and with lower radiation exposure (Conway et al. 1996).

## Nuclear Imaging (Bone Scan)

*Bone scan* is a technique whereby the emission of a injected radioactive tracer is used to construct an image of the patient. The following are characteristics of bone scans:

- Poor spatial resolution
- Nonspecific alone
- Small radiation dose
- Sensitive to early physiologic bone changes
- Relatively expensive

A bone scan indicates regions of increased metabolic activity ("hot spots") by an increased uptake of radioactive tracer. It is useful in detection of bony metastatic disease, avascular necrosis, arthritis, and Paget disease. Although very sensitive, bone scans are not very specific and need to be used in conjunction with plain films, CT, or MRI to detect the type of lesion.

## Magnetic Resonance Imaging

*MRI* is an imaging method based on the interactions of atomic nuclei with a magnetic field. Characteristics of MRI are as follows (Merritt and Bluth 1985):

- Three-dimensional sectional images in any plane
- No radiation
- Good spatial resolution
- Excellent contrast resolution
- Does not allow real-time imaging (but newer generations of MRI will)
- Allows image processing
- Lengthy test time
- Not portable
- Requires gating for cardiac and abdominal applications
- Expensive

Two main pulse sequences (T1 and T2) are used with MRI, and these have dramatic effects on the appearance of the image. These pulse-sequence weightings relate to the type of spinning the protons can do and the type of environment of the protons. A third pulse sequence called *proton density* can also be used as can a fat suppression mode to better delineate certain features. General observations for interpretation of MRIs are as follows:

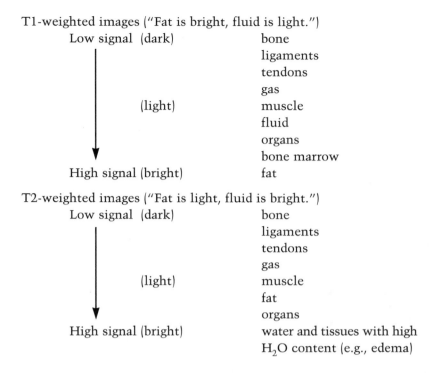

T1-weighted images ("Fat is bright, fluid is light.")

| Low signal (dark) | bone |
| | ligaments |
| | tendons |
| | gas |
| (light) | muscle |
| | fluid |
| | organs |
| | bone marrow |
| High signal (bright) | fat |

T2-weighted images ("Fat is light, fluid is bright.")

| Low signal (dark) | bone |
| | ligaments |
| | tendons |
| | gas |
| (light) | muscle |
| | fat |
| | organs |
| High signal (bright) | water and tissues with high $H_2O$ content (e.g., edema) |

MRI is the most sensitive and specific modality for detecting avascular necrosis of the hip and is therefore the modality of choice when this is suspected (Zukor and Lander 1995). MRI is also useful in detection of soft tissue lesions (including tumors), transient osteoporosis, synovial pit, bone cysts, and stress fractures, to name a few. One study has found MRI to be superior to radionuclide bone scan in the differential diagnosis of hip pain in young endurance athletes (Shin et al. 1996).

Compared to CT scan, MRI is better for imaging medullary bone and soft tissues, and CT is better for imaging cortical bone.

### Fluoroscopy

*Fluoroscopy* is a technique that uses radiography in a real-time fashion. The following are characteristics of fluoroscopy:

- Allows direct visualization of needle placements
- Moderately expensive
- As per radiography (see "Plain Film Radiography")

Fluoroscopy is particularly useful for orthopedic surgeons when relocating dislocated hip replacements and determining the mechanism of dislocation. It is also useful intraoperatively to guide pin placement when fixing femoral neck fractures and before placement of cannulated screws.

## Sonography (Ultrasound)

*Sonography* is a method that deflects sound waves from anatomic structures to delineate them from one another. The following are characteristics of ultrasound:

- Three dimensional
- No radiation
- Excellent spatial resolution
- Good-to-excellent contrast resolution
- Allows real-time imaging
- Portable
- Relatively inexpensive

Sonography is the modality of choice in evaluating the hip in patients up to 6 months of age before the femoral head has ossified. It is used routinely following hip surgery to detect for deep venous thrombosis. As the application of diagnostic ultrasound to musculoskeletal disorders expands, it may be used in diagnosis of soft tissue lesions, infection, and loosened hip prosthesis (van Holsbeeck et al. 1994).

## Arteriography and Venography

*Arteriography* and *venography* are techniques whereby contrast material is introduced in respective vessels before radiograph. Characteristics of arteriography and venography are as follows:

- Specific application at hip
- Relatively inexpensive
- As per Plain Film Radiography

Venography is considered the gold standard for detecting thrombi in the lower extremity. Arteriography can be used after pelvic trauma to diagnose hemorrhage; it can detect emboli, and it can be used to determine blood supply in surgical planning.

## Summary

Imaging of the hip complex is most helpful to the physical therapy clinician before the start of treatment to set appropriate, timely goals and to progress the patient safely and steadily. Imaging can provide information to aid the PT in determining the limits of exercise intensity, range of motion, and weightbearing status. Furthermore, imaging can identify conditions that are red flags for physical therapy.

For more information on diagnostic imaging, the reader is encouraged to read the articles cited in this chapter and the texts by Berquist (1986), Chew (1989), Forrester and Brown (1987), and Weissman and Sledge (1986), also cited in this chapter.

# 8

# Assessment of Outcomes

Timothy L. Fagerson

*Functional outcomes* is currently a buzz term in health care, and rightly so. Why should the payer spend money and the patient waste time on diagnostic procedures and treatments that do not yield appreciable positive change in patient function? This is the era of assessment and accountability (Relman 1988). We must prove our worth or perish!

Outcome assessment measures can be divided into the following groupings, which serve as the outline for this chapter:

    I. Disease specific
       A. Clinical
       B. Radiographic
       C. Survivorship
   II. Impairment specific
 III. Patient specific
 IV. Global (or generic or health status)

To yield accurate and meaningful information about treatment outcomes, high-quality measurement tools are necessary. An investigator should ensure that the outcome measure being used is valid, reliable, and responsive (Johanson 1994; Kreibich et al. 1996; Shields et al. 1995). The measurement tool should use standardized terminology and should be practical for use in the clinical setting. This chapter reviews the outcome measures used frequently in clinical practice and research related to hip patients. Not all of the measures listed have proven reliability, validity, and responsiveness.

## Disease Specific

Many of the "disease specific" scores are more "hip joint specific" than disease specific. Similarly, most of the questions in these clinical scores relate to impairments, and therefore could be termed *impairment specific*. All three of these terms (*disease specific, hip joint specific*, and *impairment specific*) are used by different authorities to describe the same scores. The term *disease specific* is the one most commonly used in the literature and is adopted here also.

## Clinical Outcome Measures

Since the 1950s, scores of disease specific outcome measures for the hip have been developed by orthopedic surgeons (Table 8-1). These measures assess for improvement in pain, motion, walking, and overall function. Physical therapists would do well to use some of these outcome instruments not only in research but also to measure clinical change in the individual patient. In selecting a particular score, however, the user should understand its biases and how it compares to other scores (Anderson 1972; Bryant et al. 1993; Callaghan et al. 1990).

With so many hip rating systems in use, it has become impossible to make comparisons of study results. To address this problem, three groups of orthopedic surgeons—the American Academy of Orthopaedic Surgeons (AAOS) Task Force on Outcome Studies, the Société Internationale de Chirurgie Orthopédique et de Traumatologie (SICOT) Commission on Documentation and Evaluation, and the Hip Society—have come together and developed, by consensus, a standardized terminology for reporting results of total hip replacement (THR). Table 8-2 outlines the components of the comprehensive evaluation system for THR suggested by the AAOS.

The AAOS system may become the gold standard for assessment of THR outcome. However, the sheer volume of data to be collected and the fact that different investigators have their own preferred method of outcome assessment decreases the appeal and practicality of the AAOS system. The AAOS realized these limitations and recommended that the standardized nomenclature be applied to existing methods (Johnston et al. 1990). Of the shorter scoring systems, Charnley's (Table 8-3) is considered by some to be the best and easiest to use (Murray 1993).

Charnley's (see Table 8-3) and Harris' (Figure 8-1) are probably the most widely used ratings worldwide. Charnley (1972) also recognized (primarily for research purposes) three categories of hip patients, which have become known as *Charnley's functional categories* (Table 8-4).

Denoting a grade with Charnley's system (see Table 8-3) is done, for example, as follows (for pain, walking, and motion, respectively):

- Right: 6.4.5
- Left: 5.4.2

**Table 8-1** Popular Hip Scores

| Popular name of hip score | Reference |
|---|---|
| Merle d'Aubigné | Merle d'Aubigné and Postel (1954) |
| Iowa | Larson (1963) |
| Harris | Harris (1969) |
| Hospital for Special Surgery | Wilson et al. (1972) |
| Charnley | Charnley (1972) |
| University of California at Los Angeles Activity Level Ratings | Amstutz et al. (1984) |
| Mayo | Kavanagh and Fitzgerald (1985) |
| American Academy of Orthopaedic Surgeons | Johnston et al. (1990)<br>Liang et al. (1991)<br>Katz et al. (1995) |

**Table 8-2** Total Hip Arthroplasty Outcome Evaluation Form of the American Academy of Orthopaedic Surgeons: Minimum Data

Outcome

    Function

        Pain

        Work activity (work history and physical requirements of work)

        Activities of daily living

        Gait

    Satisfaction and expectations of patient

    Physical examination

    Complications

Radiographic evaluation

    Cemented components

        Acetabulum

        Femur

    Uncemented components

        Acetabulum

        Femur

Source: Reprinted with permission from MH Liang, JN Katz, C Phillips, et al. (1991) The Total Hip Arthroplasty Outcome Evaluation Form of The American Academy of Orthopaedic Surgeons. *Journal of Bone and Joint Surgery [Am]* 73, 640.

**Table 8-3** Charnley Hip Score (Modified Merle d'Aubigné Hip Score)

| Pain | Function of walking | Movement (sum of all ROM arcs) |
|---|---|---|
| 1. Severe and spontaneous | 1. Few yards or bedridden<br>Two canes or crutches | 1. 0–30 degrees |
| 2. Severe on attempting to walk<br>Prevents all activity | 2. Time and distance very limited with or without canes | 2. 30–60 degrees |
| 3. Tolerable, permitting limited activity | 3. Limited with one cane (<1 hour)<br>Difficult without a cane<br>Able to stand long periods | 3. 60–100 degrees |
| 4. Only after some activity<br>Disappears quickly with rest | 4. Long distances with one cane<br>Limited without a cane | 4. 100–160 degrees |
| 5. Slight or intermittent pain on starting to walk but getting less with normal activity | 5. No cane but a limp | 5. 160–210 degrees |
| 6. No pain | 6. Normal | 6. >210 degrees |

ROM = range of motion.

Source: Adapted from J Charnley. (1972) The long-term results of low-friction arthroplasty of the hip performed as a primary intervention. *Journal of Bone and Joint Surgery [Br]* 54, 62.

Note that the middle digit is the same for left and right hips, because it refers to the general function of walking, which would be the same regardless of which side is involved. In a series of patients, the mean grade is calculated for pain, walking, and motion. The mean values recorded before intervention are then compared with the postintervention means.

The value of Charnley's functional categorization (see Table 8-4) is that, when assessing functional outcome, it is more valid to compare similar patient groups than different ones. Comparison of before and after range of motion and pain grades can be done, however, regardless of functional category.

A modern disease specific measure is the WOMAC (Western Ontario McMaster) Osteoarthritis Index. This method uses visual analog scales to doc-

| Item | Weight (score; out of 100) |
|---|---|
| I. *Pain* (44 possible points) | |
| A. None or ignores | 44 |
| B. Slight, occasional | |
| No compromise in activities | 40 |
| C. Mild pain | |
| No effect on average activities, rarely moderate pain with unusual activity | |
| May take aspirin | 30 |
| D. Moderate pain, tolerable but makes concessions to pain | |
| Some limitation of ordinary activity or work | |
| May require occasional pain medicine stronger than aspirin | 20 |
| E. Marked pain | |
| Serious limitation of activities | 10 |
| F. Totally disabled, crippled, pain in bed, bedridden | 0 |
| II. *Function* (47 possible points) | |
| A. Gait (33 possible points) | |
| 1. Limp | |
| a. None | 11 |
| b. Slight | 8 |
| c. Moderate | 5 |
| d. Severe | 0 |
| 2. Support | |
| a. None | 11 |
| b. Cane for long walks | 7 |
| c. Cane most of the time | 5 |

**Figure 8-1** The Harris Hip Score: synopsis of the evaluation system. Score interpretation: 90–100 = excellent; 80–89 = good; 70–79 = fair; <70 = poor. To determine the overall rating for range of motion (ROM), multiply the sum of the index values by 0.05. For example, if flexion is 10–100 degrees, the patient has 35 degrees in the 0–45 range, 45 degrees in the 45–90 range, and 10 degrees in the 90–110 range. Therefore, the value for flexion range of motion is $(35 \times 1) + (45 \times 0.6) + (10 \times 0.3)$. Do this for all motions specified and then add all of the totals. Multiply this total of all the index values by 0.05 (maximum ROM is 5 points). (Modified from WH Harris. [1969] Traumatic arthritis of the hip after dislocation and acetabular fractures: Treatment by mold arthroplasty: An end-result study using a new method of result evaluation. *Journal of Bone and Joint Surgery [Am]* 51, 741.)

| Item | Weight (score; out of 100) |
|---|---|
| d. One crutch | 3 |
| e. Two canes | 2 |
| f. Two crutches | 0 |
| g. Unable to walk (Specify reason) | 0 |
| 3. Distance walked | |
| a. Unlimited | 11 |
| b. Six blocks | 8 |
| c. Two or three blocks | 5 |
| d. Indoors only | 2 |
| e. Bed and chair | 0 |
| B. Activities (14 possible points) | |
| 1. Stairs | |
| a. Normally without using a railing | 4 |
| b. Normally using a railing | 2 |
| c. In any manner | 1 |
| d. Unable to do stairs | 0 |
| 2. Shoes and socks | |
| a. With ease | 4 |
| b. With difficulty | 2 |
| c. Unable | 0 |
| 3. Sitting | |
| a. Comfortably in ordinary chair 1 hr | 5 |
| b. On a high chair for 30 min | 3 |
| c. Unable to sit comfortably in any chair | 0 |
| 4. Enter public transportation | 1 |

III.  *Absence of deformity points* (4) are given if the patient demonstrates absence of all of the following:

A. Less than 30 degrees fixed flexion contracture
B. Less than 10 degrees fixed adduction
C. Less than 10 degrees fixed internal rotation in extension
D. Limb-length discrepancy less than 3.2 cm    4

**Figure 8-1** *Continued*

| Item | Weight (score; out of 100) |
|---|---|
| IV.   *Range of motion* (ROM) (Index values are determined by multiplying the degree of motion possible in each arc by the appropriate index.) | |

|  | ROM arc | Index value | 5 |
|---|---|---|---|
| A.  Flexion | | | |
| | 0–45 degrees | × 1.0 | |
| | 45–90 degrees | × 0.6 | |
| | 90–110 degrees | × 0.3 | |
| B.  Abduction | | | |
| | 0–15 degrees | × 0.8 | |
| | 15–20 degrees | × 0.3 | |
| | >20 degrees | × 0 | |
| C.  External rotation in extension | 0–15 degrees | × 0.4 | |
| | >15 degrees | × 0 | |
| D.  Internal rotation in extension | Any | × 0 | |
| E.  Adduction | | | |
| | 0–15 degrees | × 0.2 | |

Record Trendelenburg test as positive, level, or neutral.

ument five dimensions: (1) pain, (2) stiffness, (3) physical function, (4) social function, and (5) emotional function. It has been shown to be reliable, valid, responsive, and efficient as a measure of outcome for patients undergoing THR (Bellamy et al. 1988).

Most of the work regarding clinical outcomes of hip disorders has been done by orthopedic surgeons evaluating the results of THR. Physical therapists have also conducted studies on THR outcome (Roush 1985; Shields et al. 1995) and even more so on outcomes after hip fracture (Barnes 1984; Barnes and Dunovan 1987; Bohannon et al. 1990; Guccione et al. 1996; Jette et al. 1987; Kauffman et al. 1987). However, little or no research has been done on treatment outcomes for disorders of the hip not severe enough to warrant hip replacement (Cibulka and Delitto 1993).

A modification of a commonly used level of assistance scale has been found to be highly reliable, valid, and responsive (Shields et al. 1995) (see

**Table 8-4** Charnley's Functional Categories

| | |
|---|---|
| Category A | A patient with only one hip involved in whom no other condition interferes with walking |
| Category B | A patient with both hips involved, but the rest of the body is normal and therefore not responsible for any defect in ability to walk |
| Category C | A patient with some factor contributing to failure to achieve normal locomotion, such as polyarthritis, rheumatoid arthritis, senility, hemiplegia, or cardiovascular or respiratory disability |

Source: Adapted from J Charnley. (1972) The long-term results of low-friction arthroplasty of the hip performed as a primary intervention. *Journal of Bone and Joint Surgery [Br]* 54, 62.

Table 6-3). This type of scale has been used to assess the achievement of key functional milestones following hip replacement and hip fracture (Guccione et al. 1996; Kroll et al. 1994). Many impairment specific measures like these are used in physical therapy (see "Impairment Specific").

## Radiographic Outcome Measures

The outcome of THR is assessed radiographically by surgeons, in addition to clinical assessment. The AAOS provided standardized terminology for radiographic evaluation of uncemented and cemented THRs (Johnston et al. 1990).

Radiolucency at the bone-cement interface is suggestive of component loosening. The seriousness of the problem is dependent on the location, width, and extent of the radiolucent zone. To evaluate the acetabular component, the method described by DeLee and Charnley (1976) is most frequently used. For the femoral component, the method of Gruen and colleagues (1979) is widely used. Others prefer the method of Harris and colleagues (1982).

## Survivorship Analyses

Survivorship analysis has become a widely used technique for determining the success of THR. The first survivorship analysis of THR patients was described by Dobbs (1980). Between 1986 and 1992, Murray and colleagues (1993) identified 35 reports using survivorship analysis to assess the success of total knee replacement and THR. Of these 35 reports, two-thirds used the life-table method, and one-third used the product-limit method.

In the life-table method, for each year after the start of the study, the number of joints being followed and the number of failures are determined. This enables yearly failure and success rates to be calculated.

The product-limit approach is based on the actuarial analysis method described by Kaplan and Meier (1958). This method involves recalculating the success rate each time a failure occurs. The Kaplan-Meier curve that can be plotted is an effective graphical representation of the survival rate.

The reliability and validity of survivorship analysis is questionable when a large number of patients are "lost to follow-up," leaving only a small number for analysis. Survivorship analysis assumes that patients lost to follow-up are at no more risk for failure than patients who are still being followed. Other criticisms of survivorship analysis include the use of revision surgery as the measure of failure, a tendency for investigators and manufacturers to have a bias towards good results, and the attempt to predict the outcome of the surviving implants at the end of the study based on the current rate of survival (Murray et al. 1993). Despite these potential drawbacks, Dorey and Amstutz (1989) provided evidence to suggest that survivorship analysis is a valid technique for long-term outcome evaluation of THR.

## Impairment Specific

Physical therapists primarily direct their interventions at impairments and functional limitations. Disease specific clinical scores (see "Clinical") could be considered impairment specific, because they relate to impairments; however, they are classified as disease specific, because they were developed specifically for patients with hip disease. Methods of assessing impairments and functional limitation that have application to wide range of patient populations are defined here as impairment specific.

impairment specific measures of function to be considered for hip patients include the following:

- Functional capacity
  6-Minute Walk test (Guyatt et al. 1985; Laupacis et al. 1993)
- Balance
  Get-Up and Go test (Mathias et al. 1986); Timed "Up and Go" test (Podsiadlo and Richardson 1991)
  Performance-Oriented Mobility Assessment (Tinetti 1986)
  Berg Balance Measure (Berg et al. 1989)
  Functional Reach (Duncan et al. 1990)
- Functional mobility
  Functional Independence Measure (Linacre et al. 1994)

Iowa Level of Assistance Scale (Shields et al. 1995)
Independence in Key Functional Milestones (Guccione et al. 1996)
• Pain
McGill Pain Questionnaire (Melzack 1975) (see Figure 3-3)
Visual analog scale
Numeric pain rating scale (i.e., "How bad is your pain on a scale of
0–10, where 0 is no pain and 10 is the worst pain you can imagine?")
Pain drawing

## Patient Specific

Recently, it has become apparent that disease specific hip scores are based on factors that are important to an orthopedic surgeon but not always of most importance to the individual patient (Lieberman et al. 1996; Wright et al. 1994). To address this need, several patient specific scoring systems have been developed (MacKenzie et al. 1986; O'Boyle et al. 1992; Tugwell et al. 1987, 1990; Wright and Young 1997; Wright et al. 1994).

The MACTAR (McMaster-Toronto Arthritis) Patient Preference Disability Questionnaire, developed by Tugwell and colleagues (1987), is becoming a popular tool for patient specific assessment of outcome. It requires the patient to identify the five most important activities that are affected by hip disease. The MACTAR patient specific method is more sensitive to clinical change than traditional methods and is comparable to the way a clinical decision is made for an individual patient (Tugwell et al. 1987). It is an easy scale to use but has been criticized for only assessing five complaints and for giving equal weight to each of these (Wright et al. 1994).

The Patient Specific Index (PSI) (Wright and Young 1997; Wright et al. 1994) (Figure 8-2) asks a patient to give a severity rating and an importance rating to all of his or her complaints related to the hip. The PSI is comprised of 22 complaints (and any additional ones, hence the term: "ask patients what they want") that are unique to patients with hip dysfunction. The 22 complaints were chosen from seven previous hip scores and from interviews with 72 patients. There are at least four different scoring methods for the PSI, including a score out of 100 so that it can be compared with other "out of 100" hip scores. However, the easiest to use, and actually most responsive scoring method, is to simply sum together a patient's ratings of severity and importance. The generalizability of the PSI has yet to be tested with conditions other than THR, but it does have proven reliability, validity, and responsiveness with THR patients. One drawback of the PSI is that it takes

**Severity Score**

| Rate the severity of each of the following problems. | 1 (Not Severe) | 2 (Minimally Severe) | 3 (Somewhat Severe) | 4 (Moderately Severe) | 5 (Very Severe) | 6 (Extremely Severe) | 7 (Most Severe Imaginable) | NA* |
|---|---|---|---|---|---|---|---|---|
| Average daytime hip pain | | | | | | | | |
| Nighttime hip pain | | | | | | | | |
| Limp | | | | | | | | |
| Hip stiffness | | | | | | | | |
| Rate the severity of each additional problem here. | | | | | | | | |
| Rate the severity of each additional problem here. | | | | | | | | |
| **Rate the degree to which each of the following problems bothers you.** | 1 (Not Bothersome) | 2 (Minimally Bothersome) | 3 (Somewhat Bothersome) | 4 (Moderately Bothersome) | 5 (Very Bothersome) | 6 (Extremely Bothersome) | 7 (Most Bothersome Imaginable) | NA* |
| Having to take a pill for the hip | | | | | | | | |
| Having to use walking aids | | | | | | | | |
| Difference in leg lengths | | | | | | | | |
| Fear of falling because of the hip | | | | | | | | |
| Loss of independence | | | | | | | | |
| Rate the severity of each additional problem here. | | | | | | | | |
| Rate the severity of each additional problem here. | | | | | | | | |
| **Rate the degree of difficulty you have doing each of the following activities.** | 1 (Not Difficult) | 2 (Minimally Difficult) | 3 (Somewhat Difficult) | 4 (Moderately Difficult) | 5 (Very Difficult) | 6 (Extremely Difficult) | 7 (Unable) | NA* |
| Walking | | | | | | | | |
| Going up and down stairs | | | | | | | | |
| Putting on shoes or stockings | | | | | | | | |
| Sitting | | | | | | | | |
| Using public transportation (bus) | | | | | | | | |
| Driving | | | | | | | | |
| Job/housework | | | | | | | | |
| Recreational activities/hobbies | | | | | | | | |
| Sexual activity | | | | | | | | |
| Tub baths | | | | | | | | |
| Getting onto and off of the toilet | | | | | | | | |
| Bending to pick up things off of the floor | | | | | | | | |
| Standing for 5 minutes | | | | | | | | |
| Rate the severity of each additional problem here. | | | | | | | | |
| Rate the severity of each additional problem here. | | | | | | | | |

*NA=not applicable

**Figure 8-2** The Patient Specific Index. (Reprinted with permission from JG Wright, NL Young. [1997] The Patient Specific Index: Asking patients what they want. *Journal of Bone and Joint Surgery [Am]* 79, 981.)

approximately 16 minutes to complete, whereas the MACTAR takes only 3 minutes (Wright and Young 1997).

The AAOS constructed a questionnaire for THR assessment that comprises a baseline section, a history section, and a postoperative section (Katz et al. 1995). Although it collects a great deal of useful information, it is lengthy and does not involve a method of scoring. This form sheds light on the type of information that should be collected in a patient history as well as in a research database.

*Importance Score*

| Rate the importance of each of the following problems. | 1 (Not Important at All) | 2 (Minimally Important) | 3 (A Little Important) | 4 (Important) | 5 (Moderately Important) | 6 (Very Important) | 7 (Extremely Important) | |
|---|---|---|---|---|---|---|---|---|
| Daytime hip pain | | | | | | | | |
| Nighttime hip pain | | | | | | | | |
| Limp | | | | | | | | |
| Hip stiffness | | | | | | | | |
| Rate 1st additional severity item here | | | | | | | | |
| Rate 2nd additional severity item here | | | | | | | | |
| | | | | | | | | |
| Having to take a pill for the hip | | | | | | | | |
| Having to use walking aids | | | | | | | | |
| Difference in leg lengths | | | | | | | | |
| Fear of falling because of the hip | | | | | | | | |
| Loss of independence | | | | | | | | |
| Rate 1st additional bothersome item here | | | | | | | | |
| Rate 2nd additional bothersome item here | | | | | | | | |
| | | | | | | | | |
| Walking | | | | | | | | |
| Going up and down stairs | | | | | | | | |
| Putting on shoes or stockings | | | | | | | | |
| Sitting | | | | | | | | |
| Using public transportation (bus) | | | | | | | | |
| Driving | | | | | | | | |
| Job/housework | | | | | | | | |
| Recreational activities/hobbies | | | | | | | | |
| Sexual activity | | | | | | | | |
| Tub baths | | | | | | | | |
| Getting onto and off of the toilet | | | | | | | | |
| Bending to pick up things off of the floor | | | | | | | | |
| Standing for 5 minutes | | | | | | | | |
| Rate 1st additional difficulty item here | | | | | | | | |
| Rate 2nd additional difficulty item here | | | | | | | | |

**Figure 8-2** *Continued*

## Global

Global, or generic, scores are also known as *health-status instruments*. During the 1980s and 1990s, the importance of *measuring* overall improvement in health following medical interventions has become widely accepted. This is partly due to the fact that mortality-morbidity rates and disease specific measures alone provide too narrow an assessment of outcome. Additionally, providers and payers desired a broad measure of effectiveness of a wide range of interventions, such as joint replacement, coronary artery bypass, and liver transplant. The emphasis on a global view of health dates back to the 1950s when the World Health Organization defined health as "a state of complete physical, mental, and social well-being and not merely the absence of diseases and infirmity" (World Health Organization 1958).

One of the most established measures of functional status is the Sickness Impact Profile (SIP) (Bergner et al. 1981). The SIP consists of 136 items divided into 12 categories and two dimensions. It has proven reliability, validity, and responsiveness, but it is relatively time-consuming and complex to score; therefore, it is not as useful in clinical practice as shorter forms (Nelson and Berwick 1989). Using the SIP as a standard, the responsiveness of four short forms has been assessed for use with patients undergoing THR (Katz et al. 1992). Short forms with recognized reliability and validity were shown to be as responsive as the SIP and therefore were recommended for health-status measurement in joint replacement. None of the forms was found to be more sensitive than the others (Katz et al. 1992). The four measures assessed were the SF-36 (Ware and Sherbourne 1992), the Functional Status Questionnaire (Jette et al. 1986), the shortened Arthritis Impact Measurement Scales (Wallston et al. 1989), and the modified Health Assessment Questionnaire (Pincus et al. 1983).

The Medical Outcomes Trust Short-Form 36 (SF-36) has emerged as a very popular tool both in clinical practice and in research studies. The SF-36 is a shortened version of a battery of 149 questions originally used in the Medical Outcomes Study. In North America, the SF-36 has been used in hundreds of research studies, and it is also attracting attention in the United Kingdom (Ware 1993). The SF-36 consists of 36 items covering eight dimensions of health (Figure 8-3). It has proven reliability and validity, and normative data are emerging for adult populations. Its popularity is probably due to its comprehensiveness and brevity (Ware and Sherbourne 1992).

In the UK, the Nottingham Health Profile is a frequently used functional-status measure (Hunt et al. 1985).

## Summary

The intent of this chapter has been to provide an overview of outcome assessment options for hip patients and to improve comprehension when reading research reports. It should also be of benefit to the person planning a research study involving hip patients. Omitted from this chapter are cost-to-quality adjusted life-year outcome measures and utility measures, such as the standard gamble, time trade-off, and magnitude estimation (Fitzpatrick 1993).

It is recommended that a comprehensive assessment of outcome be conducted by combining different types of functional assessment (Katz et al. 1995; Laupacis et al. 1993). Nelson and Berwick (1989) called for the widespread adop-

1. In general, would you say your health is (Mark only one.)
   - ❏ Excellent
   - ❏ Very good
   - ❏ Good
   - ❏ Fair
   - ❏ Poor

2. Compared to 1 year ago, how would you rate your health in general? (Mark only one.)
   - ❏ Much better now than 1 year ago
   - ❏ Somewhat better now than 1 year ago
   - ❏ About the same as 1 year ago
   - ❏ Somewhat worse now than 1 year ago
   - ❏ Much worse now than 1 year ago

The following items are about activities you might do during a typical day. Does your health now limit you in these activities? If so, how much? (Mark one square on each line.)

|  | Yes, limited a lot | Yes, limited a little | No, not limited at all |
|---|---|---|---|
| 3. Vigorous activities, such as running, lifting heavy objects, and participating in strenuous sports? | ❏ | ❏ | ❏ |
| 4. Moderate activities, such as moving a table, pushing a vacuum cleaner, bowling, or playing golf? | ❏ | ❏ | ❏ |
| 5. Lifting or carrying groceries? | ❏ | ❏ | ❏ |
| 6. Climbing several flights of stairs? | ❏ | ❏ | ❏ |
| 7. Climbing one flight of stairs? | ❏ | ❏ | ❏ |
| 8. Bending, kneeling, or stooping? | ❏ | ❏ | ❏ |
| 9. Walking more than a mile? | ❏ | ❏ | ❏ |
| 10. Walking several blocks? | ❏ | ❏ | ❏ |
| 11. Walking one block? | ❏ | ❏ | ❏ |
| 12. Bathing or dressing yourself? | ❏ | ❏ | ❏ |

During the past 4 weeks, have you had any of the following problems with your work or other regular daily activities as a result of your physical health? (Mark one square on each line.)

13. Cut down the amount of time you spent on work or other activities?      ❏ Yes      ❏ No
14. Accomplished less than you would like?      ❏ Yes      ❏ No

**Figure 8-3** SF-36 Health Survey. (Reprinted with permission from Medical Outcomes Trust. Copyright © 1992 Medical Outcomes Trust. All rights reserved.)

15. Were limited in the kind of work or
    other activities?                              ❏ Yes        ❏ No

16. Had difficulty performing the work or
    other activities (e.g., it took extra effort)?  ❏ Yes        ❏ No

During the past 4 weeks, have you had any of the following problems with your work or other regular daily activities as a result of any emotional problems (e.g., feeling depressed or anxious)? (Mark one square on each line.)

17. Cut down the amount of time you spent
    on work or other activities?                   ❏ Yes        ❏ No

18. Accomplished less than you would like?         ❏ Yes        ❏ No

19. Didn't do work or other activities as
    carefully as usual?                            ❏ Yes        ❏ No

20. During the past 4 weeks, to what extent has your physical health or emotional problems interfered with your normal social activities with family, friends, neighbors, or groups? (Mark one square.)
    ❏ Not at all    ❏ Slightly    ❏ Moderately    ❏ Quite a bit    ❏ Extremely

21. How much bodily pain have you had during the past 4 weeks? (Mark one square.)
    ❏ None    ❏ Very mild    ❏ Mild    ❏ Moderate    ❏ Severe    ❏ Very severe

22. During the past 4 weeks, how much did pain interfere with your work (including both work outside the home and housework)? (Mark one square.)
    ❏ Not at all    ❏ Slightly    ❏ Moderately    ❏ Quite a bit    ❏ Extremely

These questions are about how you feel and how things have been with you during the past 4 weeks. For each question, please give the one answer that comes closest to the way you have been feeling. How much of the time during the past 4 weeks ... (Mark one square on each line.)

|  | All of the time | Most of the time | A good bit of the time | Some of the time | A little of the time | None of the time |
|---|---|---|---|---|---|---|
| 23. Did you feel full of pep? | ❏ | ❏ | ❏ | ❏ | ❏ | ❏ |
| 24. Have you been a very nervous person? | ❏ | ❏ | ❏ | ❏ | ❏ | ❏ |
| 25. Have you felt so down in the dumps that nothing could cheer you up? | ❏ | ❏ | ❏ | ❏ | ❏ | ❏ |
| 26. Have you felt calm and peaceful? | ❏ | ❏ | ❏ | ❏ | ❏ | ❏ |
| 27. Did you have a lot of energy? | ❏ | ❏ | ❏ | ❏ | ❏ | ❏ |
| 28. Have you felt downhearted and blue? | ❏ | ❏ | ❏ | ❏ | ❏ | ❏ |
| 29. Have you felt worn out? | ❏ | ❏ | ❏ | ❏ | ❏ | ❏ |
| 30. Have you been a happy person? | ❏ | ❏ | ❏ | ❏ | ❏ | ❏ |
| 31. Have you felt tired? | ❏ | ❏ | ❏ | ❏ | ❏ | ❏ |

32. During the past 4 weeks, how much of the time has your physical health or emotional problems interfered with your social activities (e.g., visiting with friends and relatives)?

| ❏ All of the time | ❏ Most of the time | ❏ Some of the time | ❏ A little of the time | ❏ None of the time |

How true or false is each of the following statements for you?

| | Definitely true | Mostly true | Don't know | Mostly false | Definitely false |
|---|---|---|---|---|---|
| 33. I seem to get sick a little easier than other people. | ❏ ❏ | ❏ | ❏ | ❏ | ❏ |
| 34. I am as healthy as anyone I know. | ❏ | ❏ | ❏ | ❏ | ❏ |
| 35. I expect my health to get worse. | ❏ | ❏ | ❏ | ❏ | ❏ |
| 36. My health is excellent. | ❏ | ❏ | ❏ | ❏ | ❏ |

**Figure 8-3** *Continued*

tion in clinical practice of tools that measure health and function. Based on a review of the literature, the outcome assessment tools of most clinical use for patients with hip dysfunction include: (1) the Harris hip score, because it is the most popular hip score (even though its reliability, validity, and responsiveness have not been formally tested) and is understood by orthopedists; (2) the Charnley hip score and functional class, because it is easy to use and is also well understood by orthopedists; (3) the MACTAR patient preference questionnaire, because it is patient specific, brief, and is immediately applicable to clinical practice and research; (4) the PSI, because it is comprehensive and patient specific; (5) the AAOS patient interview questionnaire, because it is thorough, complements the subjective examination, and can easily be used in a research database; (6) the SF-36, because it is emerging as the most widely accepted health-status measure for clinical use; and (7) the McGill Pain Questionnaire, because the primary problem with many patients is pain, and pain too should be measured. The reader is encouraged to review the original source or refer to an official user's guide before using any of these instruments.

Obviously, it is not practical to use all seven of these instruments on every patient. Therefore, to be pragmatic about clinical use but still maintain a comprehensive outcome assessment, I suggest using the PSI (which is not only patient specific but has components of disease specific, impairment specific, and pain assessment) and the SF-36 (a global measure) for patients with hip disorders. Additional or alternative measures should be used when warranted for specific purposes.

# References

Abraham WD, Dimon JH. (1992) Leg length discrepancy in total hip arthroplasty. *Orthopedic Clinics of North America* 23, 201–209.

Adams RC. (1993) Growing epidemic in the geriatric population: Hip fractures. *Advance for Physical Therapists* March 15, 11, 26.

Adkins HV, Baker L, Campbell J, et al. (1981) *Normal and Pathological Gait Syllabus*. Downey CA: Professional Staff Association of Ranchos Los Amigos Hospital.

Alon G. (1995) Evaluating interferential current. *Durable Medical Equipment Review* 2, 49–53.

American Physical Therapy Association. (1989) Philosophical Statement on Physical Therapy (HOD 06-83-03-05). In *Applicable House of Delegates Policies* (p. 26). Alexandria, VA: American Physical Therapy Association.

Amstutz HC, Thomas BJ, Jinnah R, et al. (1984) Treatment of primary osteoarthritis of the hip. A comparison of total joint and surface replacement arthroplasty. *Journal of Bone and Joint Surgery [Am]* 66, 228–241.

Anda S, Svenningsen S, Dale LG, Benum P. (1986) The acetabular sector angle of the adult hip determined by computed tomography. *Acta Radiologica Diagnosis (Stockholm)* 27, 443–447.

Anderson RJ. (1993) Rheumatoid Arthritis: Clinical Features and Laboratory. In HR Schumacher (ed), *Primer on the Rheumatic Diseases* (10th ed) (pp. 90–96). Atlanta: Arthritis Foundation.

Andersson G. (1972) Hip assessment: A comparison of nine different methods. *Journal of Bone and Joint Surgery [Br]* 54, 621–625.

Awbrey B. (1995) Aquatic fitness and rehab. *Biomechanics* April, 87–89.

Ballard WT, Callaghan JJ, Sullivan PM, Johnston RC. (1994) The results of improved cementing techniques for total hip arthroplasty in patients less than 50 years old. *Journal of Bone and Joint Surgery [Am]* 76, 959–973.

Barber TC, Roger DJ, Goodman SB, Schurman DJ. (1996) Early outcome of total hip arthroplasty using the direct lateral vs the posterior surgical approach. *Orthopedics* 19, 873–875.

Barnes B. (1984) Ambulation outcomes after hip fracture. *Physical Therapy* 64, 317–323.

Barnes B, Dunovan K. (1987) Physical therapy discharge outcomes after hip fracture. *Topics in Geriatrics Rehabilitation* 2, 45–51.

Barnhart ER. (1989) *Physicians' Desk Reference* (43rd ed). Ovadell, NJ: Medical Economics Data Production Company.

Barrack RL, Mulroy RD, Harris WH. (1992) Improved cementing techniques and femoral component loosening in young patients with hip arthroplasty. *Journal of Bone and Joint Surgery [Br]* 74, 385–389.

Beaton LE, Anson BJ. (1937) The relation of the sciatic nerve and of its subdivisions to the piriformis muscle. *Anatomical Record* 70, 1–5.

Behr DW. (1994) In vivo hip contact pressures generated during early postoperative rehabilitation: Comparison of two subjects. Master's thesis, Department of Physical Therapy, MGH Institute of Health Professions at Massachusetts General Hospital, Boston.

Bellamy N, Buchanan WW, Goldsmith CH, et al. (1988) Validation study of WOMAC: A health status instrument for measuring clinically important patient-relevant outcomes following total hip or knee arthroplasty in osteoarthritis. *Journal of Orthopaedic Rheumatology* 1, 95–108.

Benson H, Stark M. (1996) *Timeless Healing: The Power and Biology of Belief*. New York: Scribner.

Berg K, Wood-Dauphinee S, Williams JI, Gayton D. (1989) Measuring balance in the elderly: Preliminary development of an instrument. *Physiotherapy Canada* 41, 304–311.

Bergmann G, Graichen F, Rohlmann A. (1989, June) Five-month in vivo measurement of hip joint forces [abstract]. Presented at the Seventh International Symposium Proceedings: Adapted Physical Activity, Berlin.

Bergmann G, Graichen F, Rohlmann A. (1993) Hip joint loading during walking and running, measured in two patients. *Journal of Biomechanics* 26, 969–990.

Bergmann G, Graichen F, Rohlmann A. (1995) Is staircase walking a risk for the fixation of hip implants? *Journal of Biomechanics* 28, 535–553.

Bergmann G, Rohlmann A, Graichen F (1990a). Hip joint forces during physical therapy after joint replacement. *Transactions of the 36th Annual Meeting of the Orthopaedic Research Society* (p. 2). New Orleans: Orthopaedic Research Society.

Bergmann G, Neff G, da Silva M, et al. (1990b) Influence of ischial weight bearing orthoses on the forces at the hip joint. *Transactions of the 36th*

*Annual Meeting of the Orthopaedic Research Society* (1). New Orleans: Orthopaedic Research Society.

Bergner M, Bobbitt RA, Carter WB, Gilson BS. (1981) The Sickness Impact Profile: Development and final revision of a health status measure. *Medical Care* 19, 787–805.

Berquist TH (ed). (1986) *Imaging of Orthopaedic Trauma and Surgery*. Philadelphia: Saunders.

Berquist TH, Coventry MB. (1986) The Pelvis and Hips. In TH Berquist (ed), *Imaging of Orthopaedic Trauma and Surgery*. (pp. 181–279) Philadelphia: Saunders.

Betts RP, Watson AG. (1992) Leg load monitor for rehabilitation. *Physiotherapy* 78, 172–173.

Bissacotti JF, Ritter MA, Faris PM, et al. (1994) A new radiographic evaluation of primary osteoarthritis. *Orthopedics* 17, 927–930.

Blount WP. (1956) Don't throw away the cane. *Journal of Bone and Joint Surgery [Am]* 38, 695–708.

Bohannon RW, Kloter KS, Cooper JA. (1990) Outcome of patients with hip fracture treated by physical therapy in an acute care hospital. *Topics in Geriatric Rehabilitation* 6, 51–58.

Bohannon RW, Larkin PA, Cook AC, et al. (1984) Decrease in timed balance test scores with aging. *Physical Therapy* 64, 1067–1070.

Bonar SK, Tinetti ME, Speechley M, Cooney LM. (1990) Factors associated with short- versus long-term skilled nursing facility placement among community-living hip fracture hip patients. *Journal of the American Geriatrics Society* 38, 1139–1144.

Brown RH, Burstein AH, Frankel VH. (1988) Telemetering in vivo loads from nail implants. *Journal of Biomechanics* 15, 815–823.

Brown DE, Neumann RD. (1995) *Orthopedic Secrets*. Philadelphia: Hanley & Bulfus.

Bryant MJ, Kernohan WG, Nixon JR, Mollan RAB. (1993) A statistical analysis of hip scores. *Journal of Bone and Joint Surgery [Br]* 75, 705–709.

Burgess AR, Tile M. (1991) Fractures of the Pelvis. In CA Rockwood, DP Green, RW Bucholz (eds), *Rockwood and Green's Fractures in Adults* (pp. 1399–1442). Philadelphia: Lippincott.

Burke DW, O'Connor DO, Zalenski EB, et al. (1991) Micromotion of cemented and uncemented femoral components. *Journal of Bone and Joint Surgery [Br]* 73, 33–37.

Buschbacher R. (1994) *Musculoskeletal Disorders: A Practical Guide for Diagnosis and Rehabilitation*. Boston: Butterworth–Heinemann.

Butcher JD, Salzman KL, Lillegard WA. (1996) Lower extremity bursitis. *American Family Bursitis* 53, 2317–2324.

Cahalan TD, Johnson ME, Liu S, Chao EYS. (1989) Quantitative measurements of hip strength in different age groups. *Clinical Orthopaedics and Related Research* 246, 136–145.

Caillet R. (1988) *Soft Tissue Pain and Disability* (2nd ed). Philadelphia: Davis.

Callaghan JJ, Dysart SH, Savory CF, Hopkinson WJ. (1990) Assessing the results of hip replacement: A comparison of five different rating systems. *Journal of Bone and Joint Surgery [Br]* 72, 1008–1009.

Carlson KL. (1993) Human hip joint mechanics—an investigation into the effects of femoral head endoprosthetic replacements using in vivo and in vitro pressure data. Ph.D. thesis, Massachusetts Institute of Technology, Cambridge, MA.

Cauley JA. (1994) Epidemiology of Total Hip Replacement. In *NIH Consensus Development Conference on Total Hip Replacement, September 12–14* (pp. 19–26). Bethesda, MD: National Institutes of Health.

Ceder L, Thorngren KG, Wallden B. (1980) Prognostic indicators and early home rehabilitation in elderly patients with hip fracture. *Clinical Orthopaedics and Related Research* 152, 173–184.

Chandler HP. (1987) Postoperative Management of the Total Hip Patient. In WT Stillwell (ed), *The Art of Total Hip Arthroplasty* (pp. 371–401). Orlando, FL: Grune & Stratton.

Chandler SB. (1934) The iliopsoas bursa in man. *Anatomical Record* 58, 235–240.

Chao EYS, Cahalan TD. (1990) Kinematics and Kinetics of Normal Gait. In GL Smidt (ed), *Gait in Rehabilitation* (pp. 45–64). New York: Churchill Livingstone.

Charnley J. (1972) The long-term results of low-friction arthroplasty of the hip performed as a primary intervention. *Journal of Bone and Joint Surgery [Br]* 54, 61–76.

Charnley J. (1979) *Low Friction Arthroplasty of the Hip*. Berlin: Springer-Verlag.

Chew FS. (1989) *Skeletal Radiology*. Rockville, MD: Aspen Publishers.

Cibulka MT, Delitto A. (1993) A comparison of two different methods to treat hip pain in runners. *Journal of Orthopaedic and Sports Physical Therapy* 17, 172–176.

Cleaves EN. (1941) Observations on lateral views of the hips. *American Journal of Radiology* 39, 964–966.

Clement DB, Taunton JE, Smart GW, McNicol KL. (1981) A survey of overuse running injuries. *The Physician and Sports Medicine* 9, 47–58.

Cohn BT, Draeger RI, Jackson DW. (1989) The effects of cold therapy in the postoperative management of pain in patients undergoing anterior cruciate ligament reconstruction. *American Journal of Sports Medicine* 17, 344–349.

Conway WF, Totty WG, McEnery KW. (1996) CT and MR imaging of the hip. *Radiology* 198, 297–307.

Craik RL. (1994) Disability following hip fracture. *Physical Therapy* 74, 387–398.

Cunningham LS, Kelsey JL. (1984) Epidemiology of musculoskeletal impairments and associated disability. *American Journal of Public Health* 74, 574–579.

Curwin S, Stanish WD. (1984) *Tendinitis: Its Etiology and Treatment.* Lexington, MA: Collamore Press, DC Heath and Co.

Cyriax J. (1982) *Textbook of Orthopaedic Medicine Volume I: Diagnosis of Soft Tissue Lesions* (8th ed). London: Bailliere Tindall.

Cyriax JH, Cyriax PJ. (1993) *Cyriax's Illustrated Manual of Orthopaedic Medicine* (2nd ed). Oxford, UK: Butterworth–Heinemann.

Cyriax J, Russell G. (1980) *Textbook of Orthopaedic Medicine Volume Two: Treatment by Manipulation, Massage and Injection* (10th ed). London: Bailliere Tindall.

Daenen B, Preidler KW, Padmanabhan S, et al. (1997) Symptomatic herniation pits of the femoral neck: Anatomic and clinical study. *American Journal of Roentgenography* 168, 149–153.

Dalinka MK, Neustadter LM. (1991) Radiology of the Hip. In ME Steinberg (ed), *The Hip and its Disorders* (pp. 56–71). Philadelphia: Saunders.

Dall D. (1986) Exposure of the hip by anterior osteotomy of the greater trochanter: A modified anterolateral approach. *Journal of Bone and Joint Surgery [Br]* 68, 382–386.

Dalldorf PG, Banas MP, Hicks DG, Pellegrini VD. (1995) Rate of degeneration of human acetabular cartilage after hemiarthroplasty. *Journal of Bone and Joint Surgery [Am]* 77, 877–883.

Daniel WW, Sanders PC, Alarcon GS. (1992) The early diagnosis of transient osteoporosis by magnetic resonance imaging: A case report. *Journal of Bone and Joint Surgery [Am]* 74, 1262–1264.

Daniels L, Worthingham C. (1986) *Muscle Testing: Techniques of Manual Examination* (5th ed). Philadelphia: Saunders.

Davy DT, Kotzar GM, Brown RH, et al. (1988) Telemetric force measurements across the hip after total arthroplasty. *Journal of Bone and Joint Surgery [Am]* 70, 45–50.

Davy DT. (1994) Joint Loads in Total Hip Arthroplasty. In *NIH Consensus Development Conference on Total Hip Replacement, September 12–14* (pp. 31–34). Bethesda, MD: National Institutes of Health.

DeLee JG, Charnley J. (1976) Radiological demarcation of cemented sockets in total hip arthroplasty. *Clinical Orthopaedics and Related Research* 121, 20–31.

Dobbs HS. (1980) Survivorship of total hip replacements. *Journal of Bone and Joint Surgery [Br]* 62, 168–173.

Dorey F, Amstutz HC. (1989) The validity of survivorship analysis in total hip arthroplasty. *Journal of Bone and Joint Surgery [Am]* 71, 544–548.

Draper DO, Castel JC, Castel D. (1995) Rate of temperature increase in human muscle during 1 MHz and 3 MHz continuous ultrasound. *Journal of Orthopaedic and Sports Physical Therapy* 22, 142–150.

Draper DO, Ricard MD. (1995) Rate of temperature decay in human muscle following 3 MHz ultrasound: The stretching window revealed. *Journal of Athletic Training* 30, 304–307.

Duncan PW, Weiner DK, Chandler J, Studenski S. (1990) Functional reach: A new clinical measure of balance. *Journal of Gerontology* 45, 192–197.

Dyrek DA. (1994) Assessment and Treatment Planning Strategies for Musculoskeletal Deficits. In SD Sullivan, TJ Schmitz (eds), *Physical Rehabilitation: Assessment and Treatment* (3rd ed) (pp. 61–82). Philadelphia: Davis.

Dyrek DA. (1996) Manual therapy: Lumbopelvic region. Course notes, MGH Institute of Health Professions at Massachusetts General Hospital, Boston.

Eisenberg RL, Hedgcock MW, Akin JR. (1981) The 40° cephalad view of the hip. *American Journal of Radiology* 136, 835–836.

Ellison JB, Rose SJ, Sahrmann SA. (1990) Patterns of hip rotation range of motion: A comparison between healthy subjects and patients with low back pain. *Physical Therapy* 70, 15–19.

Engh CA, Bobyn JD. (1988) The influence of stem size and extent of porous coating on femoral bone resorption after primary cementless hip arthroplasty. *Clinical Orthopedics and Related Research* 231, 7–28.

English TA, Kilvington M. (1979) In vivo records of the hip loads using a femoral implant with telemetric output: A preliminary report. *Journal of Biomedical Engineering* 1, 111–115.

Ensberg MD, Paletta MJ, Galecki AT, et al. (1993) Identifying elderly patients for early discharge after hospitalization for hip fracture. *Journal of Gerontology* 48, 187–195.

Evans P. (1980) The healing process at cellular level: A review. *Physiotherapy* 66, 256–359.

Fagerson TL, Krebs DE, Harris BA, Mann RW. (1995) Examining shibboleths of hip rehabilitation protocols using in vivo contact pressures from an instrumented hemiarthroplasty. *Physiotherapy* 81, 533–540.

Fitzgerald JF, Fagan LF, Tierney WM, Dittus RS. (1987) Changing patterns of hip fracture care before and after implementation of the prospective payment system. *Journal of American Medical Association* 258, 218–221.

Fitzgerald JF, Moore PS, Dittus RS. (1988) The care of elderly patients with hip fracture: Changes since implementation of the prospective payment system. *New England Journal of Medicine* 319, 1392–1397.

Fitzpatrick R. (1993) Patient Satisfaction and Quality of Life Measures. In PB Pynsent, JCT Fairbank, A Carr (eds), *Outcome Measures in Orthopaedics* (pp. 45–58). Oxford, UK: Butterworth–Heinemann.

Forrester DM, Brown JC. (1987) *The Radiology of Joint Disease* (3rd ed). Philadelphia: Saunders.

Frankel VH, Burstein AH, Lygre L, Brown RH. (1971) The telltale nail. *Journal of Bone and Joint Surgery [Am]* 53, 1232.

Gapsis JJ, Grabois M, Borrell RM, et al. (1982) Limb load monitor: Evaluation of a sensory feedback device for controlling weight-bearing. *Archives of Physical Medicine and Rehabilitation* 63, 38–41.

Garden RS. (1961) Low-angle fixation in fractures of the femoral neck. *Journal of Bone and Joint Surgery [Br]* 43, 647–663.

Garden RS. (1964) Stability and union in subcapital fractures of the femur. *Journal of Bone and Joint Surgery [Br]* 46, 630–647.

Garraway WM, Stauffer RN, Kurland LT, O'Fallon WM. (1979) Limb fractures in a defined population. 1. Frequency and distribution. *Mayo Clinic Proceedings* 54, 701–707.

Geraci MC. (1994) Rehabilitation of pelvis, hip, and thigh injuries in sports. *Physical Medicine and Rehabilitation Clinics of North America* 5, 157–173.

Giannini S, Catni F, Benedetti MG, Leardini A. (1994) Terminology, Parametrization, and Normalization in Gait Analysis. In S Giannini, F Catni, MG Benedetti, A Leardini (eds), *Gait Analysis: Methodologies and Clinical Applications* (pp. 65–88). Washington, DC: IOS Press.

Givens-Heiss DL, Krebs DE, Riley PO, et al. (1992) In vivo acetabular contact pressures during rehabilitation. Part II: Postacute phase. *Physical Therapy* 72, 700–705.

Goetz DD, Smith EJ, Harris WH. (1994) The prevalence of femoral osteolysis associated with components inserted with and without cement in total hip arthroplasty. *Journal of Bone and Joint Surgery [Am]* 76, 1121–1129.

Gold RH, Nasser S, Stall SM. (1991) Conventional Roentgenography with Special Techniques for Follow-Up of Hip Arthroplasty. In HC Amstutz (ed), *Hip Arthroplasty* (pp. 121–129). New York: Churchill Livingstone.

Goodman CC, Snyder TEK. (1990) *Differential Diagnosis in Physical Therapy*. Philadelphia: Saunders.

Gore DR, Murray MP, Sepic SB, Gardner GM. (1975) Walking patterns of men with unilateral surgical hip fusion. *Journal of Bone and Joint Surgery [Am]* 57, 759–765.

Gore DR, Murray MP, Gardner GM, Sepic SB. (1977) Roentgenographic measurements after Müeller total hip replacement. Correlations among roentgenographic measurements and hip strength and mobility. *Journal of Bone and Joint Surgery [Am]* 59, 948–953.

Grabiner MD. (1989) The Hip Joint. In PJ Rasch (ed), *Kinesiology and Applied Anatomy* (7th ed) (pp. 193–207). Philadelphia: Lea & Febiger.

Greenfield S, Apolone G, McNeil BJ, Cleary PD. (1993) The importance of co-existent disease in the occurrence of postoperative complications and one-year recovery in patients undergoing total hip replacement. *Medical Care* 31, 141–154.

Grieve GP. (1983) The hip. *Physiotherapy* 69, 196–204.

Gruebel Lee DM. (1983) *Disorders of the Hip*. Philadelphia: Lippincott.

Gruen TA, McNeice GM, Amstutz HC. (1979) "Modes of failure" of cemented stem-type femoral components. *Clinical Orthopaedics and Related Research* 141, 17–27.

Guccione AA. (1991) Physical therapy diagnosis and the relationship between impairments and function. *Physical Therapy* 71, 499–504.

Guccione AA, Fagerson TL, Anderson JJ. (1996) Regaining functional independence in the acute care setting following hip fracture. *Physical Therapy* 76, 818–826.

Guyatt GH, Sullivan MJ, Thompson PJ, et al. (1985) The 6-minute walk: A new measure of exercise capacity in patients with chronic heart failure. *Canadian Medical Association Journal* 132, 919–923.

Hardcastle P, Nade S. (1985) The significance of the Trendelenburg test. *Journal of Bone and Joint Surgery [Br]* 62, 741–746.

Hardinge K. (1982) The direct lateral approach to the hip. *Journal of Bone and Joint Surgery [Br]* 64, 17–19.

Harrigan TP, Kareh JA, O'Connor DO, et al. (1992) A finite element study of the initiation of failure of fixation in cemented femoral total hip components. *Journal of Orthopaedic Research* 10, 134–144.

Harris BA, Dyrek DA. (1989) A model of orthopaedic dysfunction for clinical decision making in physical therapy practice. *Physical Therapy* 69, 548–553.

Harris SR. (1996) How should treatments be critiqued for scientific merit? *Physical Therapy* 76, 175–181.

Harris WH. (1969) Traumatic arthritis of the hip after dislocation and acetabular fractures: Treatment by mold arthroplasty: An end-result study using a new method of result evaluation. *Journal of Bone and Joint Surgery [Am]* 51, 737–755.

Harris WH. (1986) Etiology of osteoarthritis of the hip. *Clinical Orthopaedics and Related Research* 213, 20–33.

Harris WH. (1993) The Case for Cemented Fixation of the Femur in Every Patient. In M Schafer (ed), *Instructional Course Lectures 43* (pp. 367–371). Rosemont, IL: American Academy of Orthopaedic Surgeons.

Harris WH, Maloney WF. (1989) Hybrid total hip arthroplasty. *Clinical Orthopaedics and Related Research* 249, 21–29.

Harris WH, McCarthy JC, O'Neill DA. (1982) Femoral component loosening using contemporary techniques of femoral cement fixation. *Journal of Bone and Joint Surgery [Am]* 64, 1063–1067.

Harris WH, Rushfeldt PD, Carlson CE, et al. (1975) Pressure Distribution in the Hip and Selection of Hemiarthroplasty. In *The Hip: Proceedings the Third Open Scientific Meeting of the Hip Society* (pp. 93–98). St. Louis: Mosby.

Harty M. (1991) Anatomy. In ME Steinberg (ed), *The Hip and its Disorders* (pp. 27–46). Philadelphia: Saunders.

Hodge WA, Carlson KL, Fijan RS, et al. (1989) Contact pressures from an instrumented hip endoprosthesis. *Journal of Bone and Joint Surgery [Am]* 71, 1378–1386.

Hoppenfeld S. (1976) *Physical Examination of the Spine and Extremities.* East Norwalk, CT: Appleton-Century-Crofts.

Hoppenfeld S, deBoer P. (1994) *Surgical Exposures in Orthopaedics: The Anatomic Approach* (2nd ed). Philadelphia: Lippincott.

Hunt SM, McEwen J, McKenna SP. (1985) Measuring health status: A new tool for clinicians and epidemiologists. *Journal of the Royal College of General Practitioners* 35, 185–188.

Ingber RS. (1989) Iliopsoas myofascial dysfunction: A treatable case of "failed" low back syndrome. *Archives of Physical Medicine and Rehabilitation* 70, 382–386.

Isaac GH, Wroblewski BM, Atkinson JR, Dowson D. (1992) A tribological study of retrieved hip prostheses. *Clinical Orthopedics and Related Research* 276, 115–125.

Jacobs LGH, Buxton RA. (1989) The course of the superior gluteal nerve in the lateral approach to the hip. *Journal of Bone and Joint Surgery [Am]* 71, 1239–1243.

Janda V. (1983) On the concept of postural muscles and posture in man. *Australian Journal of Physiotherapy* 29, 83–84.

Jasty M, Maloney WJ, Bragdon CR, et al. (1991) The initiation of failure in cemented femoral components of hip arthroplasties. *Journal of Bone and Joint Surgery [Br]* 73, 551–558.

Jette AM, Harris BA, Cleary PD, Campion EW. (1987) Functional recovery after hip fracture. *Archives of Physical Medicine and Rehabilitation* 68, 735–740.

Jette AM, Davies AR, Cleary PD, et al. (1986) The Functional Status Questionnaire: Reliability and validity when used in primary care. *Journal of General Internal Medicine* 1, 143–149.

Johanson NA. (1994) Principles of Outcome Measures. In *NIH Consensus Development Conference on Total Hip Replacement, September 12–14* (pp. 101–103). Bethesda, MD: National Institutes of Health.

Johnston RC, Brand RA, Crowninshield RD. (1979) Reconstruction of the hip. *Journal of Bone and Joint Surgery [Am]* 61, 639–652.

Johnston RC, Fitzgerald RH, Harris WH, et al. (1990) Clinical and radiographic evaluation of total hip replacement: A standard system of terminology for reporting results. *Journal of Bone and Joint Surgery [Am]* 72, 161–168.

Johnston RC, Smidt GL. (1970) Hip motion measurements for selected activities of daily living. *Clinical Orthopaedics and Related Research* 72, 205–215.

Kaltenborn FM. (1989) *Manual Mobilization of the Extremity Joints* (4th ed). Oslo, Norway: Olaf Norlis Bokhandel.

Kapandji IA. (1970) *The Physiology of the Joints: Volume 2: The Lower Extremity*. Edinburgh, UK: Churchill Livingstone.

Kaplan EL, Meier P. (1958) Nonparametric estimations from incomplete observations. *Journal of the American Statistical Association* 53, 457.

Katz JN, Larson MG, Phillips CB, et al. (1992) Comparative measurement sensitivity of short and longer health status instruments. *Medical Care* 30, 917–925.

Katz JN, Phillips CB, Poss R, et al. (1995) The validity and reliability of a total hip arthroplasty outcome evaluation questionnaire. *Journal of Bone and Joint Surgery [Am]* 10, 1528–1534.

Kauffman TL, Albright L, Wagner C. (1987) Rehabilitation outcomes after hip fracture in persons 90 years and older. *Archives of Physical Medicine and Rehabilitation* 68, 369–371.

Kavanagh BF, Fitzgerald RH. (1985) Clinical and roentgenographic assessment of total hip arthroplasty: A new hip score. *Clinical Orthopaedics and Related Research* 193, 133–140.

Kendall FP, McCreary EK, Provance PG. (1993) *Muscles Testing and Function* (4th ed). Baltimore: Williams & Wilkins.

Kessler RM. (1983) The Hip. In RM Kessler, D Hertling (eds), *Management of Common Musculoskeletal Disorders: Physical Therapy Principles and Methods* (pp. 368–393). Philadelphia: Harper & Row.

Khan MA. (1993) Ankylosing Spondylitis. In HR Schumacher (ed), *Primer on the Rheumatic Diseases* (10th ed) (pp. 151–158). Atlanta: Arthritis Foundation.

Kiel DP. (1994) New strategies to prevent hip fractures. *Hospital Practice* February 15, 47–54.

Kisner C, Colby LA. (1990) *Therapeutic Exercise: Foundations and Techniques*. Philadelphia: Davis.

Kopell HP, Thompson WAL, Postel AH. (1962) Entrapment neuropathy of the ilioinguinal nerve. *New England Journal of Medicine* 266, 16–19.

Korr IM. (1977) *The Neurobiologic Mechanisms in Manipulative Therapy.* New York: Plenum Press.

Kotzar GM, Davy DT, Goldberg VM, et al. (1991) Telemeterized in vivo hip joint force data: A report on two patients after total hip surgery. *Journal of Orthopaedic Research* 9, 621–633.

Koval KJ, Skovron ML, Aharanoff GB, et al. (1995) Ambulatory ability after hip fracture: A prospective study in geriatric patients. *Clinical Orthopaedics and Related Research* 310, 150–159.

Krebs DE, Elbaum L, Riley PO, et al. (1991) Exercise and gait effects on in vivo hip contact pressures. *Physical Therapy* 71, 301–309.

Kreibich DN, Vaz M, Bourne RB, et al. (1996) What is the best way of assessing outcome after total knee replacement? *Clinical Orthopaedics and Related Research* 331, 221–225.

Kroll M, Ganz S, Backus S, et al. (1994) A tool for measuring functional outcomes after total hip arthroplasty. *American College of Rheumatology* 71, 78–84.

Kyle RF, Gustilo RB, Premer RF. (1979) Analysis of six hundred and twenty-two intertrochanteric hip fractures: A retrospective and prospective study. *Journal of Bone and Joint Surgery [Am]* 61, 216–221.

Kyle RF. (1994) Fractures of the proximal part of the femur. *Journal of Bone and Joint Surgery [Am]* 76, 924–950.

Larson CB. (1963) Rating scale for hip disabilities. *Clinical Orthopaedics and Related Research* 31, 85–93.

Larsson O. (1991) Get Hip! *Skiing* Jan, 63–71.

Larsson O. (1994) Get Hip: The Sequel. *Skiing* Feb, 92–95.

Laupacis A, Bourne R, Rorabeck C, et al. (1993) The effect of elective total hip replacement on health-related quality of life. *Journal of Bone and Joint Surgery [Am]* 75, 1619–1626.

Lauritzen JB, Petersen MM, Lund B. (1993) Effect of external hip protectors on hip fractures. *Lancet* 341, 11–13.

Lee D. (1989) *The Pelvic Girdle.* New York: Churchill Livingstone.

LeVeau B. (1994) Hip. In JK Richardson, ZA Iglarsh (eds), *Clinical Orthopaedic Physical Therapy* (pp. 333–398). Philadelphia: Saunders.

Lhowe DW. (1990) Intracapsular Fractures of the Femur. In CM Evarts (ed), *Surgery of the Musculoskeletal System* (2nd ed) (pp. 2549–2592). New York: Churchill Livingstone.

Liang MH, Katz JN, Phillips C, et al. (1991) The Total Hip Arthroplasty Outcome Evaluation Form of the American Academy of Orthopaedic Surgeons. *Journal of Bone and Joint Surgery [Am]* 73, 639–646.

Liang MH, Logigian MK. (1992) *Rehabilitation of Early Rheumatoid Arthritis.* New York: Little, Brown.

Lieberman JR, Dorey F, Shekelle P, et al. (1996) Differences between patients' and physicians' evaluations of outcome after total hip arthroplasty. *Journal of Bone and Joint Surgery [Am]* 78, 835–838.

Linacre JM, Heinemann AW, Wright BD, et al. (1994) The structure and stability of the Functional Independence Measure. *Archives of Physical Medicine and Rehabilitation* 75, 127–132.

Lloyd-Smith R, Clement DB, McKenzie DC, Taunton JE. (1985) A survey of overuse and traumatic hip and pelvic injuries in athletes. *Physician and Sports Medicine* 13, 131–141.

Long BW, Rafert JA. (1995) *Orthopaedic Radiography*. Philadelphia: Saunders.

Longmore RB, Gardner DL. (1978) The surface structure of aging human articular cartilage: A study by reflected light interference microscopy (RLIM). *Journal of Anatomy* 126, 353–365.

Luepongsak N, Krebs DE, Olsson E, et al. (1997) Hip stress during lifting with bent and straight knees. *Scandinavian Journal of Rehabilitation Medicine* 29, 57–64.

Macirowski T, Tepic S, Mann RW. (1994) Cartilage stresses in the human hip joint. *Journal of Biomechanical Engineering* 116, 10–18.

MacKenzie CR, Charlson ME, DiGioia D, Kelley K. (1986) A patient-specific measure of change in maximal function. *Archives of Internal Medicine* 146, 1325–1329.

Magaziner J, Simonsick EM, Kashner M, et al. (1990) Predictors of functional recovery one year following hospital discharge for hip fracture: A prospective study. *Journal of Gerontology* 45, 101–107.

Magee DJ. (1992) *Orthopaedic Physical Assessment*. Philadelphia: Saunders.

Maigne JY, Maigne R, Guerin-Surville H. (1986) Anatomic study of the lateral cutaneous rami of the subcostal and iliohypogastric nerves. *Surgical and Radiologic Anatomy* 8, 251–256.

Maitland GD. (1991) *Peripheral Manipulation* (3rd ed). Oxford, UK: Butterworth–Heinemann.

Mankin HJ. (1993) Clinical Features of Osteoarthritis. In WN Kelly, ED Harris, S Ruddy, CB Sledge (eds), *Textbook of Rheumatology, Vol. 2* (4th ed) (pp. 1374–1384). Philadelphia: Saunders.

Markos PD. (1979) Ipsilateral and contralateral effects of proprioceptive neuromuscular facilitation techniques on hip motion and electromyographic activity. *Physical Therapy* 59, 1366–1373.

Mathias S, Nayak USL, Isaacs B. (1986) Balance in elderly patients: The "get-up and go" test. *Archives of Physical Medicine and Rehabilitation* 67, 387–389.

McGann WA, Hungerford DS. (1996) Editorial comment. *Clinical Orthopaedics and Related Research* 333, 2–3.

McGrory BJ, Morrey BF, Cahalan TD, et al. (1995a) Effect of femoral offset on range of motion and abductor muscle strength after total hip arthroplasty. *Journal of Bone and Joint Surgery [Br]* 77, 865–869.

McGrory BJ, Stuart MJ, Sim FH. (1995b) Participation in sports after hip and knee arthroplasty: Review of literature and survey of surgeon preferences. *Mayo Clinic Proceedings* 70, 342–348.

McLaughlin C. (1996) Functioning on land is key outcome in documenting aquatic progress. *Advance for Physical Therapists* April, 15.

Melzack R. (1975) The McGill Pain Questionnaire: Major properties and scoring methods. *Pain* 1, 277–299.

Mennell J McM. (1964) *Joint Pain: Diagnosis and Treatment using Manipulative Techniques.* New York: Little, Brown.

Merle d'Aubigné R, Postel M. (1954) Functional results of hip arthroplasty with acrylic prosthesis. *Journal of Bone and Joint Surgery [Am]* 36, 451–475.

Merritt CRB, Bluth EI. (1985) Techniques for diagnostic imaging. *Postgraduate Medicine* 77, 56–73.

Michelson JD, Myers A, Jinnah R, et al. (1995) Epidemiology of hip fractures among the elderly. *Clinical Orthopaedics and Related Research* 311, 129–135.

Miegel RE, Harris WH. (1984) Medial-displacement intertrochanteric osteotomy in the treatment of osteoarthritis of the hip. A long-term follow-up study. *Journal of Bone and Joint Surgery [Am]* 66, 878–887.

Miller EH, Benedict FE. (1985) Stretch of the femoral nerve in a dancer: A case report. *Journal of Bone and Joint Surgery [Am]* 67, 315–317.

Mont MA, Hungerford DS. (1995) Current concepts review: Non-traumatic avascular necrosis of the femoral head. *Journal of Bone and Joint Surgery [Am]* 77, 459–469.

Moore FH. (1989) Examining infants' hips—can it do harm? *Journal of Bone and Joint Surgery [Br]* 71, 4–5.

Morrey BF. (1992) Instability after total hip arthroplasty. *Orthopaedic Clinics of North America* 23, 237–248.

Mossey JM, Knott K, Craik R. (1990) The effects of persistent depressive symptoms on hip fracture recovery. *Journal of Gerontology* 45, 163–168.

Mubarek SJ, Leach JL, Wenger DL. (1987) Management of congenital dislocation of the hip in the infant. *Contemporary Orthopaedics* 15, 29–44.

Mulligan BR. (1995) *Manual Therapy: "NAGS," "SNAGS," "MWMS" etc.* (3rd ed). Wellington, New Zealand: Plane View Services.

Murray D. (1993) The Hip. In PB Pynsent, JCT Fairbank, A Carr (eds), *Outcome Measures in Orthopaedics* (pp. 198–227). Oxford, UK: Butterworth–Heinemann.

Murray DW, Carr AJ, Bulstrode C. (1993) Survival analysis of joint replacements. *Journal of Bone and Joint Surgery [Br]* 75, 697–704.

Muthe NC. (1981) *Endocrinology: A Nursing Approach.* Boston: Little, Brown.

Nagi SZ. (1965) *Disability and Rehabilitation.* Columbus, OH: Ohio State University Press.

Naraghi FF, DeCoster TA, Moneim MS, et al. (1996) Review: Heterotopic ossification. *Orthopedics* 19, 145–152.

Nashner LM. (1990) Sensory, Neuromuscular, and Biomechanical Contributions to Human Balance. In PW Duncan (ed), *Balance: Proceedings of the APTA Forum, Nashville, TN, June 13–15, 1989* (pp. 5–12). Alexandria, VA: APTA.

National Institutes of Health. (1994) *NIH Consensus Statement, Volume 12, Number 5, September 12–14. Total Hip Replacement.* Bethesda, MD: National Institutes of Health.

Nelson EC, Berwick DM. (1989) The measurement of health status in clinical practice. *Medical Care* 27, 77–90.

Neumann DA. (1989) Biomechanical analysis of selected principles of hip joint protection. *Arthritis Care and Research* 2, 146–155.

Neumann DA, Hase AD. (1994) An electromyographic analysis of the hip abductors during load carriage: Implications for hip joint protection. *Journal of Orthopaedic and Sports Physical Therapy* 19, 296–304.

Neumann L, Freund KG, Sorenson KH. (1996) Total hip arthroplasty with the Charnley prosthesis in patients 55 years old and less. *Journal of Bone and Joint Surgery [Am]* 78, 73–79.

Norkin CC, Levangie PK. (1992) *Joint Structure and Function.* Philadelphia: Davis.

Norris CM. (1995) Spinal stabilisation. Part I. Active lumbar stabilisation—concepts. *Physiotherapy* 81, 61–64.

Oatis CA. (1990) Biomechanics of the Hip. In JL Echternach (ed), *Physical Therapy of the Hip* (pp. 37–50). New York: Churchill Livingstone.

O'Boyle CA, McGee H, Hickey A, et al. (1992) Individual quality of life in patients undergoing hip replacement. *Lancet* 339, 1088–1091.

Palmer RM, Saywell RM, Zollinger TW, et al. (1989) The impact of the prospective payment system on the treatment of hip fractures in the elderly. *Archives of Internal Medicine* 149, 2237–2241.

Parsons KO. (1945) Pain: Its significance and assessment. *Physiotherapy* 30, 71–73.

Patta CE. (1989) The Lower Extremity. In O Payton (ed), *Manual of Physical Therapy* (pp. 477–483). New York: Churchill Livingstone.

Paul JP. (1966) The biomechanics of the hip-joint and its clinical relevance. *Proceedings of the Royal Society of Medicine* 59, 943–948.

Perry J. (1992) *GAIT ANALYSIS: Normal and Pathological Function*. Thorofare, NJ: Slack.

Petty W. (1991) *Total Joint Replacement*. Philadelphia: Saunders.

Phillips TW, Messieh SS, McDonald PD. (1990) Femoral fixation in hip replacement: A biomechanical comparison of cementless and cemented prostheses. *Journal of Bone and Joint Surgery [Br]* 72, 431–434.

Pincus T, Sumney JA, Soraci SA, et al. (1983) Assessment of patient satisfaction in activities of daily living using a modified Stanford Health Assessment Questionnaire. *Arthritis and Rheumatism* 26, 1346.

Pitt MJ, Lund PJ, Speer DP. (1990) Imaging of the pelvis and hip. *Orthopedic Clinics of North America* 21, 545–559.

Podsiadlo D, Richardson S. (1991) The timed "up and go": A test of basic functional mobility for frail elderly persons. *Journal of the American Geriatrics Society* 39, 142–148.

Poss R. (1984) Current concepts review: The role of osteotomy in the treatment of osteoarthritis of the hip. *Journal of Bone and Joint Surgery [Am]* 66, 144–151.

Prentice WE. (1983) A comparison of static stretching and PNF stretching for improving hip joint flexibility. *Athletic Training* Spring, 56–59.

Prichard B. (1993) Get hip. *Golf* August, 78–79.

Puranen J, Orava S. (1988) The hamstring syndrome—a new diagnosis of gluteal sciatic pain. *American Journal of Sports Medicine* 16, 517–521.

Reid DC. (1992) *Sports Injury Assessment and Rehabilitation*. Edinburgh, UK: Churchill Livingstone.

Relman AS. (1988) Assessment and accountability: The third revolution in medical care. *New England Journal Medicine* 319, 1220–1222.

Rice CL, Cunningham DA, Paterson DH, Rechnitzer PA. (1989) Strength in the elderly population. *Archives of Physical Medicine and Rehabilitation* 70, 391–397.

Roach KE, Miles TP. (1991) Normal hip and knee active range of motion: The relationship to age. *Physical Therapy* 71, 656–664.

Robbins CE. (1995) Hip biomechanics during gait. Master's thesis, Department of Physical Therapy, MGH Institute of Health Professions at Massachusetts General Hospital, Boston.

Rose S, Draper DO, Schulthies SS, Durrant E. (1996) The stretching window part two: Rate of thermal decay in deep muscle following 1-Mz ultrasound. *Journal of Athletic Training* 31, 139–143.

Roush SE. (1985) Patient-perceived functional outcomes associated with elective hip and knee arthroplasties. *Physical Therapy* 65, 1496–1500.

Rushfeldt PD, Mann RW, Harris WH. (1981) Improved techniques for measuring in vitro the geometry and pressure distribution in the human acetabulum, II: Instrumented endoprosthesis measurement of articular surface pressure distribution. *Journal of Biomechanics* 14, 315–323.

Ruwe PA, Gage JR, Ozonoff MB, Deluca PA. (1992) Clinical determination of femoral anteversion: A comparison with established techniques. *Journal of Bone and Joint Surgery [Am]* 74, 820–830.

Rydell N. (1973) Biomechanics of the hip joint. *Clinical Orthopaedics and Related Research* 92, 6–15.

Rydell NW. (1966) Forces acting on the femoral head prosthesis: A study on strain gauge supplied prosthesis in living persons. *Acta Orthopedica Scandinavica* 37, 1–132.

Sahrmann SA. (1988) Diagnosis by the physical therapist—A prerequisite for treatment. *Physical Therapy*, 68, 1703–1706.

Sahrmann S, Woolsey N. (1992) Diagnoses of the hip-pelvic girdle region. Course notes, Program in Physical Therapy. St. Louis: Washington University School of Medicine.

Sapega AA. (1990) Current concepts review: Muscle performance evaluation in orthopaedic practice. *Journal of Bone and Joint Surgery [Am]* 72, 1562–1574.

Satterfield MJ, Dowden D, Yasumura K. (1990) Patient compliance for successful stress fracture rehabilitation. *Journal of Orthopaedic and Sports Physical Therapy* 11, 321–325.

Saudek CE. (1985) The Hip. In JA Gould III, GG Davies (eds), *Orthopaedic and Sports Physical Therapy* (pp. 365–407). St. Louis: Mosby.

Saunders HD. (1985) *Evaluation, Treatment and Prevention of Musculoskeletal Disorders* (2nd ed). Minneapolis: H Duane Saunders.

Saunders HD. (1992) *Orthopaedic Physical Therapy: Evaluation and Treatment of Musculoskeletal Disorders*. Minneapolis: H Duane Saunders.

Savage B. (1984) *Interferential Therapy*. London: Faber and Faber.

Schenkman M, Butler RB. (1989) A model for multisystem evaluation, interpretation, and treatment of individuals with neurologic dysfunction. *Physical Therapy* 69, 538–547.

Schmalzried TP, Amstutz HC, Dorey FJ. (1991) Nerve palsy associated with total hip replacement. *Journal of Bone and Joint Surgery [Am]* 73, 1074–1080.

Schmalzried TP, Jasty M, Harris WH. (1992a) Periprosthetic bone loss in total hip arthroplasty: Polyethylene wear debris and the concept of the effective joint space. *Journal of Bone and Joint Surgery [Am]* 74, 849–863.

Schmalzried TP, Kwong LM, Jasty M, et al. (1992b) The mechanism of loosening of cemented acetabular components in total hip arthroplasty. *Clinical Orthopedics and Related Research* 274, 60–68.

Schumacher HR (ed). (1993) *Primer on the Rheumatic Diseases* (10th ed). Atlanta: Arthritis Foundation.

Seinsheimer F. (1978) Subtrochanteric fractures of the femur. *Journal of Bone and Joint Surgery [Am]* 60, 300–306.

Shbeeb MI, Matteson EL. (1996) Trochanteric bursitis (greater trochanteric pain syndrome). *Mayo Clinical Proceedings* 71, 565–569.

Shields RK, Enloe L, Evans R, et al. (1995) Reliability, validity, and responsiveness of functional tests in patients with total joint replacement. *Physical Therapy* 75, 169–175.

Shin AY, Morin WD, Gorman JD, et al. (1996) The superiority of magnetic resonance imaging in differentiating the cause of hip pain in endurance athletes. *American Journal of Sports Medicine* 24, 168–176.

Shinar AA, Harris WH. (1997) Bulk structural autogenous grafts and allografts for reconstruction of the acetabulum in total hip arthroplasty. A sixteen-year-average follow-up. *Journal of Bone and Joint Surgery [Am]* 79, 159–168.

Siliski JM, Scott RD. (1985) Obturator-nerve palsy resulting from intrapelvic extrusion of cement during total hip replacement. *Journal of Bone and Joint Surgery [Am]* 67, 1225–1228.

Smidt GL. (1997) Lessons and total hip replacement [editorial]. *Journal of Orthopaedic and Sports Physical Therapy* 16, 123.

Smith-Petersen MN. (1917) A new supra-articular subperiosteal approach to the hip joint. *American Journal of Orthopedic Surgery* 15, 592.

Snyder-Mackler L. (1996) Invited commentaries. *Physical Therapy* 76, 847.

Staheli LT, Corbett M, Wyss C, King H. (1985) Lower-extremity rotational problems in children: Normal values to guide management. *Journal of Bone and Joint Surgery [Am]* 67, 39–47.

Stanish WD, Rubinovich RM, Curwin S. (1986) Eccentric exercise in chronic tendinitis. *Clinical Orthopaedics and Related Research* 208, 65–68.

Stanton PE, Purdam C. (1989) Hamstring injuries in sprinting—The role of eccentric exercise. *Journal of Orthopaedic and Sports Physical Therapy* 10, 343–349.

Strickland EM, Fares M, Krebs DE, et al. (1992) In vivo acetabular contact pressures during rehabilitation, part I: Acute phase. *Physical Therapy* 72, 691–699.

Strömberg L, Öhlén G, Svensson O. (1997) Prospective payment systems and hip fracture treatment costs. *Acta Orthopaedica Scandinavica* 68, 6–12.

Sunderland S. (1978) *Nerves and Nerve Injuries*. London: Churchill Livingstone.

Tackson SJ. (1996) Acetabular pressures during hip arthritis exercises. Master's thesis, Department of Physical Therapy, MGH Institute of Health Professions at Massachusetts General Hospital, Boston.

Thomas GJ. (1989) Swimming—An alternative form of therapy. *Clinical Management 9*, 25.

Thorngren KG, Ceder L, Svensson K. (1993) Predicting results of rehabilitation after hip fracture. *Clinical Orthopaedics and Related Research 287*, 76–81.

Tinetti ME. (1986) Performance oriented assessment of mobility problems in elderly patients. *Journal of American Geriatrics Society 34*, 119–126.

Tinetti ME, Speechley M, Ginter SF. (1988) Risk factors for falls among elderly persons living in the community. *New England Journal of Medicine 319*, 1701–1707.

Travell JG, Simons DG. (1992) *Myofascial Pain and Dysfunction. The Trigger Point Manual. Vol. 2, The Lower Extremities*. Baltimore: Williams & Wilkins.

Traycroff RB. (1991) '"Pseudotrochanteric bursitis": The differential diagnosis of lateral hip pain. *Journal of Rheumatology 18*, 1810–1812.

Tugwell P, Bombardier C, Buchanan WW, et al. (1987) The MACTAR Patient Preference Disability Questionnaire—An individualized functional priority approach for assessing improvement in physical disability in clinical trials in rheumatoid arthritis. *Journal of Rheumatology 14*, 446–451.

Tugwell P, Bombardier C, Buchanan WW, et al. (1990) Methotrexate in rheumatoid arthritis: Impact on quality of life assessed by traditional standard-item and individualized patient preference health status questionnaires. *Archives of Internal Medicine 50*, 59–62.

Turner JA, Deyo RA, Loeser JD, et al. (1994) The importance of placebo effects in pain treatment and research. *Journal of the American Medical Association 271*, 1609–1614.

Turner RR. (1996) Hip pain associated with superior gluteal nerve impingement [abstract]. *Journal of Orthopaedic and Sports Physical Therapy 23*, 62.

U.S. Congress, Office of Technology Assessment. (1994) *Hip Fracture Outcomes in People Age 50 and Over—Background Paper*, OTA-BP-H-120. Washington, DC: U.S. Government Printing Office.

van Holsbeeck MT, Eyler WR, Sherman LS, et al. (1994) Detection of infection in loosened hip prostheses: Efficacy of sonography. *American Journal of Roentgenography 163*, 381–384.

Vasey JR, Crozier LW. (1977) Basic movement patterns and their relationship to occupational physical problems. *Physiotherapy* 63, 120–123.

Vasey JR, Crozier LW. (1982) A move in the right direction. *Nursing Mirror* April 28, 42–47.

Wadsworth CT. (1988) *Manual Examination and Treatment of the Spine and Extremities*. Baltimore: Williams & Wilkins.

Wallston KA, Brown GK, Stein MJ, Dobbins CJ. (1989) Comparing the short and long versions of the Arthritis Impact Measurement Scales. *Journal of Rheumatology* 16, 1105.

Wang L, Bowen JR, Puniak MA, et al. (1995) An evaluation of various methods of treatment of Legg-Calvé-Perthes disease. *Clinical Orthopaedics and Related Research* 314, 225–233.

Ware JE. (1993) Measuring patients' views: The optimum outcome measure. SF 36: A valid, reliable assessment of health from the patient's point of view. *British Medical Journal* 306, 1429–1430.

Ware JE, Sherbourne CD. (1992) The MOS 36-Item Short-Form Health Survey (SF-36): I. Conceptual framework and item selection. *Medical Care* 30, 473–483.

Weissman BNW, Sledge CB. (1986) *Orthopedic Radiology*. Philadelphia: Saunders.

White SG, Sahrmann SA. (1994) A Movement System Balance Approach to Management of Musculoskeletal Pain. In R Grant (ed), *Physical Therapy of the Cervical and Thoracic Spine* (2nd ed) (pp. 339–357). Edinburgh, UK: Churchill Livingstone.

Williams HJ. (1993) Rheumatoid Arthritis Treatment. In HR Schumacher (ed), *Primer on the Rheumatic Diseases* (pp. 96–99). Atlanta: Arthritis Foundation.

Wilson PD, Amstutz HC, Czerniecki A, et al. (1972) Total hip replacement with fixation by acrylic cement: A preliminary study of 100 consecutive McKee-Farrar prosthetic replacements. *Journal of Bone and Joint Surgery [Am]* 54, 207–236.

Winstein CJ. (1990) Balance Retraining: Does It Transfer? In PW Duncan (ed), *Balance: Proceedings of the APTA Forum, Nashville, TN, June 13–15, 1989* (pp. 95–103). Alexandria, VA: American Physical Therapy Association.

Winstein CJ, Christensen S, Fitch N. (1993) Effects of summary knowledge of results on the acquisition and retention of partial weight bearing during gait. *Physical Therapy Practice* 2, 40–51.

Woerman AL. (1994) Evaluation and Treatment of Dysfunction in the Lumbar-Pelvic-Hip Complex. In RA Donatelli, MJ Wooden (eds), *Orthopaedic Physical Therapy* (2nd ed) (pp. 481–563). New York: Churchill Livingstone.

Woodman R. (1993) *Home Study Course: An Orthopaedic Approach to the Hip Parts I and II.* Alexandria, VA: Orthopaedic Section, American Physical Therapy Association.

Wolff R, Rohlmann A, Bergmann G, Graichen F. (1989, June) *The load upon a total hip arthroplasty during cycling* [abstract]. Presented at the Seventh International Symposium Proceedings: Adapted Physical Activity, Berlin.

World Health Organization. (1958) *The First Ten Years of the World Health Organization.* Geneva: World Health Organization.

World Health Organization. (1980) *International Classification of Impairments, Disabilities, and Handicaps (ICIDH).* Geneva: World Health Organization.

Wright JG, Rudicel S, Feinstein AR. (1994) Ask patients what they want: Evaluation of individual complaints before total hip replacement. *Journal of Bone and Joint Surgery [Br]* 76, 229–234.

Wright JG, Young NL. (1997) The patient-specific index: Asking patients what they want. *Journal of Bone and Joint Surgery [Am]* 79, 974–983.

Wroblewski BM. (1978) Pain in osteoarthrosis of the hip. *Practitioner* 1315, 140.

Younger TI, Bradford MS, Magnus RE, et al. (1995). Extended proximal femoral osteotomy. *Journal of Arthroplasty* 10, 1–10.

Zuckerman JD. (1996) Hip fracture. *New England Journal of Medicine* 334, 1519–1525.

Zukor D, Lander P. (1995) Appropriate imaging studies and their interpretation. *Canadian Journal of Surgery* 38, 6–12.

# Index

Note: Page numbers followed by f indicate figures; page numbers followed by t indicate tables.

Gemellus inferior muscle
   description and function of, 19t, 20–21
   origin, insertion, and nerve supply to,
      19t
Gemellus superior muscle
   description and function of, 19t, 20–21
   origin, insertion, and nerve supply to,
      19t
Gender, as factor in
   ankylosing spondylitis, 47–50
   avascular necrosis, 54
   developmental dysplasia of hip, 79
   hip fractures, 58
   osteoarthritis, 40
   osteoporosis, 51
   rheumatoid arthritis, 44
   slipped capital femoral epiphysis, 87
   trochanteric bursitis, 67
Genitofemoral nerve, in nerve supply to
      muscles of hip, 13
*Get Hip*, 205
Gill sign, in hip evaluation, 129
Gluteal artery(ies), in blood supply to hips,
      13
Gluteal bursitis, 66–68. *See also* Bursitis,
      trochanteric
Gluteal nerve
   in nerve supply to muscles of hip, 14
   superior, disorders of, differential diag-
      nosis of, 151t
Gluteus maximus muscle
   description and function of, 16
   origin, insertion, and nerve supply to,
      17t
Gluteus medius lurch, 28–29
Gluteus medius muscle
   description and function of, 19–20
   disorders of, differential diagnosis of,
      155t, 158t
   origin, insertion, and nerve supply to,
      18t
Gluteus minimus muscle
   description and function of, 19–20
   disorders of, differential diagnosis of,
      159t
   origin, insertion, and nerve supply to,
      18t
Gracilis muscle, description and function
      of, 19
Greater sciatic foramen, 14–15
Greater trochanter, 5–6
Greater trochanteric bursa, 11f, 12
Guarding, in postoperative physical ther-
      apy, levels of, 267–268, 268t

Hamstring muscle, disorders of, differential
      diagnosis of, 155t–156t
Hamstring syndrome, 77–78
Hand-hold assist, described, 267, 268t
Harris Hip Score, 317f–319f
Health, general, in hip evaluation, 109
Health-status instruments, 324–325
Heat, in hip dysfunction treatment, 208
Hemiarthroplasty, 233–234
   drawing of, 239f
Hernia(s), inguinal, 74–75
Heterotopic ossification, 57
   classification of, 57
   defined, 57
   epidemiology of, 57
   incidence of, 57
   management of, 57
   risk factors for, 57
Hilgenreiner line, as alignment issue in
      radiographic assessment of
      hip, 84f,
Hilton's law, 13
Hip(s). *See also* Biomechanics; *specific part,
      e.g.,* Femur *and under*
      Anatomy
   abduction at, 25
   accessory mobilizations at, 183, 188,
      188f–190f
   adduction at, 25
   anatomy of, 1–23. *See also* Anatomy, of
      hip
   apposition of muscles of, 21
   biomechanics of, 23–37. *See also* Bio-
      mechanics, of hip
   capsular pattern of, 24
   "classic" capsular pattern for, 179
   close-packed position of, 24
   congenital dysplasia of. *See* Develop-
      mental dysplasia of hip
   deltoid of, described, 20
   dermatomes of, 124f
   developmental dysplasia of, in children,
      79–85. *See also* Developmen-
      tal dysplasia of hip, in chil-
      dren
   diagnostic imaging of, 291–311. *See
      also* Diagnostic imaging, of
      hip
   disorders of, 39–95. *See also
      specific disorder, e.g.,*
      Osteoarthritis (degenerative
      joint disease)
      age-related, 40t
      arthritis, 40–50

Hip(s)—*continued*
bone, 50–57
in children, 79–94. *See also* Children, hip disorders in
differential diagnosis of, 149t–159t
dislocations, 61, 62t
fractures, 58–61
nerve entrapment syndromes, 75–79
physical therapy for, 161–211. *See also* Physical therapy, for hip dysfunction
soft tissue, 66–75
evaluation of, 97–158. *See also* Evaluation, of hip
fractures of, 58–61. *See also under* Fracture(s)
in gait, 26–33. *See also* Gait
kinematics of, 24–26
loose-packed position of, 24
lower quarter segments of, evaluation of, 97–146
motion of, anatomic structures limiting, 141, 141t
normal, radiography of, 294, 295f–296f
open-packed position of, 24
osteology of, 1–7
pain in. *See under* Pain, hip
peripheral nerves of, sensory distribution of, 123f
range of motion of, normative, 182t–183t
resting position of, 24
surgeries of, 213–246. *See also* Surgery(ies), of hip
Hip abduction orthoses, 275
Hip abductor, weakness of, as factor in hip surgery outcome, 279–280
Hip counterrotation, for skiing, 206
Hip extension, forces and pressures at hip during
isometric, 34t
prone, 34t
resisted, 34t
Hip extensor gait, 29
Hip flexion and adduction test, in hip evaluation, 145t–146t
Hip fracture. *See also* Fracture(s), of hip
Hip fracture internal fixation, approaches for, 240–241
Hip fusion, as alternative to hip replacement, 242, 243f
Hip grind test, in hip evaluation, 144t–145t
Hip joint
accessory motions of, 143–146

alignment of, changes in, assessment of, 126–129, 127f
anterior glide in prone, 189f
arthrokinematics of, assessment of, 143–146
described, 1
differential tests of, 138t–148t
end-feels of
abnormal, 142
normal, 142
extension of, 25
flexion of, 25
fluid in, radiographic signs of, 300–301
long-axis distraction, 183, 188f
loose body in, differential diagnosis of, 153t
osteoarthritis of, pain patterns in, 106–107, 107t
posterior glide in supine, 190f
range of motion at, 24–26
shape of, changes in, assessment of, 126–129, 127f
soft tissue of, changes in, assessment of, 129–142
swelling in, in hip evaluation, 121
three degrees of freedom of, 23, 23f
Hip pointer, 73
Hip replacement, *see also* Total hip arthroplasty
alternatives to, 237–245
acetabular fracture reconstruction, 244–245
core decompression, 241–242
hip fracture repair, 238–240, 239f
hip fusion, 242, 243f
osteotomy, 237–238
resection arthroplasty, 242–244
nerve palsy after, 78
Hip rotation. *See* Rotation
Hip spica brace, 275
Hip strength, normative, 197, 198t, 199, 200t
Hip surgery
assistive devices after, 266–267
discharge planning after, 278–282, 280f–281f
falls after, prevention of, 286, 287t–289t
frequently asked questions after, 287t–288t
functional mobility scale after, 264
gait faults after, 271
hip-joint loads after, minimization of, 282–284
leg discrepancy after, 284